Fetal Medicine

Chinmayee Ratha • Ashok Khurana

Fetal Medicine

Insights for Clinicians

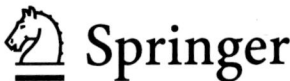

Chinmayee Ratha
Resolution Fetal Medicine Centre and
Research Institute
Hyderabad, India

Ashok Khurana
The Ultrasound Lab
New Delhi, India

ISBN 978-981-19-6101-4   ISBN 978-981-19-6099-4   (eBook)
https://doi.org/10.1007/978-981-19-6099-4

© Springer Nature Singapore Pte Ltd. 2022
This work is subject to copyright. All rights are reserved by the Publisher, whether the whole or part of the material is concerned, specifically the rights of translation, reprinting, reuse of illustrations, recitation, broadcasting, reproduction on microfilms or in any other physical way, and transmission or information storage and retrieval, electronic adaptation, computer software, or by similar or dissimilar methodology now known or hereafter developed.
The use of general descriptive names, registered names, trademarks, service marks, etc. in this publication does not imply, even in the absence of a specific statement, that such names are exempt from the relevant protective laws and regulations and therefore free for general use.
The publisher, the authors, and the editors are safe to assume that the advice and information in this book are believed to be true and accurate at the date of publication. Neither the publisher nor the authors or the editors give a warranty, expressed or implied, with respect to the material contained herein or for any errors or omissions that may have been made. The publisher remains neutral with regard to jurisdictional claims in published maps and institutional affiliations.

This Springer imprint is published by the registered company Springer Nature Singapore Pte Ltd. The registered company address is: 152 Beach Road, #21-01/04 Gateway East, Singapore 189721, Singapore

Preface

Fetal medicine is the branch of clinical medicine dedicated to the health conditions of the fetus in utero. This is a relatively new clinical specialty where the focus of health care shifts toward the unborn fetus in a given pregnancy and hence poses a unique challenge to Obstetricians who have been used to considering only the pregnant lady, or "mother," as their primary patient. Yet, the final outcome of a pregnancy is deemed successful when both mother and the baby/babies are safe and healthy. The importance of fetal health care has now become evident with better understanding of the cause and effect of fetal conditions. Many of these events remained obscure in the yesteryears when there was neither the technology to visualize the fetus at different stages of life nor the understanding of pathogenetic mechanisms of its problems. Today it has become imperative to consider fetal outcomes as a parameter of perinatal health with such clarity that the fetus itself is treated as a separate patient in a pregnancy. It has now been understood that every pregnancy merits screening and managing fetal issues like risk of chromosomal aneuploidies, structural abnormalities, and fetal growth problems. The complexity in the Obstetric paradigm has also increased with a rise in the average maternal age, environmental teratogens, ability of women with medical conditions to conceive, and of course assisted reproduction in general. This creates a bigger scope to investigate and detect fetal problems which need special attention. In such times, clinicians need a thorough understanding of the remit of fetal medicine. This book intends to provide such an understanding to every clinician who will deal with fetal problems either directly or indirectly.

The fact that even preconceptional health of the parents can affect the well-being of the fetus opens the scope of fetal medicine into almost every clinical specialty. The authors hope that this book will help create a bridge of understanding of fetal medicine which will empower clinicians to address yet another patient who may be yet to be born or even conceived.

The style of this book is descriptive and clinically oriented to give readers a ready perspective for practical, clinical application. References for further reading have been provided for readers looking for in-depth theoretical information. This book will serve as a foundation of understanding the concepts of fetal medicine for students of obstetrics and gynecology, pediatrics, radiology, and even internal medicine as this subspecialty is going to be an integral part of their day-to-day practice. Other branches of clinical medicine will also benefit from the simple language of description of fetal conditions because every clinician today needs to be aware of potential fetal effects of the conditions they are managing as well as the management modalities they are using.

There was a need for one comprehensive book which can form the base of understanding of fetal medicine. This can be used as a textbook for foundation years as well as a handbook for clinical practitioners. We wish the readers a happy journey in the path of understanding fetal medicine.

Hyderabad, India Chinmayee Ratha
New Delhi, India Ashok Khurana

Contents

1 **Introduction to Fetal Medicine** 1

2 **History Taking in the Fetal Medicine Clinic**................ 5
   2.1   At the First Antenatal Visit........................... 5

3 **Timeline of Fetal Evaluation in Normal Pregnancy** 7
   3.1   4–6 Weeks of Gestation 7
   3.2   6–11 Weeks of Gestation 8
   3.3   11–14 Weeks of Gestation 8
   3.4   14–16 Weeks of Gestation 8
   3.5   16–18 Weeks of Gestation 9
   3.6   18–20 Weeks of Gestation 9
   3.7   20–28 Weeks of Gestation 9
   3.8   28–32 Weeks of Gestation 10
   3.9   32–40 Weeks of Gestation 10
   3.10 Beyond 40 Weeks of Gestation 10

4 **Principles and Methods of Screening for Fetal Aneuploidies** ... 13
   4.1   What Is Screening? 13
   4.2   The Concept of "Intermediate Risk" 15
   4.3   Which Pregnant Woman Should Be Offered
         Screening for Fetal Aneuploidies?...................... 16
   4.4   Which Are the Tests Available for Screening for Fetal
         Aneuploidies? 16
   4.5   First Trimester Combined Screening Test 17
   4.6   Second Trimester Maternal Serum Biochemistry
         (Quadruple Test) 19
   4.7   Cell-Free Fetal DNA Test 20
   4.8   The Midtrimester Genetic Sonogram.................... 20
   Suggested Reading 21

5 **Basics of Imaging for Fetal Evaluation**..................... 23
   5.1   Fetal MRI.. 26
   5.2   Safety of Ultrasound 28
   5.3   Some Good Practice Points 28
   5.4   Ethical Considerations............................... 28

6	**Evaluation of Fetal Biometry**	31
	6.1 Ultrasound Biometry in Early Pregnancy	31
	6.2 Significance of Early Pregnancy Biometry	34
	6.3 "Dating Is a New Beginning!!"	34
	6.4 Fetal Biometry in Second and Third Trimester	35
	6.5 Biparietal Diameter	35
	6.6 Head Circumference	36
	6.7 Abdominal Circumference	38
	6.8 Measurement of Fetal Femur Length	39
	6.9 Calculation of Estimated Fetal Weight on Ultrasound	39
	6.10 Supplementary Biometry: The Transcerebellar Diameter	40
	Suggested Reading	41
7	**Midtrimester Fetal Anomaly Scan**	43
	7.1 Prerequisites to Performing a Fetal Anomaly Scan	43
	7.2 Fetal Number and Viability	45
	7.3 Orientation of the Fetus (Assessment of Situs)	46
	7.4 Fetal Anatomy Assessment	47
	7.4.1 Fetal Skull	47
	7.4.2 Fetal Brain	48
	7.4.3 Fetal Face	49
	7.4.4 Fetal Neck	49
	7.4.5 Fetal Thorax	51
	7.4.6 Fetal Heart	51
	7.4.7 Fetal Abdomen	53
	7.4.8 Fetal Spine	54
	7.4.9 Fetal Limbs	55
	7.4.10 Genitalia	56
	7.4.11 Other Parameters Assessed at the MTAS	56
	7.5 Scope of the Midtrimester Anomaly Scan	57
	7.6 Planning Further Care After Detecting Fetal Anomaly	58
	Suggested Reading	58
8	**Basics of Doppler Imaging and Application in Fetal Medicine**	59
	8.1 Fetal Circulation	62
	8.2 Umbilical Artery Doppler	64
	8.3 Fetal Middle Cerebral Artery Doppler	64
	8.4 Fetal Ductus Venosus Doppler	65
	8.5 Uterine Artery Doppler	67
	8.6 Safety Issues with Fetal Doppler	68
	Suggested Reading	69
9	**Fetal Growth Disorders**	71
	9.1 Fetal Growth Restriction	72
	9.1.1 Etiology and Classification of Fetal Growth Restriction	73
	9.1.2 Diagnosis and Evaluation of Fetal Growth Restriction	74
	9.1.3 Management of Fetal Growth Restriction	77
	9.2 Fetal Overgrowth Conditions	78
	Suggested Reading	80

10	**The "First Trimester (11–14 Weeks) Scan"**		81
	10.1	Reconfirmation of Fetal Viability and Dating	82
	10.2	Detailed Fetal Structural Assessment at the 11–14 Weeks' Scan	85
	10.3	Screening for Spina Bifida by IT (Intracranial Translucency)	95
	10.4	Markers for Fetal Aneuploidy Screening in the 11–14 Weeks' Scan	96
		10.4.1 Fetal NT	96
		10.4.2 Fetal Nasal Bone	96
		10.4.3 Tricuspid Blood Flow	98
		10.4.4 Ductus Venosus Blood Flow	98
	10.5	Basic Workup of Multifetal Pregnancy at the 11–14-Week Scan	100
	10.6	Evaluation of Uterine Artery Doppler in First Trimester Scan	102
	10.7	Evaluation of Maternal Cervix in First Trimester Scan	103
	Suggested Reading		104
11	**Multiple Pregnancy Evaluation in Fetal Medicine Clinic**		105
	11.1	Establishing the Diagnosis and Chorionicity of Multifetal Pregnancy	105
	11.2	Dating of a Multifetal Pregnancy	107
	11.3	Systematic Labeling of Fetuses in Multifetal Gestation	108
	11.4	Aneuploidy Screening in Multifetal Pregnancy	109
	11.5	Screening for Fetal Anomalies in Multifetal Pregnancy	111
	11.6	Planning a Rational Follow-up for Serial Monitoring of Multiple Pregnancy	112
		11.6.1 DICHORIONIC DIAMNIOTIC Twins	112
		11.6.2 MONOCHORIONIC DIAMNIOTIC Twins	114
	11.7	Twin Reversed Arterial Perfusion (TRAP) Sequence	117
	11.8	Monochorionic Monoamniotic (MCMA) Twins	120
		11.8.1 Conjoined Twins	120
	11.9	Higher-Order Multiples (Triplets, Quadruplets, and So on)	121
	Suggested Reading		121
12	**Placenta, Cord, Amniotic Fluid, and Cervix**		123
	12.1	Evaluation of the Placenta in Pregnancy	124
	12.2	Placenta in Second Trimester	125
	12.3	Location and Edges	125
	12.4	Size	128
	12.5	Morphology of the Placenta	129
	12.6	Umbilical Cord Insertion	132
	12.7	Assessment of Umbilical Cord Morphology	132
	12.8	Single Umbilical Artery	134
	12.9	Persistent Right Umbilical Vein	134
	12.10	Amniotic Fluid	137
	12.11	Assessment of Cervix	139
	Suggested Reading		141

13	**Basics of Genetics in Fetal Medicine** 143
	13.1 Fluorescence in Situ Hybridization (FISH) 147
	13.2 Quantitative Fluorescent PCR (QfPCR) 149
	13.3 Multiplex Ligation-Dependent Probe Amplification (MLPA). 151
	13.4 Clinical Exome Sequencing (CEX). 152
	13.5 Targeted Mutation Analysis 153
	Suggested Reading 154
14	**Recurrent Fetal Problems: Looking for Solutions**. 155
15	**Invasive Prenatal Diagnostic and Therapeutic Procedures**. 161
	15.1 Indication 161
	15.2 Pretest Counseling 162
	15.3 Rhesus Status Check 162
	15.4 Maternal HIV and Hepatitis B Screening 162
	15.5 Consent 162
	15.6 Amniocentesis 163
	15.7 Chorionic Villus Sampling (CVS) 164
	15.8 Fetal Blood Sampling 165
	15.9 Invasive Prenatal Threapeutic Procedures 166
16	**Rhesus Isoimmunization and Fetal Infections** 167
	16.1 Rhesus Isoimmunization 167
	16.2 Fetal Infections. 170
	Suggested Reading 173
17	**Potential for Assessing Maternal Morbidity in Fetal Medicine Clinics** 175
	17.1 Uterine Artery Doppler Studies Predict Risk of Preeclampsia 175
	17.2 Hyperglycemia in Pregnancy 178
	17.3 Maternal Autoimmune Diseases 178
	Suggested Reading 180
18	**Essentials of Counseling in Fetal Medicine**. 181
	18.1 Pretest Counseling 181
	18.2 Pretest Counseling for Fetal Scans 181
	18.3 Posttest Counseling for Fetal Scans. 182
	18.4 Pretest Counseling for Fetal Screening Tests. 182

About the Authors

Chinmayee Ratha, MS (ObGyn), FRCOG, FIMSA, FICOG is the Director and Lead Consultant—fetal medicine at the Resolution Fetal Medicine Centre and Research Institute, Hyderabad. She runs a fetal medicine practice catering to the needs of patients and clinicians from all over Telangana and even adjoining states. She is a passionate teacher and an FMF (UK) approved trainer for fetal medicine scans. She runs a clinical fellowship program for subspecialty trainees in fetal medicine in India, including the ICOG-certified fetal medicine course, since 2018. She has spent the last two decades increasing the awareness of fetal problems and available solutions not only among clinicians but also among the public through various information dissemination platforms. She is a popular orator and is known for the simplicity and clarity of her thoughts during her presentations. She has published papers in peer-reviewed, indexed journals and has received several awards and prizes for presentations of her research projects and audits at various state, national, and international seminars. She is a member of several prestigious professional bodies like FOGSI, SFM, FMF, RCOG, and ISUOG, in addition to local bodies and has served in official positions in many of these organizations. She is currently the Chairperson of the FOGSI Perinatology Committee (2021–2024) and the President of SFM Telangana Chapter (2022–2024).

Ashok Khurana commenced his medical studies at All India Institute of Medical Sciences, New Delhi, India. Apart from running a private medical facility with the vision of providing world-class ultrasound services, Dr Ashok Khurana has to his credit several academic and technological firsts in the city, including transrectal scans, transvaginal scans, color Doppler, 3D and 4D ultrasound, and ultrasound-guided surgical procedures. He has authored two medical textbooks, one on 3D and 4D ultrasound and the other on breast ultrasound. He has contributed several articles on ultrasound in prestigious medical journals. This includes pioneering work in cancer of the uterus. Dr Khurana is currently the Secretary of the Society of Fetal Medicine. He is a member of several academic societies where he has lectured extensively, conducted training workshops, and chaired several scientific sessions. These include the International Society for Ultrasound in Obstetrics and Gynecology, Indian Radiological and Imaging Association, Indian Medical Association, Federation of Obstetric and Gynecological Societies of India, Indian Academy of Human Reproduction, and the Indian Federation of

Ultrasound in Medicine and Biology. He is also a member of the FOGSI Genetic and Fetal Medicine Committee for which he conducts several academic exercises. His ultrasound facility is accredited by FOGSI for training programs. Dr Khurana is also the former Clinical Director of the Test-Tube Baby facility of the Institute for Fertility Fulfilment, former President of the Indian Federation of Ultrasound in Medicine and Biology, Delhi Chapter, and former Secretary, Indian Radiological and Imaging Association, Delhi branch.

Introduction to Fetal Medicine

Fetal medicine is a branch of medicine dealing with screening, diagnosing, and treating health issues of the fetus—*the unborn patient*. What started as a refinement of fetal imaging has now transformed into a complete speciality dealing with all aspects of fetal health. As the mother and the fetus are always together, fetal medicine is closely entwined to maternal medicine. As a natural consequence, majority of the present-day fetal medicine specialists are basically obstetricians who have concentrated their training and practice into health issues of the fetus.

The practice of fetal medicine thus requires a thorough insight into the concepts of fetal imaging and fetal physiology, explaining the variety of findings on imaging along with maternal well-being, and planning delivery under optimal circumstances to help the "fetus" in utero smoothly progress into a "newborn" that is received satisfactorily by the neonatologist in the best possible circumstances (Fig. 1.1). Also, several fetal conditions need specialized newborn care, or some maternal conditions can dictate the need for delivering a preterm fetus or even otherwise, the neonatologist becomes the natural caretaker of the fetus after birth such that there is an emergence of the concept of "perinatology" which is a cusp of fetal-maternal medicine, obstetrics, and neonatology.

For centuries, pregnancy care had been focused on the mother and even "obstetrics" was more of a parturition related science to begin

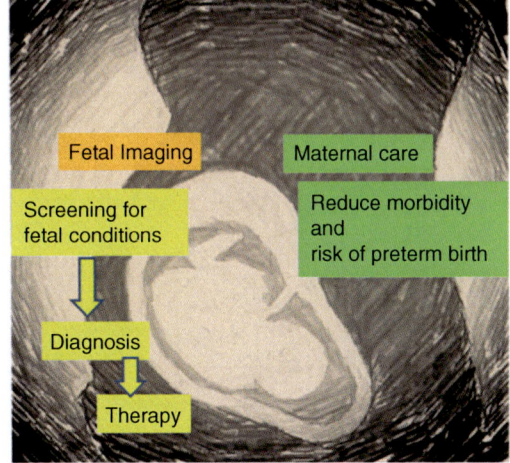

Fig. 1.1 Concept of fetal medicine

with. Just as the role of "antenatal" care became as important as "intrapartum" care in the present-day obstetrics—the role of "fetal medicine" has emerged as the major "discovery" in the last quarter of a century when every practitioner effectively realized few important facts as listed below:

1. The final outcome of pregnancy is both a healthy mother *and* a healthy baby.
2. The complexity of pregnancy care is increasing with maternal morbidity being better handled and these morbidities can affect the fetus.

© Springer Nature Singapore Pte Ltd. 2022
C. Ratha, A. Khurana, *Fetal Medicine*, https://doi.org/10.1007/978-981-19-6099-4_1

3. The concept of "fetal origin of adult disease" became more acceptable in the face of unequivocal evidence that optimizing prenatal health could help reduce the burden of adult disease.
4. "Screening" for fetal aneuploidies and anomalies became a logical part of antenatal care spectrum.
5. Advances in genetics and ultrasound enabled safe and effective "prenatal diagnosis" of fetal aneuploidies and genetic problems.
6. Mutifetal pregnancies are increasing in incidence and are posing fetus-specific challenges to management.
7. Neonatology is evolving so that limits of viability have been pushed to earlier gestation and "intact survival" requires precise fetal surveillance and optimizing time of delivery.
8. Awareness and management of structural anomalies has improved, and again proper fetal workup seems to be the vital measure in optimizing outcome.
9. "Fetal therapy" has evolved with better understanding of fetal physiology and improvisation in instruments and anesthesia.
10. Finally, a risk of liability has emerged if fetal problems have been missed and the overall perinatal outcome is compromised for any reason.

Every pregnancy is now understood as a "maternal-fetal" situation. All obstetricians have redefined pregnancy care and allocated an equal measure of attention and resources to the fetus. Fetal evaluation starts in early pregnancy and at every stage some vital information about the fetus is obtained through tests.

Present-day clinicians have accepted the emergence of "fetal medicine" as a separate branch of obstetrics. The major speciality that justifies fetal medicine as a subspecialty seems to be obstetrics as the primary patient is the mother who houses the fetus within her. There is, however, a significant role of an imaging specialist and neonatologist in all cases along with a case-based role of subspecialists like pediatric neurologists, pediatric surgeons, pediatric cardiologists in specific situations, and maternal medicine subspecialists as the case may be. Therefore, it is a fact that fetal medicine is a multidisciplinary science with multiple stakeholders with the primary aim of delivering a healthy baby of a healthy mother.

The most important aspect of fetal medicine is the acknowledgment that the fetus in utero deserves full medical attention and that too not only while it is physically formed but well in advance in cases where maternal morbidity indicates the possibility of fetal problems in future pregnancies or where previous pregnancy issues indicate a risk of recurrence. It is now imperative for all subspecialists to be aware that their patients are not merely taking medicines to cure or manage their ailments, but also these people are part of a reproductive process that may get affected due to the primary condition and its treatment. For example, a girl with SLE will achieve a pregnancy if she is under a good rheumatologist but unless her medications are "fetus safe" in pregnancy or the anti-Ro/anti-LA antibody levels have been optimized—we may deal with fetal complications that could have been potentially avoidable! So it would be useful for rheumatologists treating women of reproductive age to have appropriate "preconception" counseling and workup with maternal-fetal medicine specialists. The same holds true for women with cardiac diseases who are on warfarin or women on antiepileptic medications—success of medical therapy and obstetrics till the last few decades was measured in terms of ability to carry on a pregnancy in this case; medical care in this century is not just about "survival" but rather about "intact survival" and hence the focus has shifted on fetal medicine.

While screening and diagnosing remained the mainstay of fetal care for many decades, it is remarkable that advances in technology especially endoscopy and better understanding of fetal physiology along with great contributions from pediatric surgery colleagues, the scope of fetal "therapy" has enhanced a lot. From needle-based procedures to insertion of shunts to fetoscopy-guided surgery and finally open fetal surgery is all part of realistic fetal care although the permeation is patchy at the global level.

Nevertheless, hope for successful therapy for fetal problems which was dismal earlier is looking brighter day by day.

Many doctors equate obstetric scanning with fetal medicine, and it is important to understand that while scanning is extremely important in examining a fetus, imaging is only one part of the entire fetal health evaluation. Obstetricians who plan to practice fetal medicine have to learn the basics of ultrasound scans and their application in fetal imaging. Similarly, radiologists who wish to concentrate on fetal health have to understand the background embryological development and obstetric physiology and epidemiology of fetal problems to be able to contribute meaningfully to fetal care. It is heartening to see the emergence of interest and avenues of such interdisciplinary training and collaboration at all levels such that the beneficiary is primarily the fetus in utero, and finally the society at large.

In epitome, fetal medicine (Fig. 1.2) is a conglomeration of all aspects of medicine and technology that can help to screen, examine, evaluate, and treat the fetus in utero to ensure that it receives the best healthcare that present-day technology and clinical evidence can provide.

Fig. 1.2 Multidisciplinary setup for FM

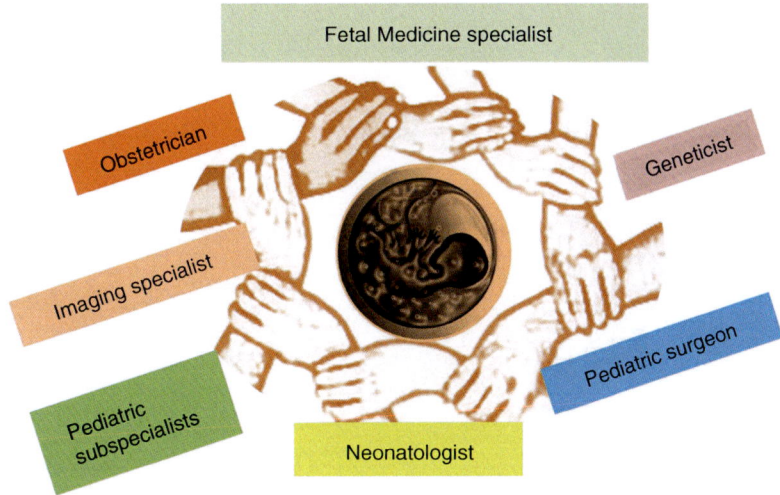

History Taking in the Fetal Medicine Clinic

The aim of antenatal care is to ensure the birth of a healthy baby at term while maintaining maternal well-being throughout pregnancy and puerperium. This aim, if well achieved, has far-reaching consequences in ensuring the overall health of the society, and it is so important that both maternal and infant morbidity and mortality indicators have become the benchmark parameters of a good healthcare system. Anticipating complications is the first step toward planning better management.

All obstetricians are mentally alert and technically equipped to address maternal issues and do an extensive antenatal care plan layout usually during the first antenatal visit. However, the ultimate success of any pregnancy management plan is when *both* the mother and her fetus(es) make it safely through pregnancy and remain healthy after the delivery. It is imperative therefore to make a specific care plan for the fetus in each pregnancy. A timeline for fetal evaluation would be one of the preliminary steps for the same.

2.1 At the First Antenatal Visit

It is natural for every obstetrician to take a detailed clinical history at the time of the first antenatal visit of the expectant mother. At this opportunity, specific issues that may necessitate modification of the care plan for further fetal evaluation and assessment may be made.

A thorough history for potential fetal problems is a MUST at the first antenatal visit for every pregnant woman. It is surprising that in many cases that actually come to fetal medicine clinics, there is a lot of basic information yet unexplored in the patient's history. The points to be definitely covered are the following:

1. **Age of the mother**—Although most women nowadays are very sure of their age, in some societies, women do not know there exact date of birth and provide a number which may not be accurate! Based on clinical situations if the doctor is not convinced, spending a few extra minutes in obtaining this information is very useful—reconfirm dates by any reliable documents if available or even correlate her lifetime events to some well-known dates like a political event, sports event, or contemporary life events of another person in the family with a confirmed date of birth! This may sound hilarious to some readers who are fortunate to have a more enlightened patient population, but in many parts of the developing countries, such ignorance is still common and needs to be addressed.

2. **The mother's blood group and rhesus status**—Testing the mother's blood group and rhesus type provides a very basic medical information and is of unquestionable importance in obstetric population; thus, it is imperative that a pregnant woman MUST have a

© Springer Nature Singapore Pte Ltd. 2022
C. Ratha, A. Khurana, *Fetal Medicine*, https://doi.org/10.1007/978-981-19-6099-4_2

documented report of her blood group and rhesus status. One would be surprised how many pregnant women present at the tertiary care fetal medicine centers for evaluation and do not have this basic report. Worse still, some women just quote an answer without actually knowing the importance, so one must insist that a documented blood group report is available in her obstetric notes at all times.

3. **Mode of conception**—This is important in fetal medicine for many reasons: induced ovulation results in changes in biochemical parameters used for aneuploidy screening; in ART procedures if "donor gametes" are used, then age correction for aneuploidy screening has to be done accordingly; and similarly the risk of inheritance of genetic problems will vary in such cases, so the need for prenatal testing has to be reviewed accordingly.

4. **Menstrual regularity and last period date**—This is important in evaluating the accuracy of dating a pregnancy. If a woman has longer menstrual cycles, say 35-day periods, then we expect that the ovulation will be 5–7 days later in her case than the usually expected 28-day cycles—this in turn will affect the expected date of conception and hence the expected gestational age of the fetus has to be readjusted accordingly.

5. **Obstetric history**—Previous births: mode, gestational age, and birth weights, any pregnancy complications, any special issues with the children like congenital anomalies detected before or after birth, and developmental history of the children in particular are important as they can have a bearing on the fetus in the present pregnancy. In cases of fetal or neonatal losses, detailed recollection of facts and, if possible, review of notes are also important. It is sad that many families do not preserve medical records of fetal and neonatal losses due to sentimental and superstitious reasons, but we must start sensitizing our patients toward the importance of keeping a detailed record of every detail in the cases that have adverse outcomes so that future workup is facilitated.

6. **Family history**—Any specific medical condition affecting several members of a family is very important as it may indicate a heritable genetic disorder and the scope and feasibility of prenatal diagnosis can be explored. Similarly, history of consanguinity is important to look for clues regarding presence of any genetic conditions in the family which may be inherited in the "autosomal recessive" manner. Such problems can affect fetuses of apparently healthy parents and may not always present as structural abnormalities but may have very severe adverse effect on quality of life of babies like severe neurodevelopmental delays or in some cases even death in the newborn period due to metabolic abnormalities which remains elusive and often classified as "unexplained" neonatal deaths

7. **General medical/surgical history**—Preexisting maternal medical conditions like hypothyroidism, diabetes mellitus, epilepsy, or cardiac disease can all have impact on the pregnancy as well as the fetus. Some conditions require medications which are potentially teratogenic (e.g., anti-epileptics), while in many conditions, the disease itself may cause fetal problems like hyperglycemia in peripartum period thereby increasing chances of structural defects in the fetus or when anti-Ro/anti-LA antibodies can cause congenital heart blocks in the fetus.

The abovementioned checklist may not be "complete" in all cases as there will be specific issues that may have significance in individual cases, but it is a comprehensive list of "never to miss" points during history taking in a fetal medicine clinic. Unless a proper history has been taken, the context of fetal imaging remains obscure and the final goal of solving that patient's specific concerns will not be fulfilled. A memory aid for the points in history taking is shown in Fig. 2.1 as a simple alphabetical mnemonic of ABCDEFG.

A- Age
B- Blood group /Rh
C- Conception type
D- Dates
E- Each past pregnancy
F- Family history
G- General Medical/Surgical history

Fig. 2.1 Memory aid for basic history taking in the FM clinic

Timeline of Fetal Evaluation in Normal Pregnancy

3

A normal pregnancy is a journey of a zygote through 37–40 weeks while it develops into a complete human being from a single totipotent cell! Most women would suspect that they are pregnant when they miss a normal menstrual period and then confirm their pregnancy by the urine pregnancy tests.

They usually then visit the doctor either immediately or after a couple of weeks to seek antenatal care. At every stage of pregnancy, a definite evaluation of the fetus is part of the "total" antenatal care scheme. Depending on what period of gestation the woman presents at the antenatal clinic, specific tests can be offered to check the well-being of the fetus growing within her womb.

A "timeline" for fetal evaluation is expressed in Fig. 3.1 and further elaborated in this chapter.

3.1 4–6 Weeks of Gestation

This is the period when most women discover their pregnancy and are very excited about it. In most cases, it would be prudent to plan the first fetal evaluation only after 2 weeks of a confirmed pregnancy test so that at least a definite gestational sac could be seen. Very often, women get a scan done as soon as they have a pregnancy test positive and then get very anxious if the pregnancy viability remains doubtful, even if the reason may be totally physiological!

In some cases where there is a worrying symptom like lower abdominal pain or bleeding per vaginam or where there is a history of ectopic pregnancy or factors predisposing to such an occurrence, an early pregnancy assessment at 4–6 weeks of gestation may be done, best by

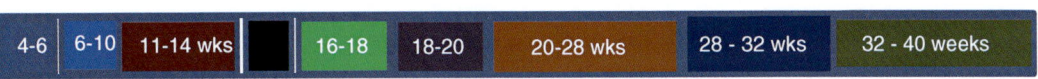

Fig. 3.1 Timeline for fetal evaluation in a normal pregnancy

© Springer Nature Singapore Pte Ltd. 2022
C. Ratha, A. Khurana, *Fetal Medicine*, https://doi.org/10.1007/978-981-19-6099-4_3

transvaginal ultrasound, with the primary aim of detecting an intrauterine pregnancy and ruling out an extrauterine gestation.

The primary aim is to establish the presence of a pregnancy sac, and if viability is doubtful, it is better to reassess the woman after 1 week rather than declaring a pregnancy failure.

3.2 6–11 Weeks of Gestation

At 6–11 weeks, fetal evaluation is usually done to ensure the presence, viability, size, and even multiplicity of the pregnancy. By 6 weeks, a definite fetal pole MUST be seen, and if the crown-rump length of the fetus is 7 mm or more, a definite cardiac activity MUST be seen in a viable pregnancy.

Early pregnancy evaluation should include a documentation of the CRL as this is also an accurate method of dating the pregnancy. In case of multiple pregnancies, documentation of more than one fetal poles and an early assessment of number of sacs and placenta can be done although in some cases, the findings may not be very clear till about 9–10 weeks and thus a repeat evaluation around this gestation may be planned to clarify such doubts.

Assessment of the uterine contour to rule out any uterine anomalies and examination of the adnexa to rule out extrauterine gestation of other adnexal masses is an important aspect of the early pregnancy ultrasound scan.

3.3 11–14 Weeks of Gestation

This is the time frame for the first comprehensive fetal evaluation. The ultrasound scan done in the 11–14 weeks of gestation (fetal CRL between 45 and 84 mm) has become one such investigation which has enhanced its scope to predict many pregnancy complications—both maternal and fetal.

A detailed fetal anatomy assessment is possible at the first trimester scan such that it has become widely recognized and accepted as the "first fetal anomaly scan" or an "early TIFFA" in common practice. A "head-to toe" evaluation for major developmental milestones in fetal anatomy is possible and is imperative to be done by anyone who scans a fetus at this stage. A detailed description of all that can be performed at this stage is given in the Chap. 10. All obstetricians should try and check these details on the first trimester scan report to ensure that an optimal fetal assessment has been done. In fact, the checklist given in the first trimester scan protocol is designed to help the obstetrician plan her pregnancy care better and start necessary interventions to avoid problems later. For example, detection of a major anomaly like anencephaly which warrants termination can be addressed right away as the process of first trimester termination is always safer and less traumatic both physically and emotionally than later.

The fetal nuchal translucency has been firmly established as a marker for risk of fetal chromosomal abnormalities, and along with other markers, the "NT scan" has become a very effective screening tool for fetal aneuploidies. The details of the NT assessment and its implications are given later in the book in the chapter on "screening or fetal aneuploidies."

Any findings that are suspicious of fetal problems can help to triage the fetuses for further testing at the right time to ensure a good perinatal outcome.

This period of gestation has been now identified as the base of the "inverted pyramid of antenatal care" such that efforts to screen for maternal problems like preeclampsia are also possible.

3.4 14–16 Weeks of Gestation

If all the above said investigations and workup have been done correctly, this period of pregnancy does not warrant any specific testing for the fetus. In fact, there is very little that can be offered based on current evidence at this gestation. Ideally, we would expect women to have booked for antenatal care earlier and had the workup as delineated above, but just in case that has not happened, then for women who present for the first time at this gestation or for those who for some reason did not have the tests earlier, a fetal evaluation scan can be done at this stage with the purpose of identifying the viability, number, and basic anatomy of the fetus and ruling out any obvious adnexal pathology to the extent possible now.

In terms of screening for aneuploidies, there are no obvious scan-based parameters validated in this window, but the option of cell-free DNA testing is available in appropriately counseled cases. If parents want conventional screening, then the option is available after 16 weeks.

3.5   16–18 Weeks of Gestation

Again, this evaluation is not routinely scheduled for a fetus if appropriate first trimester workup has been done, but if the woman books for antenatal care at this gestation or has missed her earlier workup, then the fetal evaluation starts from now on. A basic fetal anatomy evaluation along with confirmation of viability, number, and biometry can be done to check dating of the pregnancy. However, if a proper first trimester scan has been done and documented, then the dating established in early scans should not be changed based on the biometry now. If there is a discrepancy, then the cause should be evaluated rather than conveniently changing dates.

Sometimes, a 16–18-week evaluation may be scheduled for an early anomaly scan in case there is very high risk for structural defects in the fetus, e.g., pregestational diabetes or intake of teratogens in the first trimester. Another indication for a scheduled fetal evaluation at this gestation could be for the second trimester biochemical screening (quadruple test) for assessing the risk for fetal aneuploidies or a genetic sonogram based on ultrasound markers for aneuploidies.

3.6   18–20 Weeks of Gestation

This is usually a scheduled appointment for a fetal anomaly scan—popularly also known as the TIFFA (Targeted Imaging for Fetal Anomalies). This period of gestation is an optimal window for the detailed midtrimester anomaly scan especially in countries where the law is strict about not allowing termination of pregnancy for fetal indications beyond 20 weeks. A normal anomaly scan is very reassuring, whereas any markers/anomalies detected on the scan allow some time for workup and results prior to the legal deadline for decisions regarding continuation of pregnancy.

The protocol for the anomaly scan involves a systemic evaluation of fetal viability, structure, biometry, and general evaluation of activity and other intrauterine factors. These issues have been explained in relevant chapters that follow in this book. Some standard formats for reporting an anomaly scan have also been given in later chapters.

Some conditions warrant a detailed fetal echocardiography and that can be performed well at this gestation, but if views are limited, it is acceptable to review the fetus for a fetal echo at around 24 weeks.

3.7   20–28 Weeks of Gestation

If all the previously mentioned fetal evaluation sessions have been accomplished successfully, there is usually no routine indication for a fetal checkup in this window in a normal pregnancy. However, some specific indications may necessitate a fetal checkup.

As mentioned earlier, some women may be recalled for a fetal echocardiography due to specific indications. In some units, there is a recall at 22 weeks for uterine artery Doppler evaluation for screening for preeclampsia, but with recent emerging evidence of the preponement of preeclampsia screening to first trimester, and initiating prophylactic medications earlier, there is little use of this extra visit at the fetal medicine clinic.

In case there is a high risk for preeclampsia and fetal growth restriction, the first "growth scan" is recommended at 26 weeks. Similarly, some fetuses with special needs like those having correctable anomalies may be reviewed in this window with individualized protocols specific to their situation.

3.8   28–32 Weeks of Gestation

This is the time frame for the first "routine" growth scan in a normal pregnancy. Even if all is apparently going well with the mother, there is evidence to support at least one growth assessment for the fetus in the third trimester so that any deviation from the normal growth patterns can be detected early and followed up optimally.

Till many years back, this one growth scan being normal would suffice for the remainder of the pregnancy, but with emerging evidence about "late-onset fetal growth restriction," it is now imperative to suggest a "late growth scan" closer to term.

3.9   32–40 Weeks of Gestation

A late growth scan has now become an acceptable practice in most setups since the identification of the concept of the "late-onset fetal growth restriction." Fetal biometry is ideally represented in "centiles for gestation" and plotted on charts such that trends of fetal growth can be assessed and significant fall or rise in centiles will alert the clinician to growth disorders. While the late growth scan is an important landmark opportunity to detect fetal growth restriction, it is also the ideal time to detect "macrosomia" that is a common occurrence due to suboptimal glycemic control in late pregnancy and may help in optimizing perinatal care to avoid fetal injury due to peripartum complications of maternal hyperglycemia.

Another important aspect of late term fetal evaluation is confirmation of fetal lie and placental position—both these parameters at this time period are closely related to final obstetric decisions regarding mode of delivery.

3.10   Beyond 40 Weeks of Gestation

Although fetal monitoring at this stage is largely by CTG and clinical methods, there may be specific indications to scan for amniotic fluid levels or the fetal biophysical profile to take crucial decisions regarding continuation of pregnancy versus induction of labor or decision to deliver.

As is evident, the bulk of the activity in terms of fetal evaluation is actually concentrated in the first part of pregnancy (Fig. 3.2), and thus the traditional thinking of obstetricians needs a radical modification such that women are referred to fetal medicine clinics earlier than later if any meaningful fetal workup is expected. Although a third trimester scan yields a lot of information, fetal growth evaluation may be meaningless without a first trimester confirmation of dates. Similarly, if the crucial first trimester risk assessment for aneuploidies is missed, a golden opportunity is lost, and since all the markers may be gestation specific, they may disappear and there may be no other reason to be alerted to the possibility of a fetal aneuploidy. Even evaluation of fetal structure is extremely difficult in the third trimester, and thus the anomaly scan must be offered in the midtrimester. In settings where the onus is on the woman and her family to accept or decline tests, the correct action on the part of the clinician is to suggest the right test at the right time. This suggestion must be backed up with relevant information and support material. Fetal medicine has expanded its scope tremendously over the decades, but nothing can be achieved successfully unless the patient, i.e., the "fetus," actually gets to meet the fetal medicine care team at the right time!!

3.10 Beyond 40 Weeks of Gestation

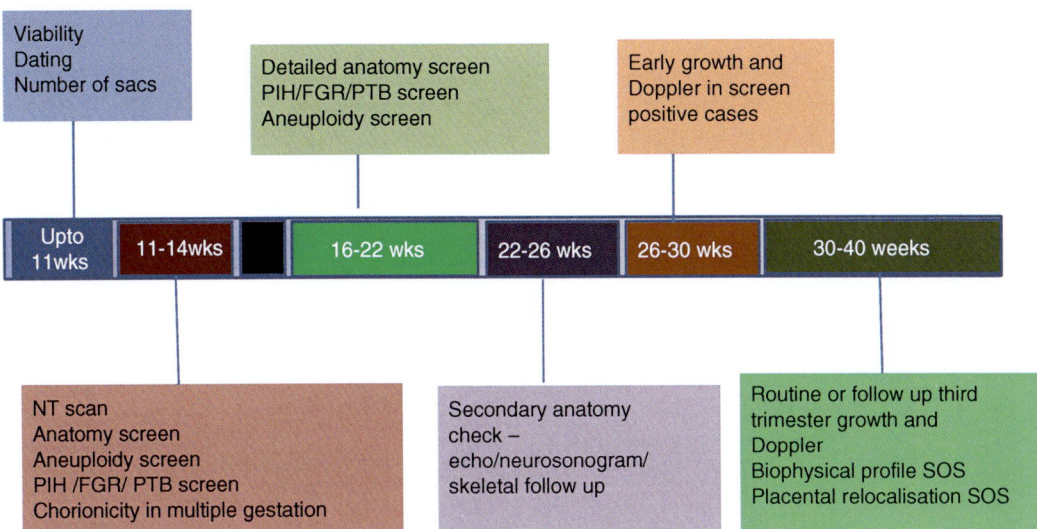

Fig. 3.2 Possibility of fetal evaluation in the first, second, and third trimester

Principles and Methods of Screening for Fetal Aneuploidies

4

Screening for fetal problems is a vital aspect of fetal care as our knowledge in background literature and even each clinician's individual experience tells us that most problems actually happen in pregnancies which were traditionally thought of as the "low-risk" group. Every obstetrician now feels uncomfortable in declaring a "low-risk" pregnancy because essentially this is a retrospective diagnosis! It is therefore imperative that we spend optimum time and resources in "screening" for problems in pregnancy, stratify risk categories based on the screening tests and then institute appropriate care modification to the high-risk group such that the final perinatal outcome is improved. Pregnancy care is essentially preventive care aimed at optimizing maternal and fetal outcome. Screening for potential problems in the mother and the fetus during pregnancy is therefore an important issue as it helps to pick up a "high-risk" group who can then be offered special care to help reduce the incidence, morbidity, and complications of the particular condition for which they have screened "positive."

Fetal aneuploidies are conditions where there is an "abnormal number" of chromosomes in the fetus. This abnormality happens most commonly due to "nondisjunction" during meiosis which is the "reduction" division of cells leading to formation of gametes. This process occurs every time a gamete is released, and technically, it is acceptable to say that every pregnancy has a potential "risk" or "probability" for fetal aneuploidy. This "risk" or "probability" appears to increase with increasing maternal age, but really, there is no age at which a woman "cannot" have an aneuploidic gamete so over the years, it has been clearly understood that every pregnancy has a risk of fetal aneuploidy.

4.1 What Is Screening?

- Screening is a process applied on apparently healthy individuals to detect the risk of any particular problem. It is offered to a general population, and the results of screening will determine whether the individual is at "high risk" or "low risk" for a given condition (Fig. 4.1). So the results of a screening test are "screen positive," i.e., "high risk" for a condition, or "screen negative," i.e., "low risk" which indicates low probability of having that condition.
- SCREENING IS NOT THE SAME AS DIAGNOSIS. Hence, the results of screening tests can only guide us to the need for conducting diagnostic tests. *Screening tests do not confirm or rule out the condition* completely. They only allocate the "risk" or "probability" for a certain condition. Someone who is "high risk" may not have the condition (false positive). Similarly, a "low risk" also may have the condition (false negative). Hence, "screening" is NOT a "diagnosis."

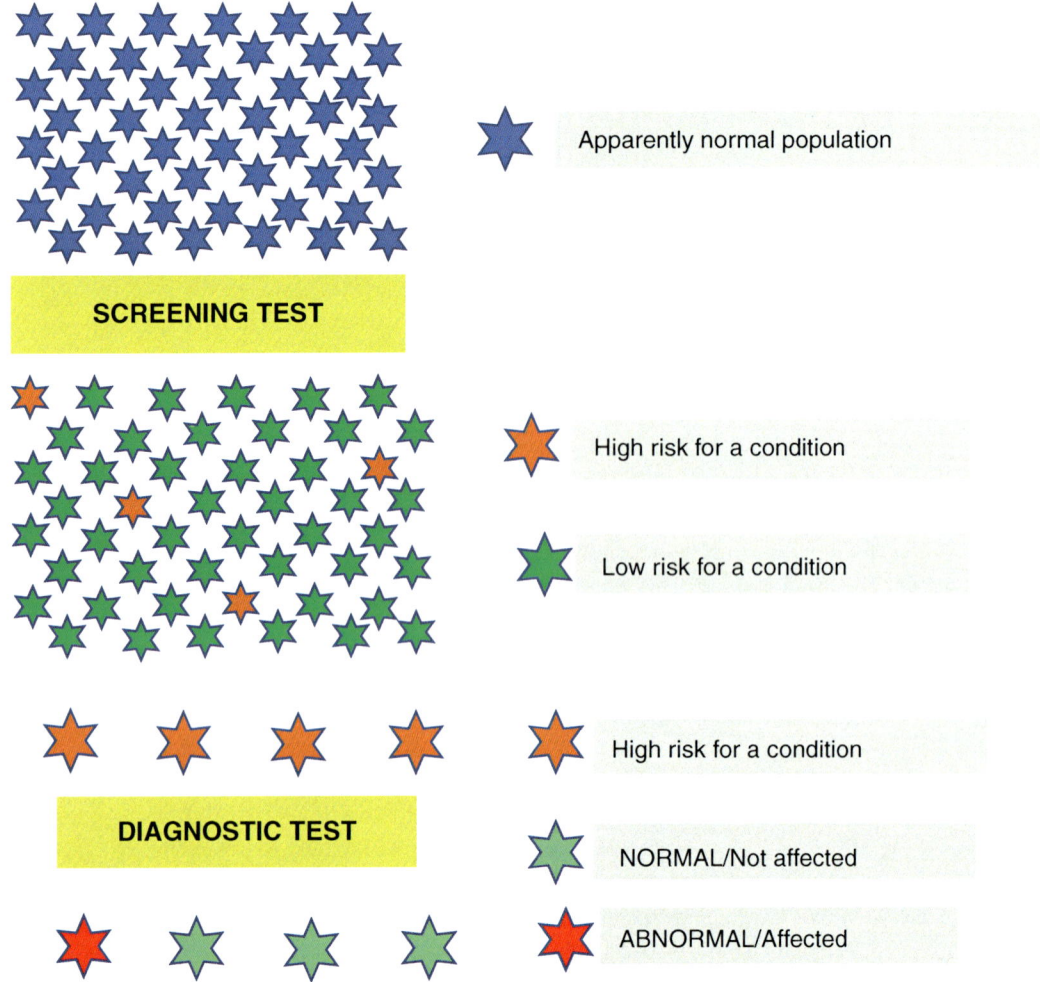

Fig. 4.1 Screening concept

When we talk about screening for fetal chromosomal abnormalities, we need to first understand that every pregnant woman carries a risk of having a fetus with chromosomal abnormalities—this risk is called the "background risk" or a priori risk and depends on maternal age and some factors in her medical history. This risk can be reassessed based on screening tests to "high" or "low" risk.

Clinicians often find the whole concept of screening as "confusing" and as an added "burden" to their clinical schedules. So it is a well-known fact that many clinicians do not offer screening for fetal aneuploidies as part of their regular antenatal care. As the incidence of these problems is rather low, as an individual practitioner, seeing a limited number of cases, one may not encounter these problems much in daily practice and may remain oblivious to their potential presence. Then one fine day when there is a birth of a baby with aneuploidy in their patient group, they suddenly get disturbed by the aftermath of this case. In some cases, clinicians are so hassled with the explanation of the results of screening tests that the discussion that ensues often scares the patients so much that they may even discontinue a pregnancy based on a "high-risk" result on screening alone! Since quantitative assessment of human behavior or attitude will remain controversial, we may never be able to generate "evidence" for the fact that it is the "understanding and attitude" of the clinician which is a primary determinant in the success of a screening program. A very common, real-life example of a "screening" test is the "baggage screening" that happens in airports when we travel through them. *Every piece of baggage is screened*, which implies "screening is universal"—or in other words, only universal screening can help achieve the purpose of screening at all!! The purpose of this screening is to detect and prevent any possible unsafe material being carried on board. "Cutoffs" are fixed based on either "size," "weight," "metal detection," or "sharpness," etc., and only articles that are within these "cutoffs" are screened as "low risk" and allowed through the screening center. In any case of the baggage being "suspicious," it is taken to another place and "opened" or checked with different "invasive" methods. The first-level screening is simpler, caters to a large quantity of article, and is "noninvasive." Those who are "screen negative" are allowed to continue along their normal routes. Those who are "screen positive" are subjected to "invasive" testing like opening the bags or dismantling an equipment—and if found safe ("false positives"), they too are allowed to continue to boarding but if found truly dangerous ("true positives") are removed from the boarding process an dealt with through a different channel individually.

The design of a "screening test" is such that it will pick up any case with a possibility of the problem as "high risk," and hence this group will contain not only the cases which really have the condition (true positives) but also some cases which actually are normal but have been picked up in the high-risk category (false positives) due to the "high sensitivity" of a screening test which determines its ability not to miss "true positives." The natural fallout in this process is that there will be a certain number of "false positives" in every screening test. Since a good screening test is unlikely to miss "true positives," women with "low risk" can be reassured, while those with "high risk" can be offered confirmatory tests to check fetal chromosomes. The tests to confirm fetal chromosomes are generally "invasive tests" which carry a risk of miscarriage, and hence they are justifiably undertaken only if the risk of finding a chromosomal abnormality in the fetus is high based on the results of the screening test. Therefore, a screening test helps in optimizing the need for invasive testing while increasing the pickup rate for fetal chromosomal problems (aneuploidies).

4.2 The Concept of "Intermediate Risk"

The post-screening test classification yields a quantitative "risk" for every woman and this number may be "high risk" or "low risk" depending on the "cutoff" set for that population. It is a challenge to set this "cutoff" as at every level, an optimum trade-off between "detection rate" and "false positives" has to be set. The detection rate will improve if the test is refined, but increased complexity of a test is a limiting factor for population-based implementation. Therefore, the idea of having an "intermediate-risk" group (Fig. 4.2) helps increasing the final "detection rate" while reducing the need of very refined tests only for a limited subgroup.

The "cutoffs" for these risk levels can be fixed as per local protocols. Some units may use fixed numerical cutoffs for the whole population, for example, "low-risk" group is less than 1 in 1000, "high-risk" group is more than 1 in 50, and the group with risks between 1 in 50 and 1 in 1000 is the intermediate-risk group. Similarly, some units follow another protocol like using a fixed cutoff for the "high-risk group," e.g., 1 in 300, while the intermediate-risk group is related to the maternal age risk. Say a woman age-related risk for trisomy 21 is 1 in 1200 and her risk after primary screening is 1 in 700, she falls in the intermediate-risk group, but if her age-related risk is 1 in 400 and final risk is 1 in 700, then she falls in the low-risk group.

Screening protocols have evolved over the years with better understanding of what is acceptable and implementable in populations along with better technology in the tests available. It will be correct to say that the exact protocols as we have them today are likely to change in future, but the "concept" of screening for fetal aneuploidies will remain the same.

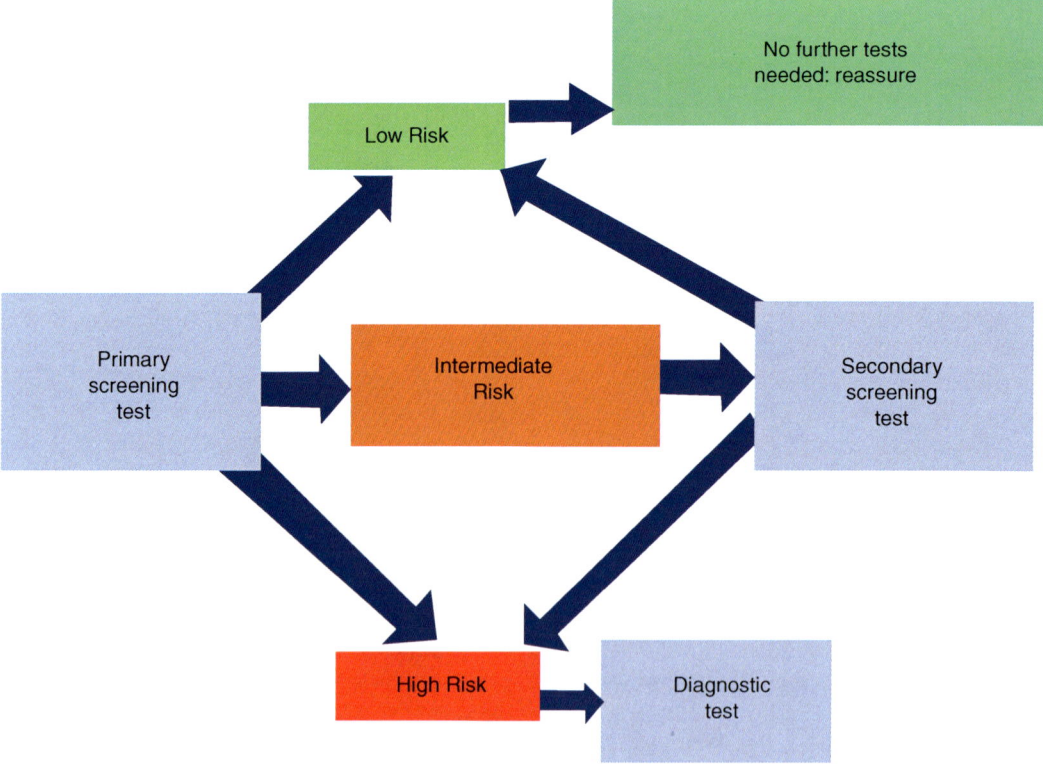

Fig. 4.2 Concept of intermediate risk

4.3 Which Pregnant Woman Should Be Offered Screening for Fetal Aneuploidies?

Every woman has a risk of having a fetus with aneuploidy—this risk varies with her age and history of previous aneuploidic pregnancies, but there is no age at which there is a "zero risk" of fetal chromosomal abnormality. Therefore, *every pregnant woman should be offered a screening test for fetal aneuploidies*. It is important here to remember few points about screening tests:

1. As a concept, screening for fetal aneuploidies should be offered to all pregnant women.
2. Adequate pretest counseling must be done (*details of counseling are dealt with in the Chap. 18 later in this book*).
3. Accepting or declining the test is a woman's prerogative as long as she makes an informed choice.
4. If she declines such tests, this fact must be duly documented in her notes.
5. If she accepts screening tests, then the optimal test should be offered and the results should be explained to her in a session dedicated to "posttest counseling."
6. In cases of artificial reproduction if "frozen self-eggs" or "donor ova" are used for fertilization, then the age of the mother at the time of egg retrieval or the age of the "donor" at the time of egg retrieval must be used as baseline "age risk" for fetal aneuploidies.

4.4 Which Are the Tests Available for Screening for Fetal Aneuploidies?

There are several tests available for screening for fetal aneuploidies in pregnancy. The components of these tests vary, and it is important for clinicians to understand each of these tests well so that they apply it logically and appropriately to their patients and get the desired results. The following tests can be offered to any pregnant woman who opts for "fetal aneuploidy screening":

1. First trimester combined screening test
2. Second trimester quadruple test
3. Cell-free fetal DNA test
4. Second trimester genetic sonogram

4.5 First Trimester Combined Screening Test

This test involves the nuchal translucency scan (11–14 weeks) and a blood test with biomarkers that help in assessing the risk for aneuploidies. Traditionally, two biomarkers were part of the combined test—free beta-hCG (human chorionic gonadotropin) and PAPP-A (pregnancy-associated plasma protein-A). Nuchal translucency is defined as the sonographic appearance of the subcutaneous collection of fluid behind the fetal neck in the first trimester in pregnancy. Increased nuchal translucency has been associated with increased risk of fetal aneuploidies. The details about the NT scan are available in the chapter on "first trimester scan." The biomarkers are chemicals produced in the "fetoplacental" unit, and their relative levels vary in aneuploidic pregnancies in a statistically significant manner such that these values can be used to generate a quantitative risk allocation for aneuploidies in a given pregnancy.

Human chorionic gonadotropin (hCG) is a hormone produced by the developing fetus and then large quantities by the placenta. The free beta subunit of hCG is used in first trimester screening. Concentrations of serum hCG usually rise rapidly in the mother's circulation for the first 8–10 weeks and then decrease and stabilize at a lower level for the rest of the pregnancy. The values of free beta hCG are found to be almost twice the normal values in the first trimester in fetuses with trisomy 21 as compared to euploid fetuses. In fetuses with trisomy 13 or 18, the free beta hCG levels are very low as compared to euploid fetuses. The absolute value of these biomarkers is expressed in "multiples of median" (MoM) for that gestation, and for the ease of comparison and as "median" is a measure of "central tendency," it is easier to understand and remember that the "normal" value would be close to 1 MoM. Any deviations from this value is expressed as increased (e.g., 3.5 MoMs is 3.5 times higher than expected) or decreased MoMs (e.g., 0.2 MoMs is almost a fifth of what is expected at that gestation).

PAPP-A is a protein produced first by the outer layer of the developing trophoblast and then by the growing placenta. During a normal pregnancy, PAPP-A levels increase in the mother's blood until delivery. Fetuses with aneuploidy tend to be associated with low levels of PAPP-A production in placenta, and thus this is used as a parameter for risk assessment for the same.

The "double marker" test can be offered anytime from 9 to 14 weeks of gestation, but the "NT scan" for risk assessment of aneuploidies can be done only in the time frame when the fetal CRL is between 45 and 84 mm. This is usually between 11 and 14 weeks of gestation. The sensitivity of the "combined test" is much better than the individual performance of first trimester biochemistry or the NT scan alone in screening for aneuploidies. As there are two tests involved and logistically it may not be possible for all fetal medicine clinics to provide *both* results on the same day, different protocols could be used based on a unit's infrastructure and facilities. Variations in arranging logistics and patient acceptability have necessitated different protocols (Table 4.1) for conducting the first trimester combined test.

The sensitivity of the "combined test" is about 90–95% for a false-positive rate of 5% with this performance yield limited to "FMF-accredited" sonographers and labs. Unless the criteria which were used in evaluation and validation of these methods are followed, this efficacy cannot be expected.

The first trimester combined test can be used even for twin pregnancies as long as the "chorionicity" is confirmed. Further screening issues with multiple pregnancies are dealt with in the chapter on "multiple pregnancy assessment" later.

As the scope of the first trimester screening is increasing and the spectrum of care provided at the first trimester clinic widens, there is a drive toward achieving more goals from tests at this

Table 4.1 Different protocols for performing the combined first trimester screening

	Protocol	Advantages	Limitations
Module 1 "One-stop clinic"	Patient visits once between 11 and 14 weeks (fetal CRL is between 45 and 84 mm); blood test is taken—patient waits in the clinic and both results are combined to give her the "combined test" result on the same day	1. Single visit for patient	1. Needs intensive in-house-accredited lab support
		2. Ability to offer results and counseling in one visit—better acceptability for both components of the "combined test"	2. May increase the cost of the test
			3. Although "convenient" for the patient, she gets lesser time to think about the test and may not understand everything well
Module 2 Two visits—biochemistry first/early biochemistry	Patient attends twice for the screening test. In the first visit, she gives the biochemistry test sample and schedules the NT scan appointment after a few days. On the day of the scan, the "combined" result is communicated to her.	1. Can be provided even in centers that do not have in-house-accredited labs	1. Two visits required—chances of noncompliance increase
	It is important to remember that "risk calculation" is done ONLY after BOTH scan and biochemistry results are available—not individually	2. Pretest counseling can be done at first visit and she gets enough time to understand the concept and ask questions about the process—better overall patient satisfaction	2. In few cases where there will be a fetal miscarriage, patient dissatisfaction over a seemingly "unnecessary" test creates some problems in counseling for the care provider
Module 3 Two visits—scan first followed by biochemistry	Patient attends twice for the screening test. In the first visit, she has the NT scan and then counseled about the biochemistry to help improve the sensitivity of the screening test. She then gives the sample for the blood test and returns for posttest counseling in a few days when results are ready.	1. Can be provided even in centers that do not have in-house-accredited labs	1. Two visits required—chances of noncompliance increase
	It is important to remember that "risk calculation" is done ONLY after BOTH scan and biochemistry results are available—not individually	2. Pretest counseling can be done at first visit and she gets enough time to understand the concept and ask questions about the process—better overall patient satisfaction	2. Even after a "normal" scan, there is a possibility of high-risk result on the combined test, and it sometimes makes the patient anxious and may warrant extensive counseling
		3. In few cases where there are gross abnormalities on the scan, the final care plan may have to be modified irrespective of the biochemistry results so it allows to avoid that test in these specific cases. *Such issues are important in settings where patients pay for their tests and would like to save on unnecessary tests*	

stage of pregnancy. Addition of certain placental biomarkers to the first trimester biochemistry protocol is opening up opportunities for screening for maternal preeclampsia too, and these issues are dealt with in the chapter on "screening for maternal disorders in the fetal medicine clinic" later on in this book.

Table 4.2 Analytes assessed in quadruple test and variations expected in trisomy 21

Analyte	Expected variation in trisomy 21 pregnancies as compared to pregnancies with euploid fetuses
HCG	Increased
Inhibin A	Increased
AFP	Decreased
Unconjugated estriol	Decreased

4.6 Second Trimester Maternal Serum Biochemistry (Quadruple Test)

The composition of certain "fetoplacental" chemicals can be tested in the maternal serum between 15 and 22 weeks to establish the risk for fetal aneuploidies. The relative proportion of these chemicals change in pregnancies associated with chromosomal abnormalities, and this is the rationale of evaluating the quantity of these substances and comparing them in terms of "multiples of median (MoM)" for that stage of gestation.

Traditionally, the triple serum test was performed which elevated maternal serum alfa-fetoprotein, hCG, and unconjugated estriol to assess the risk for Down syndrome. Triple test had a sensitivity of 60–70% for a false-positive rate of 10–15%. With the addition of one more analyte—inhibin A—to the triple test, the quadruple marker test has been designed, and this is known to have a better sensitivity (80–85%) with a lower false-positive rate (10%), and hence this has become the preferred modality of second trimester maternal serum biochemistry. The analytes involved in quadruple test and their expected changes in trisomy 21 are expressed in Table 4.2.

The composite algorithm for calculating risks based on these analytes is done by approved software, and the crucial points remain baseline maternal age and correct estimation of gestational age. This quadruple test can therefore be offered to women who have missed the first trimester screening for any reason and want a good risk reassessment in the second trimester. Dating the pregnancy is important and hence early pregnancy dating methods remain the most accurate method of dating. For all practical purposes, the EDD established during early pregnancy assessment can be used for dating throughout pregnancy to avoid confusions. Many labs use the second trimester BPD and reallocate dates even in cases of confirmed first trimester dating, and that is not desirable as gestational age allocation should be done once in early pregnancy and should not be changed repeatedly. In case there is no first trimester fetal assessment and the mother has booked late or her dates are unreliable, then the most reasonable option remains to use the second trimester biometry—especially the BPD for dating although it comes with the caveats of discrepancy due to early IUGR or fetal anomalies. In case the BPD is used for dating, the labs generally use a range of 30–50 mm for the quadruple test, and similarly if the EDD is used, a window of 15–22 weeks is acceptable although 16–18 weeks of gestation is optimal.

Another important point with risk allocation in the second trimester screening is to consider the first trimester screening results in case they are available. Ideally, if the first trimester combined screen is "low risk," there is no need to conduct a second trimester biochemistry as this test has a lower sensitivity than the FTS.

The quadruple test is also a "screening test" and the results generally indicated a "low risk" or "high risk" for fetal aneuploidies. The "low-risk" patients can be reassured, and the "high-risk" patients are explained that they need to be further evaluated to establish the need for definitive diagnostic tests to confirm fetal karyotype.

4.7 Cell-Free Fetal DNA Test

This is a SCREENING test for major fetal aneuploidies with very high sensitivity (99%). It is based on analysis of "cell"-free fetal DNA which is circulating in the mother's blood due to passage of DNA fragments into maternal circulation through the fetoplacental vessels after apoptosis of fetal cells in the placental bed.

It is based on a maternal blood test which can be done after 10 weeks of gestation. The "fetal fraction" of DNA is analyzed and if that fraction is more than 4%, then the results are valid for fetal screening. Assuming that the mother is euploid and there is no other source of "nonmaternal" DNA in the maternal blood stream, the results are likely to indicate fetal DNA-based results and are hence highly sensitive with more than 99% sensitivity reported for chromosome 21 trisomy assessment. The results are again like "high risk" or "low risk" for aneuploidies and high-risk results warrant invasive test. The "low-risk" cases can be reassured as the negative predictive value (with good fetal fraction) of this test is very good, but in cases of "high-risk" results, confirmation of fetal chromosomal status with amniocentesis is indicated. There are some causes that can contribute to false-positive results like confined placental mosaicism, maternal chromosomal mosaicism, maternal neoplasia-related karyotypic aberrations, etc. Hence, this is NOT a diagnostic test and "high-risk" results on cell-free fetal DNA test must be followed up with a diagnostic test.

The greater sensitivity of this test is definitely "tempting" to the clinician who is hassled often with the extensive counseling for "false positives" and lower detection rates of standard screening tests. However, the cell-free fetal DNA does not prove to be very useful or cost-effective as a "primary screening test." The added benefits of the first trimester scan for issues well beyond aneuploidy screening still place it as a better tool for primary screening as the "combined test" in first trimester.

4.8 The Midtrimester Genetic Sonogram

This is a systematic ultrasound evaluation of the fetus to look for any obvious "markers" for fetal aneuploidy in midtrimester (16–24 weeks). There are "major markers" or "minor markers" that can be seen at the time of the scan. The major markers are major structural anomalies which definitively increase the risk for associated chromosomal abnormalities and hence justify the need for invasive testing to confirm fetal karyotype. The "minor markers" are subtle features which can be detected by trained sonographers, and although they may not cause any functional implications to the fetus as such, their presence or absence alters the risk for fetal aneuploidies. There are many "minor" or soft markers associated with risk of fetal aneuploidies when detected in the midtrimester scan, e.g., absent/hypoplastic nasal bone, ventriculomegaly, aberrant right subclavian artery, intracardiac echogenic foci, echogenic bowel, fetal renal pyelectasis, short femur or humerus, etc. Individual markers and their importance have been mentioned in the chapter of system-wise midtrimester scan evaluation.

This alteration occurs based on the "likelihood ratio" of that particular minor marker with relation to fetal aneuploidy. This ratio (LR) is calculated by the "likelihood" of finding this marker in an aneuploid fetus versus the "likelihood" of finding this marker in normal euploid fetuses. Thus, a marker which is present commonly in euploid fetuses and is also seen in aneuploid fetuses will have a lower likelihood ratio than a marker which is seldom seen in normal fetuses.

An important concept here to understand is that just like the presence of a particular marker that increases the risk of trisomy 21 based on its isolated positive likelihood ratio, the absence of other markers also reduces the risk of trisomy 21 based on their collective negative likelihood ratios. Thus, any report which mentions presence of one soft marker must also mention presence/absence of other soft markers. The final risk of trisomy 21 will depend on the composite calculation of positive and negative likelihood ratios. From time to time, the individual markers vary in importance as more and more data accumulates based on the prevalence of these markers in normal population as compared to aneuploid fetuses. It is thus imperative for all fetal medicine practitioners to keep themselves updated on the latest protocols for such screening.

In summary, there are a range of tests available for screening and each has its own merits and limitations. All tests are not meant to be offered to all patients as it will lead to tremendous confusion and defeat the purpose of the tests!! Each unit has to adopt a screening protocol that fits best to their local practices, but it must be backed up by methods that carry evidence-based sanction for use. Literature is plenty about "combined" screening, "sequential" screening, "contingent" screening, or "integrated" screening. Each model can be applied in a unit depending on the overall availability of resources, efficiency, and patient satisfaction. In many cases, one has to have a plan for "opportunistic" screening models as healthcare seekers may not present uniformly at a certain gestation or may come with several past confusing reports—that is the reality in many sectors where practices are yet to be standardized. While the drive to uniform and evidence-based care should be a continuous forward movement, clinicians have to understand and adapt practices befitting their local population so as to at least sensitize the population toward fetal screening in the first place. The final goal would be to provide an ideal screening solution to every pregnant woman.

Key Learning Points in Screening for Fetal Aneuploidies

1. Screening for aneuploidies should be offered UNIVERSALLY to all pregnant women.
2. The options of tests available and their efficacy and limitations must be discussed in a PRETEST counseling.
3. Screening is voluntary and those who opt out of the process have a right to do so—the decision should be well informed and documented.
4. Screening protocols should be up to date considering constant advancement of science, technology, and contemporary guidelines.
5. Screening test results should be explained to women in a POSTTEST counseling session to help alleviate doubts and concerns.
6. A rational approach to screening strategies can help provide a very satisfying experience to women and is a good adjunct to pregnancy healthcare.

Suggested Reading

Agathokleous M, et al. Meta-analysis of second-trimester markers for trisomy 21. Ultrasound Obstet Gynecol. 2013;41:247–61.

Benn P, et al. Position statement from the chromosome abnormality screening committee on behalf of the board of the international society for prenatal diagnosis. Prenat Diagn. 2015;35(8):725–34.

Cuckle HS, Wald NJ. Principles of screening. In: Wald N, Leck I, editors. Antenatal & neonatal screening. 2nd ed. Oxford: Oxford University Press; 2000. p. 3–22.

Nicolaides KH. A model for a new pyramid of prenatal care based on the 11 to 13 weeks' assessment. Prenat Diagn. 2011;31:3–6.

Nicolaides KH, et al. First-trimester contingent screening for trisomies 21, 18 and 13 by biomarkers and maternal blood cell-free DNA testing. Fetal Diagn Ther. 2013;35:185.

Basics of Imaging for Fetal Evaluation

Imaging of the fetus is one of the most important aspects of evaluating the fetus who is the "patient" in the science of fetal medicine. Just like the protocol of any clinical examinations that starts with "inspection," even in fetal medicine, "inspecting" the fetus starts the actual examination. Now unlike other specialities, our patient in fetal medicine comes to us hidden from our view, positioned inside the mother! Therefore, in order to visualize the fetus, we have to use techniques to overcome the barrier of maternal tissues, and the "ultrasound" has become our "magic eye" which helps us see the fetus through the mother's abdomen rather "noninvasively."

Doctors generally get intimidated by the concepts of physics that are the basis of this ultrasound technology, and we think it is impossible for us to understand this heavy theoretical physics stuff!! However, it is important not only to understand the basics but also to be aware of the potential and limitations of this brilliant technology because it is a revolutionary tool and its applications are increasing day by day.

Sound waves are mechanical waves that have the property of getting reflected when they encounter an obstacle. Ultrasound is conducted as "waves" and the "frequency" is defined as the number of vibrations (cycles) per second. The unit of frequency is Hertz (Hz). Ultrasound waves have a frequency of greater than 20,000 Hz and cannot be heard by the human ear (*20–20,000 Hz approximately is the range of the human hearing!!*). Obstetric ultrasound employs frequencies of 2–15 megahertz (MHz). The higher the frequency of the ultrasound wave, the better is the resolution, but penetration depth is lesser than a lower-frequency wave. Thus, in fetal imaging, an optimal compromise has to be made between resolution and penetration to get the best possible information required for fetal evaluation.

An ultrasound machine has a transducer or "probe" which is used to transmit and receive signals from the area of investigation, a processor in the machine which processes this information into images that is relayed on the "screen" which we view as "images," and a "control panel" that helps in coordinating commands in the entire process (Fig. 5.1).

The probe or transducer has several "piezoelectric" crystals mounted together. These crystals can produce a mechanical wave when electric pulse is applied to them, and inversely, when pressure is applied to the surface of certain crystals, an electric current is produced. This "piezoelectric effect" and its inversion lead to formation of images on the scanning machine which we are able to decipher to understand fetal anatomy and physiology.

The ultrasound waves pass into the tissues in their path and get reflected back from tissue interfaces. Reflection takes place at the interfaces of media with different acoustic densities and is proportionate to the acoustic density differences in the sampled area. If the acoustic density differ-

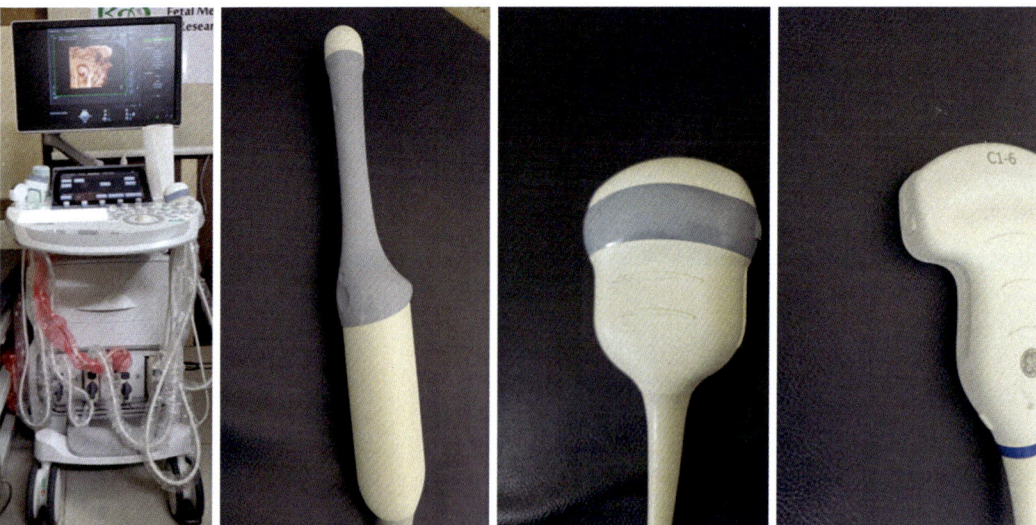

Fig. 5.1 Ultrasound probe, machine electricity source

Fig. 5.2 Hyperechoic and hypoechoic

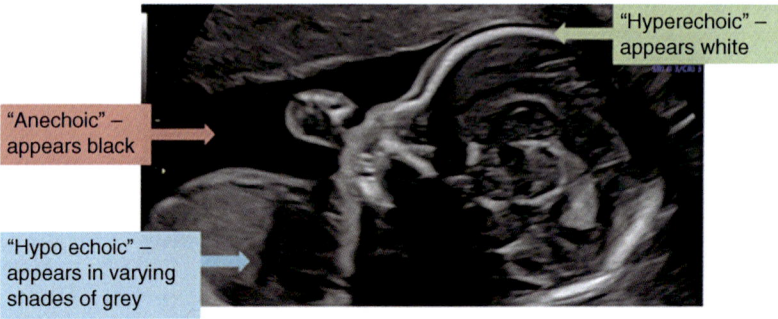

ences are low, low level echoes result. If the acoustic densities are all identical as in homogeneous fluids like blood, amniotic fluid, and urine, the entire wave is transmitted and none is reflected resulting in a "hypoechoic" image. When the acoustic densities are markedly different such as when dense tissue like bone is encountered, the image is "hyperechoic" (Fig. 5.2).

The information contained in the returning waves is converted back into electrical impulses and fed into the computer for processing into an ultrasound image. The processor computes the location (depth) of the signal based on time differences between transmitting and receiving. Echoes reflected back from tissues close to the transducer come in earlier than those from tissues deeper in the field. The ultrasound picture as computed by the processor is then displayed on the computer monitor (screen). The velocity of sound waves is constant at 1540 m/s and is determined by the wavelength and frequency. The higher the frequency, the shorter the wavelength. Higher-frequency transducers have a better spatial resolution. This means that they can better differentiate two closely located side-by-side spots in the region of interest. The penetration of high-frequency waves is, however, limited. Therefore, high-frequency probes are used to look at near structures and lower-frequency probes are used to study tissues at depth. Abdominal transducers use a frequency of 2–6.5 MHz and transvaginal transducers use frequencies of 5–15 MHz.

The most common form of ultrasound scan used for fetal studies today is a real-time grayscale "B-mode" study. B-mode studies indicate

5 Basics of Imaging for Fetal Evaluation

reflections arranged along two axes in the region of interest. They use a grayscale which reflects the intensity of the signal and imparts texture to the image.

In fetal evaluation, the image on the screen has to be interpreted by the operator in terms of the fetal parts being represented, and thus it is important to keep in mind the "orientation" of the part being scanned. Many times operators do not use the entire display screen and struggle to see structures on the screen without magnifying the image. Most machines have the ability to "zoom" the image, and it is imperative to magnify the area of interest to use the screen optimally and visualize better.

The "gain" on the machine can be adjusted to alter the brightness and contrast features of the image. As a rule, when highly echogenic structures like bone are visualized, the "gain" is usually reduced so that the margins become sharply defined. However, when better soft tissue delineation is expected, the gain has to be increased.

The picture (Fig. 5.3) here demonstrates the effects of gain alteration in obtaining pictures of the fetal head. When the gain is low, the skull margins are sharply delineated but the intracranial structures are not clearly seen. When the gain is increased, better visualization of the brain matter is achieved at the cost of some "fuzziness" in bony margins.

The other attribute of B-mode studies is real-time. When ultrasound was first used, the image was static. It has now for many decades moved into the real-time mode where the image moves in the same manner as the region of interest moves in real life, similar to the difference between a photograph and a video. To this can be added the concept of depth or the third dimension. This is made possible by a special transducer and computer software arrangement and is referred to as 3D ultrasound. This has further advanced to real-time 3D ultrasound which is known as 4D ultrasound. 3D/4D imaging has taken the potential of fetal imaging another step forward such that apart from mere imaging planes, "volume" analysis is possible and better delineation of fetal anatomy, placental planes, etc. can be achieved. Figure 5.4 shows a comparative display of 2D and 3D pictures—the fourth dimension in "4D" ultrasound is actually "time" such that real-time imaging in 3D is actually called 4D imaging.

The term M-mode refers to a motion mode in B-mode studies. This is currently employed in obstetrics to assess fetal cardiac motion to assess heart rate and rhythm as well as for studying the

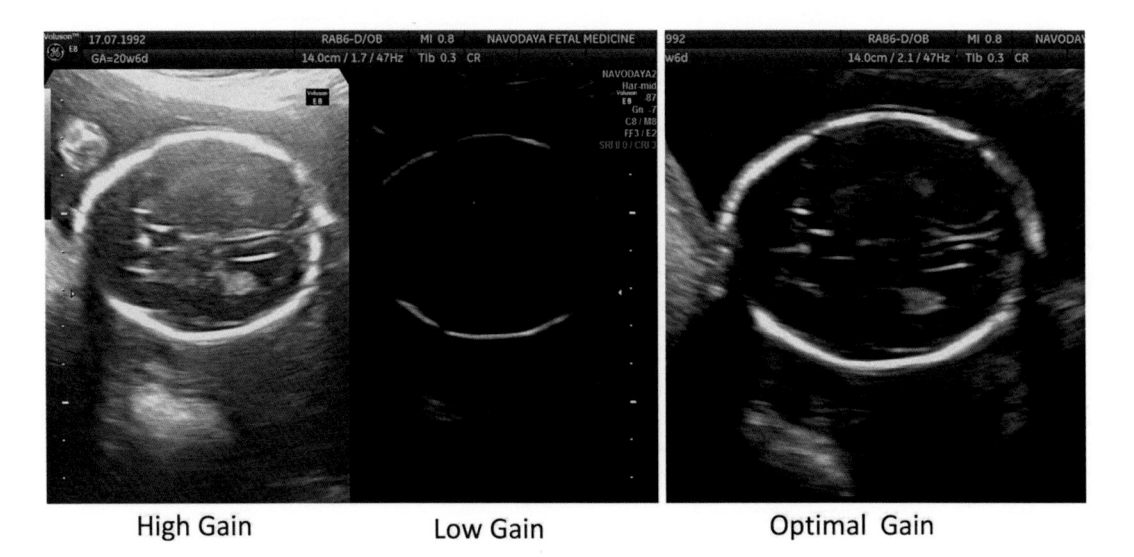

Fig. 5.3 Gain settings: high and low

Fig. 5.4 2D/3D pictures

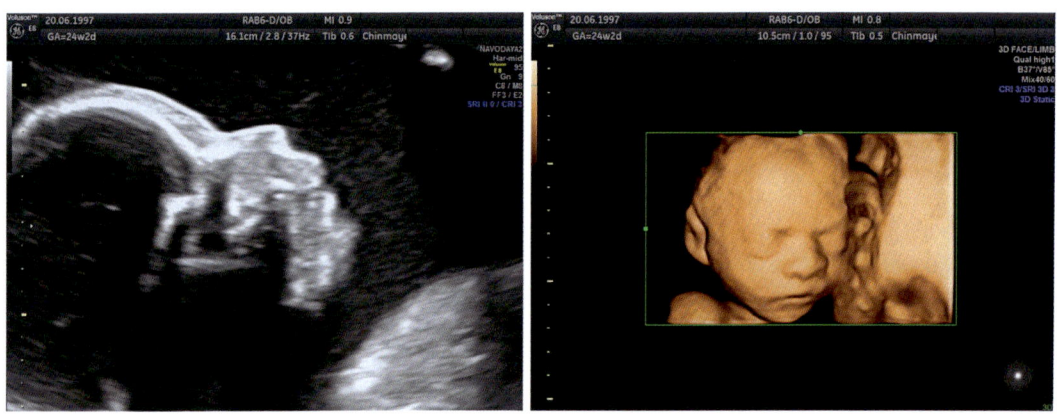

2D fetal face profile

3D fetal face surface rendering

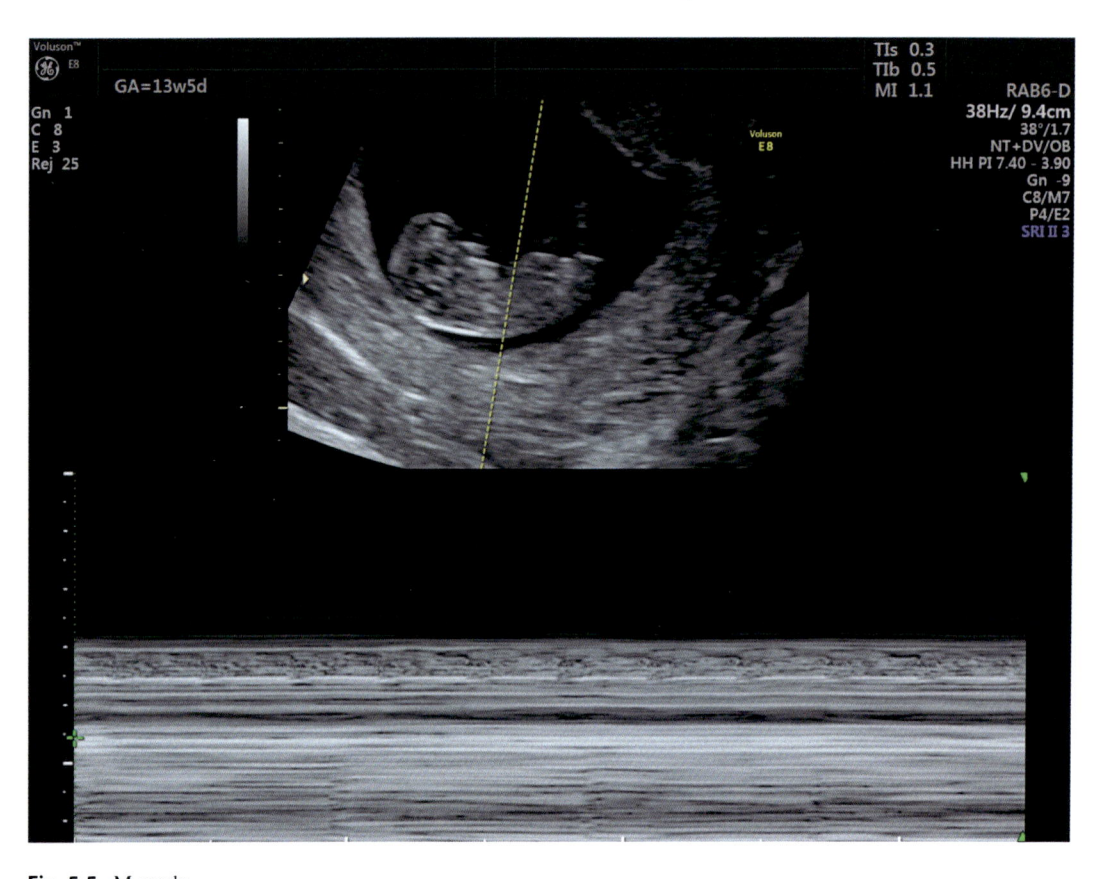

Fig. 5.5 M-mode

excursions of the valves and the myocardium. Figure 5.5 shows an M-mode study of the fetal heart rate. The cursor runs across a section of tissues and any motion is detected by pulses on the image corresponding to the region of the moving object.

5.1 Fetal MRI

In very limited indications, fetal MRI can be used to augment findings of the ultrasound and help in refining the diagnosis. Over the years, MRI has corroborated findings of ultrasound, and especially in fetal CNS malformations, the role of MRI has been accepted in view of better delineation of soft tissue arrangements. There were some initial studies which suggested a definite advantage of MRI over ultrasound, but considering the improvement both in ultrasound technology and in the expertise of fetal ultrasound, the practical utility of fetal MRI remains rather limited. Fetal movement is a hindrance to good image acquisition on MRI, and sometimes the efforts to achieve fetal quiescence can increase the time taken for MRI, hence increasing the cost and time inputs further (Fig. 5.6).

MRI can provide useful information about fetal CNS malformations in the third trimester, but by then the obstetric plans cannot change much. Safety of 1.5 T MRI without contrast has been accepted in all trimesters of pregnancy. Sometimes getting an MRI helps in reconfirming the findings of ultrasound and better documentation and demonstration for sharing a medicolegal responsibility in case the ultrasound findings are questioned. Thus, an MRI is not a replacement for ultrasound in fetal imaging but has some adjunctive role which can be justified in select cases with rational indications.

In a nutshell, plan 2D ultrasound remains the most important method of fetal imaging which is easily complemented by Doppler techniques. Additional multiplanar imaging (3D/4D) is done for surface rendering, better storage of imaging data, and post-storage processing options which help in learning and teaching. Fetal MRI has a limited role as an adjunct modality for corroboration of ultrasound findings when in doubt especially in CNS malformations where soft tissue delineation is vital.

A pictorial representation of all imaging modalities in fetal medicine is given in Fig. 5.7.

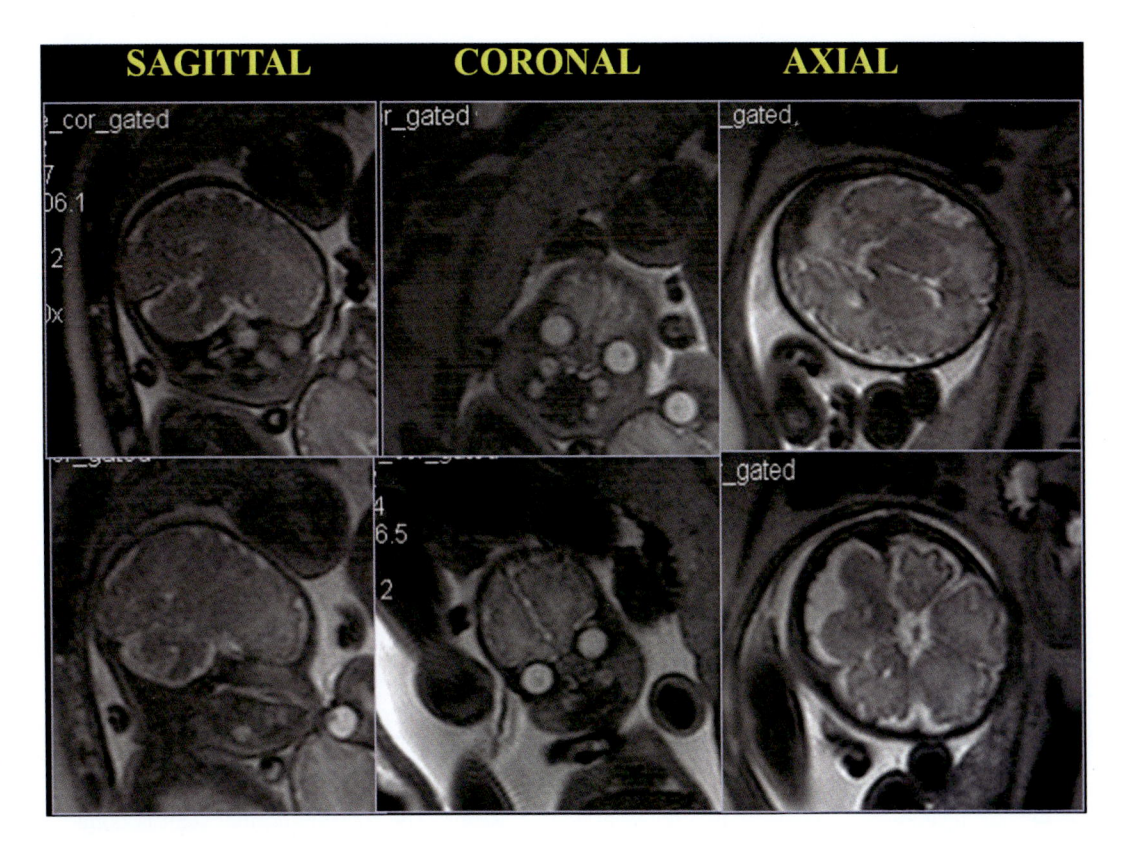

Fig. 5.6 Fetal MRI

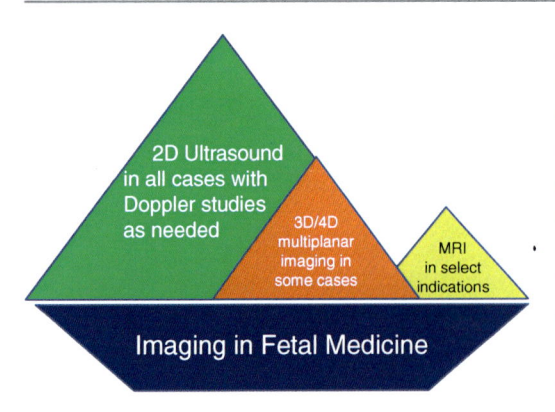

Fig. 5.7 Imaging in fetal medicine

5.2 Safety of Ultrasound

Ultrasound remains one of the safest methods of fetal evaluation, and despite its use through decades, there are no confirmed biologic effects on patients and their fetuses from the use of diagnostic ultrasound evaluation. The benefits to patients exposed to the prudent use of this modality outweigh the risks if any. Most research and monitoring bodies have corroborated this fact and have laid down safety guidelines to further minimize any potential damage that can be foreseen. It is wise, therefore, as for any medical test, to perform the examination only when clearly indicated. The operator performing the examination should exercise due care to use appropriate energies and keep a track of the duration of the study in order to comply with the ALARA principle. This principle simply states that the use of technicalities should be optimized to obtain quality images with frequencies, power, and duration as low as reasonably achievable.

5.3 Some Good Practice Points

While ultrasound itself is a safe method of fetal evaluation, the ultrasound machine needs to be kept in optimum condition to get the best results of fetal imaging. The machine should be placed in a room with a temperature regulation facility to maintain a stable room temperature as there can be significant heat generated while the scanner is functioning. A stable, uninterrupted power supply should be connected to prevent potentially dangerous voltage fluctuations. The probes must be handled carefully to prevent any mechanical damage. After the scan is over, the surface of the probe should be wiped clean using a soft tissue or cloth to remove any remnants of the coupling gel.

- It is important to "freeze" the probe when it is not being used to prevent unnecessary heating of its piezoelectric crystals. Most machines are mounted on wheels that can be locked and unlocked to facilitate movement of the unit. Training the scan room assistant staff members in the correct handling of the machine and probes will go a long way in increasing the longevity of the scan machine by minimizing the avoidable wear and tear problems.

5.4 Ethical Considerations

It is important to remember that the woman undergoing an ultrasound examination is a human being and not a laboratory specimen. She may already be well informed and have undergone several examinations in the past but is equally likely to be a first-timer with the attendant anxiety, ignorance, and apprehension. She should be reassured about the "painlessness" and safety, particularly in the context of the fetus. A brief overview of the information wanting to be obtained by the clinician should be conveyed. An appropriate review of clinical features should be carried out, and appropriate clinical information and consent forms should be completed as per institutional and legal norms. Since the procedure involves an invasion of privacy, however legal, care should be taken to restrict the flow of medical personnel into and out of the examining suite. Where possible, an attempt should be made to keep those parts of the anatomy covered that do not need to come in contact with the transducer. Since ultrasound gel and bleeding can be messy, it is considerate to offer the patient a gown to change into.

Fasting is not required for fetal scans and must be stated prior to wall women waiting for their scans. The transabdominal scan is done in a supine position. In advanced pregnancy, this might compromise venous return to the heart from the lower limbs. The patient could feel faint or vaguely uncomfortable and should be put into a lateral position for a few minutes before resuming the scan. Transvaginal scans do not require a lithotomy position or suspension of the feet in stirrups. A foldaway table is useful to help angulate the vaginal transducer. If the luxury of this is not available, a cushion under the pelvis is useful. A condom could be used to cover the transducer if special probe covers are unavailable. Operators must use gloves for a transvaginal procedure and disposable probe covers are mandatory. Air-drying of transducers is adequate for destroying the human immunodeficiency virus but inadequate for several other microbes. Some centers additionally use transducer dipping in microbicidal solutions. Manufacturers' recommendations need to be followed for this, and there are specialized probe decontamination instruments available too. Ultrasound gel should be used as necessary to permit smooth transducer movements. This gel is rather cool and can be uncomfortable sometimes so it should be warmed in winter months. When using this gel for assisting in ultrasound-guided procedures, it is useful to sterilize it to prevent infections.

After the completion of the fetal scan, the finalization of the report and conveying the same to the parents should be done with utmost sensitivity and confidentiality. When the results are normal, a fetal scan should be a very satisfying experience for the parents. In situations where a fetal anomaly is detected, measures should be taken in confirming the facts and preparing a multidisciplinary care plan so that the parents have understood the problem and have clarity toward the next step.

Imaging in fetal medicine is therefore a very vital part of fetal evaluation but is only one aspect of the entire concept of fetal care. The purpose of this chapter was to introduce the reader to the basics of instruments and technology used for fetal imaging which will help produce the images as explained in the following chapters.

Evaluation of Fetal Biometry

6

Bios stands for *life*, and metros for measurement—so "biometry" is a term used for an activity where we are "measuring" living things. In fetal medicine, biometry is the activity of measuring certain parts of the fetus such that an assessment of growth can be made and with some combination of measurements, fetal weight can be estimated.

Measurements are taken on images magnified on the screen of the ultrasound machine, and these "absolute" values are then expressed as "centiles" for that stage of gestation based on data amalgamated through large population studies—both cross-sectional and longitudinal. These measurements or "biometry" is an integral part of any fetal evaluation because the status of fetal growth—whether appropriate or aberrant—is one of the basic parameters of establishing normalcy of the fetus. Even in the absence of any detectable anomaly, a fetus whose growth is lagging behind its expected gestational age parameters (small for dates—SGA) or one which shows an accelerated pace of growth (large for dates—LGA) has a worse prognosis than an appropriately grown fetus. What is the "normal parameter" is defined based on reference charts and standard graphs derived from population-based studies, and the concept of "fetal growth" will be dealt with in detail in a separate chapter in this book. The present chapter concentrates on the technique of measuring fetal parts that are used to derive the assessment of fetal size at every stage of pregnancy.

At different stages of fetal development, the biometry parameters are different and have been validated for correlation with gestational age such that growth assessment can be done.

6.1 Ultrasound Biometry in Early Pregnancy

The most important aspect of early pregnancy ultrasound is to establish an intrauterine pregnancy and its viability followed by biometry. The "gestational sac" first becomes visible on TVS during the fifth week appearing as a small sonolucent area surrounded by an echogenic ring of chorionic villi. The yolk sac appears during sixth week and is seen as a hypoechoic ring with echogenic margin. By the end of sixth week, the fetal pole is visible on TVS as a 2–8 mm pole with embryonic cardiac activity.

On TAS these landmarks are visible 1 week later than on TVS. With ultrasound equipment improving in quality of resolution and penetration, every year these limits are bound to get redefined (Fig. 6.1).

The biometric parameters in early pregnancy ultrasound are mentioned in Table 6.1.

© Springer Nature Singapore Pte Ltd. 2022
C. Ratha, A. Khurana, *Fetal Medicine*, https://doi.org/10.1007/978-981-19-6099-4_6

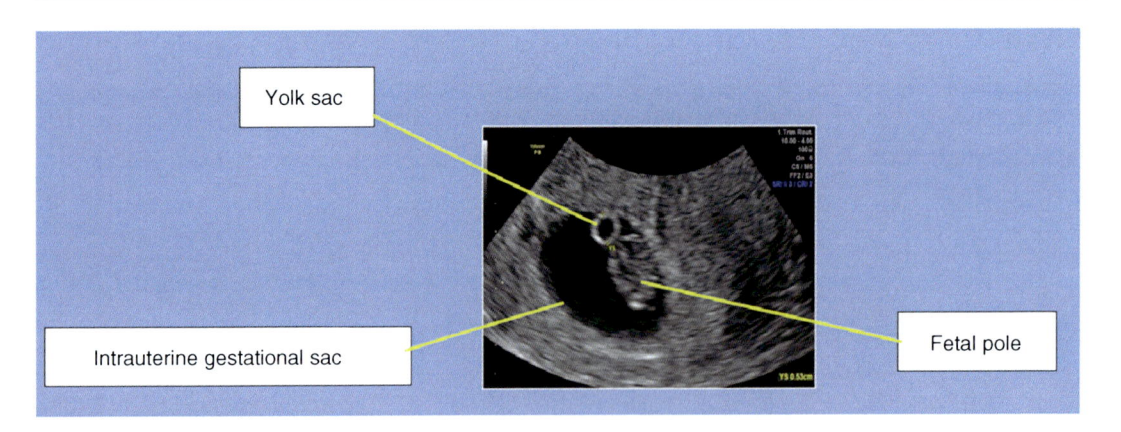

Fig. 6.1 Early pregnancy scan

Table 6.1 Biometric parameters in early pregnancy ultrasound

	What and how to measure	Picture
Fetal pole	Length: The fetal pole is measured as the longest measurement along its longitudinal axis excluding the yolk sac and extremities and expressed as crown-rump length (CRL) in millimeters (mm) or centimeters (cm)	
Yolk sac	Diameter: The longest diameter of the yolk sac is measured as a straight line	

6.1 Ultrasound Biometry in Early Pregnancy

Table 6.1 (continued)

	What and how to measure	Picture
Gestational sac	Mean sac diameter (MSD): The longitudinal diameter of the GS is measured in three orthogonal planes and then divided by 3	
Fetal heart rate	Beats per minute: Measured using calipers on an M-mode tracing of the fetal cardiac activity	
Any adnexal structure (e.g., maternal ovaries or any other mass like cysts, etc.)	Dimensions: Linear measurements at least in two perpendicular planes	

6.2 Significance of Early Pregnancy Biometry

CRL is measured as the largest dimension of embryo in its longitudinal axis, and it is used as a primary measure of gestational age between 6 and 14 weeks (or up to a CRL of 84 mm). This concept of dating a pregnancy based on the crown-rump length of the fetal pole was suggested by Hugh Robinson in a seminal paper in 1975, and it is indeed one of those "time tested" facts that even today continues to be accepted, quoted, and referenced even in the most recent publications on dating of human pregnancies. Since it is widely acknowledged that maternal recall of last menstrual period dates may be inaccurate for the purpose of dating in almost 40% cases due to a number of reasons, ultrasound-based dating is the most accurate estimation of gestational age in early pregnancy. Studies have accepted that as long as the ultrasound dating and LMP-based dating are concordant within a week's time, it is acceptable to use either method, but if the disparity is more than a week, it is better to redate based on the USG in early pregnancy.

In multifetal gestations, where there are more than one fetuses, the CRL of the larger fetus is taken into account to date the pregnancy. The rationale behind this is that while there are known causes of early fetal growth restriction, it is highly unlikely for macrosomia to set this so early and hence the larger fetus probably represents the normal growth pattern. In multiple pregnancies, especially with ART and delayed embryo transfers, these concepts are getting further refined. This aspect will be dealt with in detail in the chapter on "multiple pregnancy."

6.3 "Dating Is a New Beginning!!"

This "dating" is of utmost importance in the overall management of pregnancy as major obstetric and perinatal decisions are led by the estimation of gestational age. The phrase "dating is a new beginning" has been coined with the idea of establishing how "dating" the pregnancy helps in properly planning further care—it is as good as a new beginning to the whole gamut of maternofetal evaluation in pregnancy. Table 6.2 enumerates some important issues which are based on proper dating of the pregnancy.

This leads us to the fact that by the end of the first trimester, there should be an unequivocal clarity about the dating of the pregnancy. As we have understood that the LMP is not the most accurate method and hence after checking both LMP and the CRL of the first trimester scan, an expected date of delivery or "EDD" should be allocated to the pregnancy. Thereafter, in that pregnancy, the patient must be explained to quote her EDD every time she comes for an obstetric evaluation as women are traditionally accustomed to quote their LMP and this leads to significant confusion in maternofetal evaluation. EDD once allocated in first trimester should not be changed subsequently in the same pregnancy.

Table 6.2 Importance of "dating" a pregnancy

1. Assessment of appropriateness of fetal growth
2. Timing of fetal aneuploidy and anomaly screening scans
3. Timing and interpretation of serum biochemistry-based aneuploidy/PIH screening
4. Planning invasive prenatal diagnostic tests
5. Decisions to deliver in cases of PPROM/IUGR/complications of fetal anomalies/multiple gestations, etc.

6.5 Biparietal Diameter

All obstetricians and fetal medicine practitioners should remember to "date" a pregnancy BEFORE starting to evaluate the fetus. This will automatically dispel most confusions regarding growth problems. A detailed discussion on growth evaluation will be done in Chap. 9 ("Fetal Growth Disorders").

6.4 Fetal Biometry in Second and Third Trimester

The standard fetal biometric measurements reported on second and third trimester ultrasound are:

- Biparietal diameter (BPD)
- Head circumference (HC)
- Abdominal circumference (AC)
- Femur length (FL)

These measurements when calculated together based on formulas give the estimated fetal weight. Most modern ultrasound machines have these formulae included in their basic calculation software such that one need not memorize these, but it is important to understand their derivation.

6.5 Biparietal Diameter

This is the length between the two parietal eminences in the fetal skull measured in an axial plane—either a transventricular plane or a transthalamic plane.

This is measured perpendicular to falx cerebri at the broadest part of the skull, either from the outer margin of proximal parietal bone to either the inner margin of distal parietal bone or the outer margin of the same (Fig. 6.2). The academic debate between which method should be used remains unanswered as in reality there is not much a difference in the actual measurement either ways.

The rationale of using one method over the other is based on the fact that in the age of the earlier scan machines, it was easier to define the inner margin of the distal parietal bone—this is hardly an issue with the excellent resolution abilities of the present-day machines.

The proponents of the "outer-to-outer" measurement claim that this is clinically better justified because when the head circumference is measured after birth, it is always along the outer margin of the skull, so logically the same approach should be followed antenatally. Table 6.3 enumerates the important points to be considered while measuring the fetal BPD.

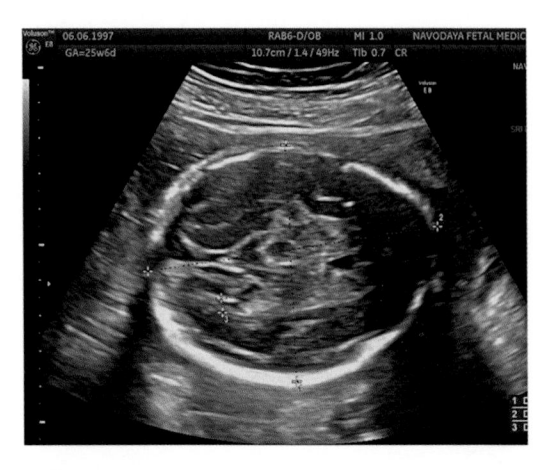

Fig. 6.2 BPD

Table 6.3 Measurement of fetal biparietal diameter (BPD)

Axial view of the skull along transventricular/transthalamic plane
Low gain settings to get sharper margins of the bone
CSP should be well visualized interrupting the falx cerebri. Cerebellum should NOT be seen in this view
Largest diameter between the parietal eminences is measured perpendicular to the falx
One may measure either O-O or O-I but it is important that the same protocol be used in all serial measurements of a particular fetus

6.6 Head Circumference

It is measured at the outer edges of calvarium. The anatomical slice required to measure the HC is the same as that for the BPD. The HC may be directly measured with an ellipse (see Fig. 6.3a, b) or can be derived from the BPD and the occipital-frontal diameter (OFD).

The BPD is measured as explained above, and the OFD is obtained by placing the calipers in the middle of the bone echo at both the frontal and occipital skull bones.

After taking two mutually perpendicular measurements, the head's circumference is computed using the formula: HC = (BPD + OFD) × 1.62.

In some cases, the OFD is longer than usual which is compensated by a smaller BPD and the cross section of the fetal head looks somewhat oval as shown in Fig. 6.4a, a condition called dolichocephaly. This may be a normal variant in many cases especially when the fetus is in breech presentation in utero but rarely may be part of a dysmorphology sequence and hence needs a detailed evaluation.

Similarly at times, the head shape is somewhat squarish with a smaller OFD compensated by a larger BPD leading to brachycephaly (Fig. 6.4b). This may be a normal variant but is associated with some fetal anomalies and trisomy 21.

The ratio between the biparietal diameter and the occipitofrontal diameter is known as the "cephalic index," and it is calculated using the formula: CI = BPD/OFD × 100.

In normal cases, it ranges between 75% and 78% in the second and third trimesters with a gradually increasing trend in pregnancy such that fetuses at term and in cephalic presentation have higher CI than preterm fetuses or those in breech presentation.

The advantage of the ellipse method is its ease of application, but it may not work very well in cases where there is significant distortion of the perimeter either due to inherent anomalies or a deeply engaged head when it is difficult to get a complete view of the fetal head. Independent measurements of two perpendicular axes are helpful in such situations.

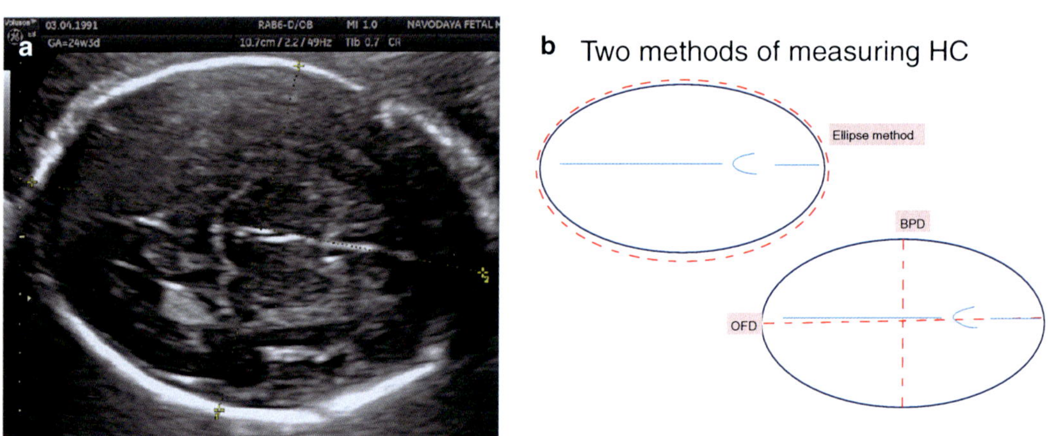

Fig. 6.3 (**a**) HC. (**b**) Methods to measure HC

6.6 Head Circumference

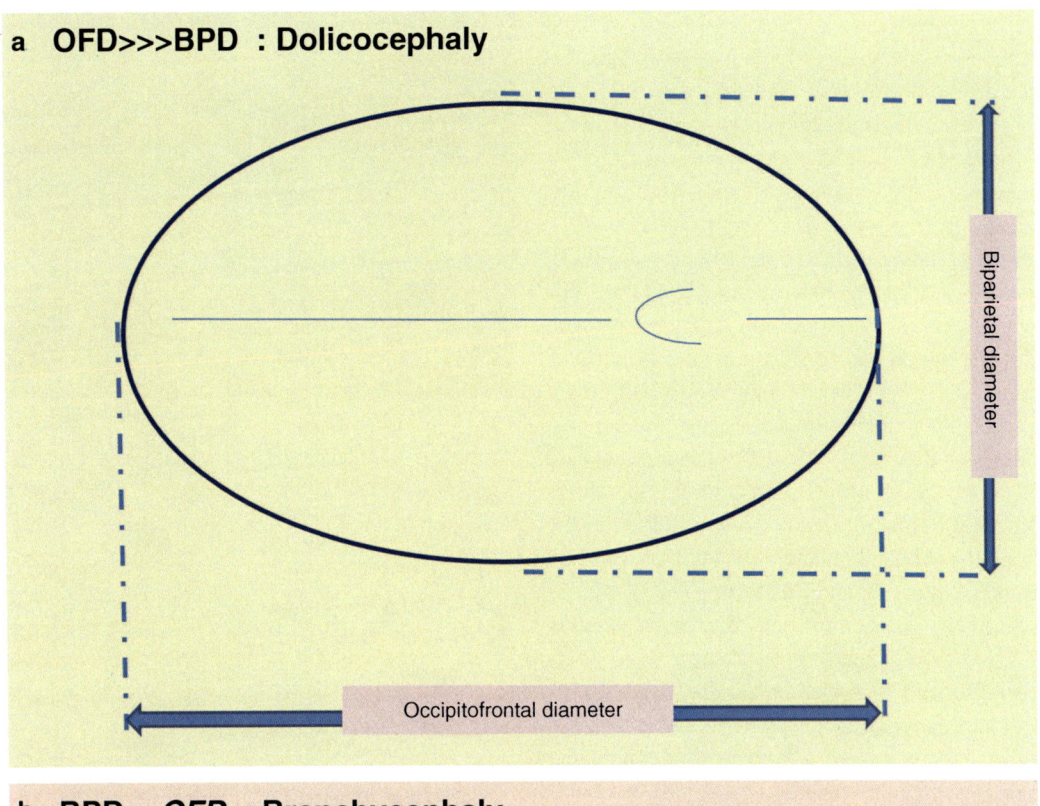

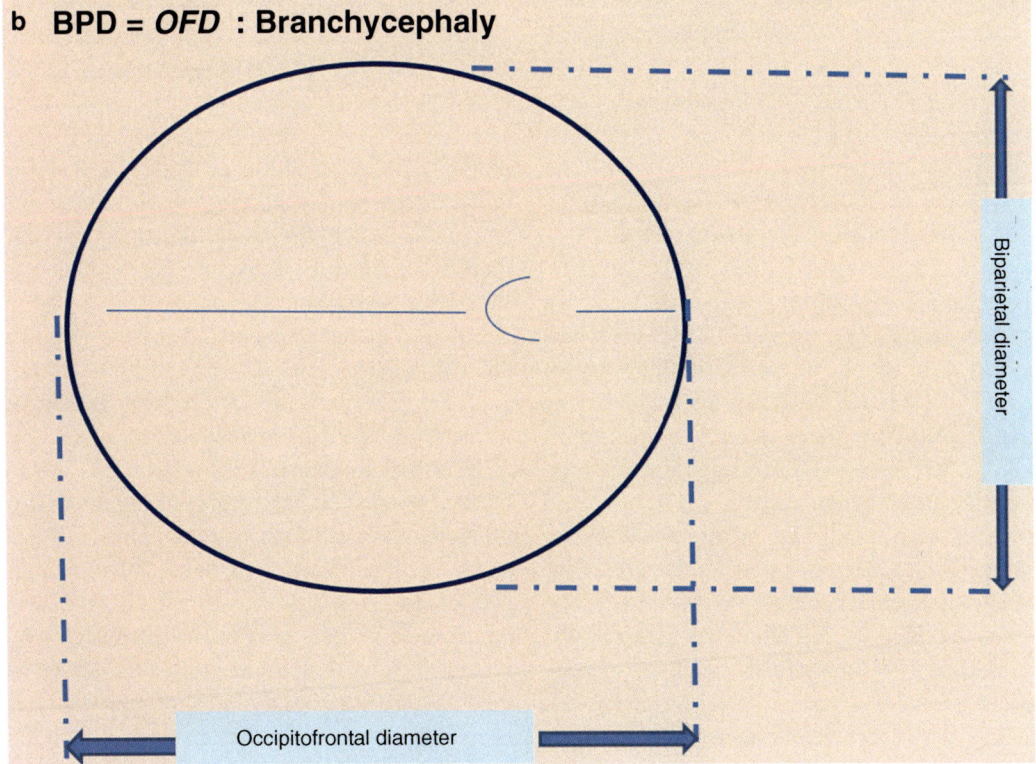

a OFD>>>BPD : Dolicocephaly

b BPD = *OFD* : Branchycephaly

Fig. 6.4 (**a**) Dolichocephaly. (**b**) Brachycephaly

Both these methods are acceptable in clinical practice and most users have a personal preference of one or the other. What is important is to maintain similar measurement protocols to avoid confusion in comparison in serial evaluations.

Accurate measurement of fetal head circumference is important as it is acceptable as a method of dating in the second trimester for those where first trimester dating is unavailable. For every stage of gestation, biometry charts are available which can convert numerical measurements into "centiles," and a measurement between 5th and 95th centile is considered appropriate for dates. In case the HC measurements are below the 5th centile (microcephaly) or above 95th centile (macrocephaly), one is alerted to the possibility of a fetal anomaly, and it warrants detailed evaluation and follow-up.

Biometry can be represented in centiles, or as ±2.5 SD from mean or as Z-score deviations depending on which method adheres to local protocol and the comfort level of the users. The use of Z-scores in recent publications depicts that there is a distinct advantage especially for comparison, but as most conventional users are well versed with the concept of "centiles," it is still the most prevalent method of clinical explanation of fetal biometry.

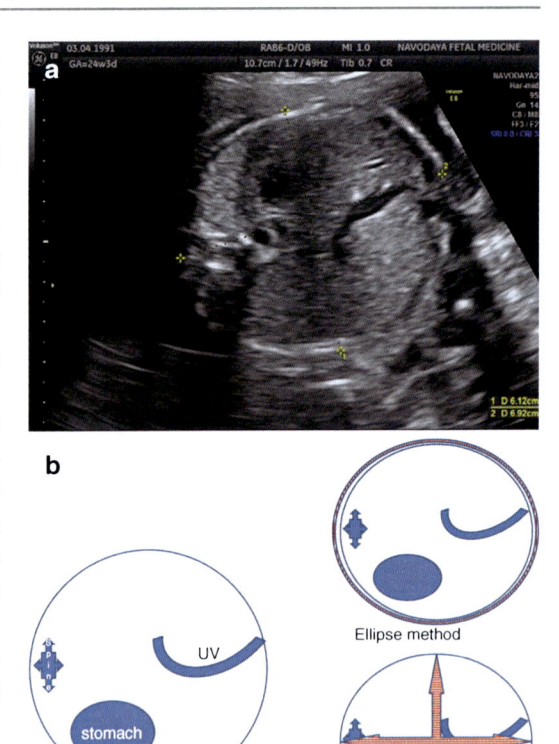

Fig. 6.5 (**a**) AC. (**b**) Different methods of AC measurement

6.7 Abdominal Circumference

This is measured on the transverse section of the abdomen as the outer margin of the plane where the stomach bubble is seen and the entry of umbilical vein to DV is seen as a J shape curving toward right with a single rib on each side. Again, like the HC, AC can be measured as an ellipse along the outer margins of the plane described above or as a composite measurement of the transverse and anteroposterior diameters at the same level as shown in Fig. 6.5a, b.

The AC is measured along the external skin line, either with the "ellipse" method or using two perpendicular linear measurements—the anteroposterior abdominal diameter (APAD) and transverse abdominal diameter (TAD) as shown in Fig. 6.5b. The APAD is the linear distance between the skin over the anterior abdominal wall to the back of the spine, while the transverse diameter is the widest distance perpendicular to the APAD in the same section.

The AC is then calculated using the formula: AC = π(APAD + TAD)/2 = 1.57(APAD + TAD).

The important considerations while taking AC measurements are given in Table 6.4.

The fetal abdominal circumference is one of the first parameters that is altered in growth disorders like IUGR or macrosomia. This is related to the fact that most of the fetal abdominal circumference is due to the size of the fetal liver which is the storehouse of fetal energy. A growth-restricted fetus will have a smaller abdomen much before restriction of size of the fetal head or long bones start and thus changes in fetal AC are sensitive indicators of fetal growth.

6.9 Calculation of Estimated Fetal Weight on Ultrasound

Table 6.4 Important points while measuring the fetal AC

Axial view of the fetal abdomen is obtained with the abdominal segment of the umbilical vein seen at the level of the portal sinus
Medium gain settings to get soft tissue shadows in addition to the bony rib margins
Normally, the stomach bubble should be seen in this view but NOT the fetal kidneys
AC can be measured as an ellipse along the outer margin of this view
Alternatively, TAD and APAD can be measured separately as described in the text
It is better to measure the AC in a view such that the spine is laterally placed—at 3 o'clock or 9 o'clock position rather than directly anterior or posterior
Excessive pressure on the maternal abdomen can distort the AC and lead to erroneous measurement.

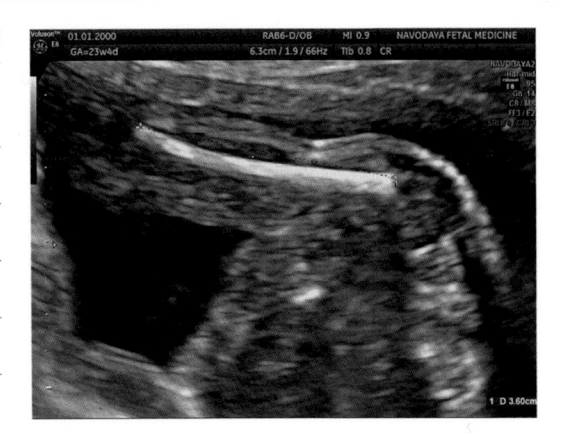

Fig. 6.6 Femur length

6.8 Measurement of Fetal Femur Length

In second and third trimesters, fetal femur length is taken as an important component of the formula that helps in estimating the fetal weight through ultrasonographic measurements. All long bones are examined in low gain settings to get a sharper definition of the edges and are measured end to end, excluding the epiphysis. The femur is thus measured along its long diameter, while the image is optimally magnified and the bone is placed at an angle of insonation of 45–90°. Care is taken to exclude the distal femoral epiphyses and only the ossified diaphysis is measured. The angle of insonation should be optimal lest it may foreshorten or lengthen the bone shadow leading to inaccurate measurements (Fig. 6.6).

The bone length is plotted on the reference chart and the centiles are followed on serial growth estimation. Bone length is a familial trait and sometimes in families with low average adult height, the fetal long bones may appear to be along the lower centiles. As long as the shape and echogenicity are normal and there is definite positive interval linear growth in 2–3-week intervals, it is expected to be a normal pattern. However, if the femur length is well below the 5th centile in addition to abnormal shape or curvature of the shaft, then there is a likelihood of skeletal dysplasia and that required detailed testing and workup. The femur closer to the probe is measured to avoid artifacts and inaccuracy.

In routine biometry, it is not necessary to measure all long bones individually, and a general visualization of the presence and symmetry of the limbs is sufficient. However, whenever the femur length is discrepant for gestational age, it is imperative to measure all long bines and thoracic circumference to check whether the problem is isolated or generalized.

6.9 Calculation of Estimated Fetal Weight on Ultrasound

Using the biometric parameters described above, the fetal weight can be estimated by several formulae. There are more than 30 such formulae suggested in literature claiming various degrees of accuracy, but in common usage, the Hadlock formulae are used and in these the composite (AC-FL-HC-BPD):

- Hadlock 1: Log 10 (weight) = 1.304 + 0.052 81*Ac + 0.1938*FL − 0.004*AC*FL
- Hadlock 2: Log 10 (weight) = 1.335 − 0.003 4*AC*FL + 0.0316*BPD + 0.0457*AC + 0. 1623*FL
- Hadlock 3: Log 10 (weight) = 1.326 − 0.003 26*AC*FL + 0.0107*HC + 0.0438*AC + 0. 158*FL

- Hadlock 4: Log 10 (weight) = 1.3596 − 0.00386*AC*FL + 0.0064*HC + 0.00061*BPD*AC + 0.0424*AC + 0.174*FL

The estimation of fetal weight is accurately up to 90% and errors creep in at larger sizes and larger gestational ages. The estimated fetal weight is a marker for fetal "size," but fetal growth can only be determined by a temporal assessment of progressive increase in this size. Hence, growth is commented upon only after serial measurements of size over at least 2–3-week intervals. Fetal growth and its related concepts will be dealt with separately in Chap. 9.

6.10 Supplementary Biometry: The Transcerebellar Diameter

While all the abovementioned parameters are routinely used to assess fetal size and dates, the transcerebellar diameter is also measured in the second and third trimester as a corroborative evidence of fetal dating. TCD is measured in a plane identified by obtaining an oblique view through posterior fossa that included visualization of midline thalamus, cerebellar hemispheres, and cisterna magna. The longest diameter across the cerebellar peduncles is measured and the values are compared to the nomograms for that gestation. Fetal cerebellum can be visualized as early as 10–11 weeks by USG. From second trimester onward, it grows with a linear correlation with gestational age. In cases of IUGR, the cerebellum is the least affected parameter maintaining its size in case of fetal growth restriction; hence, accurate GA can be predicted with TCD (Fig. 6.7).

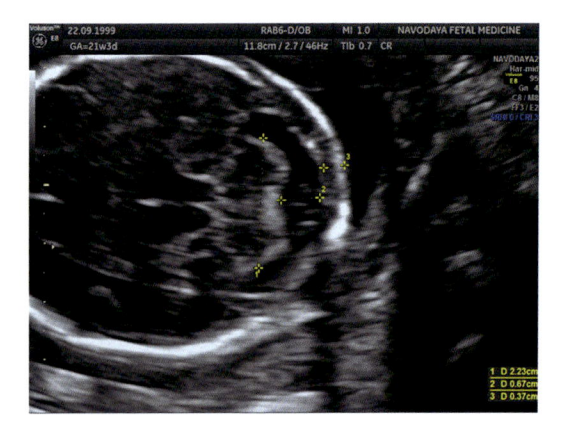

Fig. 6.7 Tanscerebellar diameter

The cerebellum is located in the posterior cranial fossa surrounded by the dense petrous ridges and the occipital bone making it withstand the deformation caused by extrinsic pressure, and this makes it possible for assessing GA even in third trimester by this measurement. Thus, it is a good practice to include TCD measurements as part of the regular biometry protocol for fetal evaluation.

The above biometry parameters are used commonly to assign size of a fetus. Several other parameters can be assessed and measured in the fetus. Such parameters may be relevant in specific circumstances and need not be included in each and every fetal assessment. A common example is the measurement of all fetal long bones whenever the femur length appears shorter than expected or measuring the interorbital distance when the facial evaluation suggests dysmorphism or asymmetry. In these situations, objective measurements help in quantifying the problem or ruling out one as may be the case. The purpose of this chapter is to provide a basic overview of fetal biometry for the "generalist" who wants a clearer understanding of the basics. We have not included such extended biometry in this chapter to avoid confusion.

Having understood basic fetal biometry, it is equally important to realize that biometry only assigns the "size" of a fetus and does not necessarily correspond to "growth." To comment on growth, at least one baseline confirmation of dates is needed and even better to have serial fetal biometry readings which can help in commenting on the pattern of growth. We will deal with fetal growth issues in detail in a separate chapter.

Key Learning Points in Fetal Biometry
1. Ideally, a pregnancy should be "dated" in early gestation—maximum by the end of the first trimester, a confirmed EDD should be allocated.
2. Up to 14-week CRL can be used for dating pregnancies (i.e., up to a CRL of 84 mm); thereafter, HC should be used for dating if needed.
3. Once an EDD is allocated in early pregnancy, it should not be changed.
4. BPD, HC, AC, and FL are used for calculation of EFW.
5. TCD may be measured to help corroborate dates ad growth in difficult cases.
6. Measurements should be compared with standard nomograms based on centiles/SD or Z-scores.
7. Biometry is the measurement of the "size" of a fetus—"growth" assessment requires serial biometry.

Suggested Reading

Hadlock FP, et al. Estimation of fetal weight with the use of head, body, and femur measurements--a prospective study. Am J Obstet Gynecol. 1985;151(3):333–7.

ISUOG. Practice Guidelines: ultrasound assessment of fetal biometry and growth. Ultrasound Obstet Gynecol. 2019;53:715–23.

Robinson HP, Fleming JEE. A critical evaluation of sonar "crown-rump length" measurements. BJOG. 1975;82(9):702–10.

Midtrimester Fetal Anomaly Scan

A systematic evaluation of fetal anatomy is of paramount importance in planning fetal healthcare. The most commonly performed scan for fetal evaluation is usually the midtrimester anomaly scan. Although the science of fetal medicine is advancing, the first trimester evaluation of anatomy is gaining importance; the midtrimester anomaly scan cannot be dispensed with because many anatomical parameters just cannot be assessed in the first trimester based on their physiological nondevelopment at that stage. The details of first trimester fetal evaluation are given in Chap. 10. This chapter will concentrate on the second trimester fetal anatomy evaluation.

This "targeted" anomaly scan is done for routine screening of fetal anatomy in the second trimester and must be offered to all pregnant women. This evaluation can reassure most parents about normal anatomy of the fetus and just in case any fetal structural abnormality is detected, appropriate modification of care can be planned.

It is a known fact that fetal structural anomalies can occur in about 2–3% of pregnancies even in an apparently "low-risk" population. The potential to detect these abnormalities has increased manifold over the decades with better resolution of ultrasound machines and better understanding of the fetal anatomy and physiology. Over the years, with more and more clinical units including this evaluation as part of routine care, sensible, reproducible, and practical protocols for conducting the scan have also emerged. Such protocols help in standardizing the conduct of the scan and moderating the expected results thereof. The midtrimester fetal anomaly evaluation is by far the most "potential" opportunity to detect most of the fetal congenital anomalies and that too at a time when meaningful decisions regarding the course of the pregnancy can be made.

While confirming normal fetal anatomy is extremely reassuring for the parents and doctors, the diagnosis of any fetal anomaly warrants an intensive workup to establish prognosis and institute modifications in antenatal, perinatal, and postnatal care of the fetus based on the specific issues surrounding the fetal anomaly. A detailed description of all anomalies is beyond the scope of this book, but this chapter will outline the remit of systematic evaluation of the fetal anatomy as expected in standard settings and will also provide a brief preview into common anomalies and their expected workup plans.

7.1 Prerequisites to Performing a Fetal Anomaly Scan

The fetal anomaly scan is a highly specialized method of screening fetal anatomy with the aim of detecting fetal structural anomalies. It requires specialized training to develop the skill of fetal imaging and interpretation to get the expected results of fetal evaluation. A good resolution ultrasound machine is also a necessary prerequisite to performing a fetal anomaly scan along with some technical capacity to acquire and store images for documentation. There are several types of ultrasound machines available in the market and many new fancy features keep getting added to the usual basic software almost every year due to tremendous progress in science and technology. While new features always add more clarity in acquisition and demonstration of images, they also add to the cost of the equipment, often significantly. It is unreasonable to expect state-of-the-art equipment in every obstetric scanning unit all over the world. Therefore, some basic cutoff is needed to set a bar uniformly at which level it is acceptable to perform a fetal anomaly scan. The International Society of ultrasound in Obstetrics and Gynecology (ISUOG) has prescribed some important features to be present in any machine used for satisfactory fetal anatomy evaluation. Table 7.1 enumerates these features.

As is evident from the above list, the requirements are very basic and expected to be present in most standard machines which are affordable to average obstetric scan units. The next most important requirement is a skilled operator who can make accurate diagnosis of fetal anomalies. This skill can be acquired by structured training and certification and honed further by constant practice.

After fulfilling the prerequisites, the plan for the midtrimester anomaly scan (Fig. 7.1) includes a general survey of the fetus in utero to assess fetal number, viability, biometry, and anatomy along with the placenta, cord, and cervix.

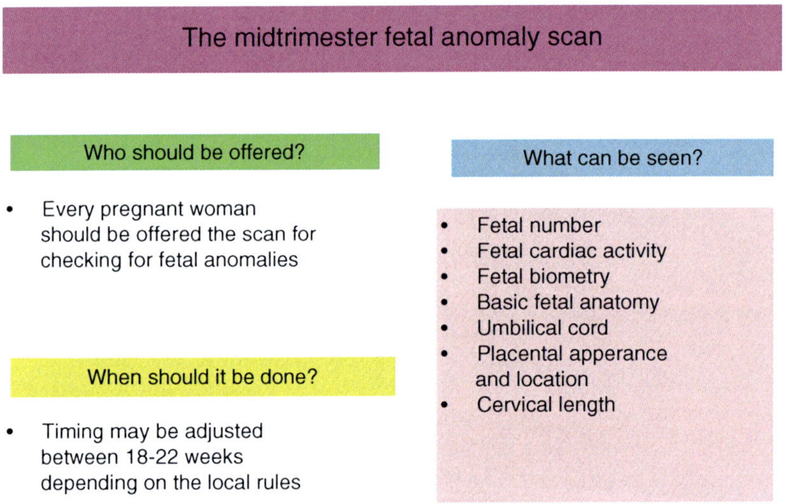

Table 7.1 Machine requirements to perform a fetal anomaly scan

• Real-time, grayscale imaging
• Transabdominal transducer 3–5 MHz
• Adjustable acoustic power output controls with output display standards
• Freeze frame capabilities
• Electronic calipers
• Capacity to pin/store images
• Regular maintenance and servicing for optimum performance

Fig. 7.1 Remit of the midtrimester fetal anomaly scan

The midtrimester fetal anomaly scan

Who should be offered?
- Every pregnant woman should be offered the scan for checking for fetal anomalies

When should it be done?
- Timing may be adjusted between 18-22 weeks depending on the local rules

What can be seen?
- Fetal number
- Fetal cardiac activity
- Fetal biometry
- Basic fetal anatomy
- Umbilical cord
- Placental apperance and location
- Cervical length

7.2 Fetal Number and Viability

This chapter will deal specifically with the assessment of fetal anatomy as the other aspects have been addressed in other chapters of this book. The checklist for fetal anatomy would include the structures enumerated in Table 7.2.

Table 7.2 Checklist for fetal ultrasound evaluation at the MTAS

• Start scan by checking fetal number, viability, and situs assessment before a detailed anatomy check	
Fetal anatomy:	Others:
• Skull	• Placenta
• Brain	• Umbilical cord
• Face	• Amniotic fluid
• Neck	• Cervical length
• Thorax	• Uterine artery Doppler
• Heart	
• Abdomen	
• Spine	
• Limbs	
• *Genitalia (local legal limits apply)*	

A general survey of the gravid uterus will reveal the number of fetuses and one must be always alert to the possibility of multifetal gestation especially with the rising numbers of the same. In most cases nowadays, women would have had first trimester scans and the diagnosis of multifetal pregnancy would have been established early, but in case this is her first fetal ultrasound evaluation in pregnancy, it would not be unreasonable to assume an undetected multiple gestation.

In case of multifetal pregnancy, the number of fetuses and chronicity/amnionicity assessment must be performed followed by detailed anatomical assessment of each fetus.

Majority of pregnancies are singleton and this should be established and documented in the report of a fetal anomaly scan.

Fetal viability is determined by an actively beating fetal heart. This can be seen in real-time ultrasound as movements of heart valves and chamber muscles rhythmically. It is however a good idea to document the same by taking one measurement of the fetal heart rate. In the second trimester, this is usually done by using spectral wave gate across any of the heart valves (Fig. 7.2),

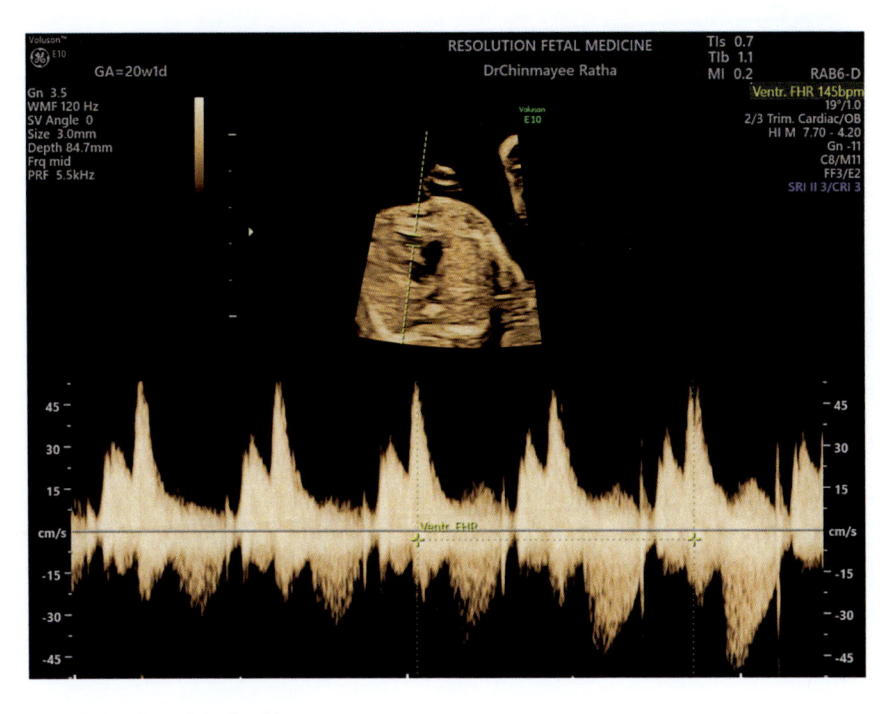

Fig. 7.2 Rhythmic beating of the fetal heart

and the expected normal heart rate is anything between 120 and 160 bpm.

7.3 Orientation of the Fetus (Assessment of Situs)

Fetal situs determines how the visceral organs are arranged inside the fetal body. Before embarking upon a detailed anatomy scan, it is useful to assess fetal situs and ensure that the organs are arranged as expected in "normal" anatomical arrangement. Just like before starting a long journey, one must review the navigation parameters and orient oneself to the expected route, and establishing fetal situs before doing the anatomy scan is of utmost importance. Sometimes, the stomach and the heart may be situated in opposite sides of the fetus (Fig. 7.3), and then it is important to find out which one is on the left and which one on the right.

We know that the fetal heart points toward the left and that the fetal stomach is also normally found in the left upper abdomen, but if we assume left laterality of the heart or stomach by default, then one may miss major abnormalities like dextrocardia or dextrogastria where the arrangements are reversed. It is therefore important first to understand which side is left and which side is right while performing ultrasound scan on a fetus and then checking that organs expected to be on that side are situated in their correct position.

A popular method used as an aid to determine fetal situs is the "right-hand thumb" rule described by Bronstein et al. for assessing fetal situs during transabdominal scans. In this method, the palm of the right hand represents the face of the fetus, and the fetal heart and stomach are on the same side of the examiner's thumb. The operator can thus place his right hand in supine position for dorsoposterior orientation and prone for dorsoanterior orientation.

Many machines have inbuilt guides for orientation of the operator with the fetal lie which is useful for beginners. It may also be a practically useful exercise to keep a doll in the scan room and place it in the fetal position in case one is confused with other methods of determining situs.

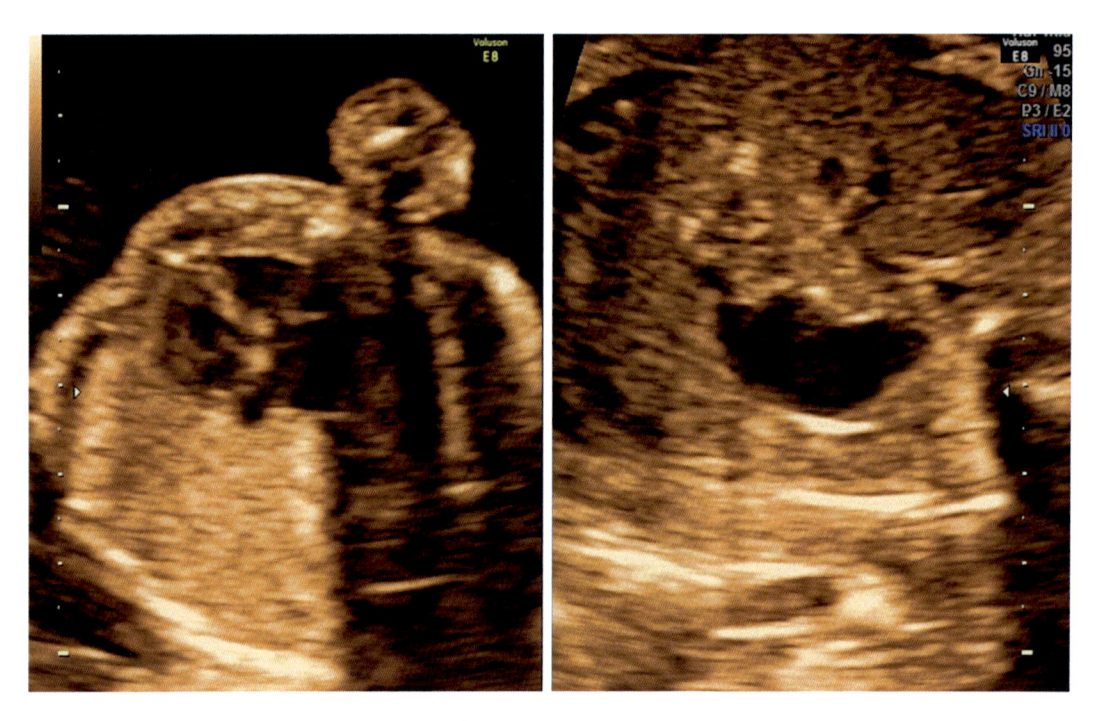

Fig. 7.3 Stomach and heart on opposite sides—situs anomaly

Many methods have been suggested to check fetal situs and each has its own merit. By far the most reliable method is to imagine yourself in the fetal position once you see the fetus on the screen. The left and the right of the screen show different landmarks of the fetus, and if one notes the position of the fetal head and spine, it is simple to imagine yourself lying in that position and establish right-left laterality. This can be applied to the fetus in that position and the position of the fetal stomach and heart apex can be then noted to confirm that they are on the left side as expected; this is the simplest method of determining situs and works well in whichever position the fetus is, whether the operator is left-handed or right-handed.

7.4 Fetal Anatomy Assessment

7.4.1 Fetal Skull

The presence of the fetal skull along with its normal shape and contours is noted (Fig. 7.4). The skull bones are assessed for size, shape, integrity, and bone density. The skull bones are arranged in a manner to form an appropriate "casing" for the brain and cranial nerves which are so important in the general functioning of the individual. The normal appearance of these skull bones with the expected "gaps" at the anatomical suture lines is highly reassuring. The measurement of fetal head circumference and biparietal diameter is done as explained in the Chap. 6. The normal shape of the fetal skull in axial view is oval with possible variations due to familial, genetic, or ethnic characteristics like brachycephaly, dolichocephaly, etc. However, major abnormalities in shape may be indicative of underlying structural malformations, e.g., "lemon-shaped" skull in spina bifida or "cloverleaf" skull in craniosynostosis, etc.

As the fetal skull houses the fetal brain, it is of utmost significance that it provides a strong case along with adequate space and capacity for the brain to grow in time. Abnormal protrusions from the fetal skull are seen in cases of encephaloceles, and poor mineralization of skull bones (e.g., in osteogenesis imperfecta) indicates association of genetic defects. Some common anomalies seen associated with the fetal skull are absence of the skull vault or acrania and premature fusion of the sutures (craniosynostosis) leading to abnormal shape of the skull. Figure 7.5 shows images of some of these conditions.

Absence of fetal skull or acrania is uniformly lethal in postnatal life and there is no

Fetal Skull checklist at anomaly scan

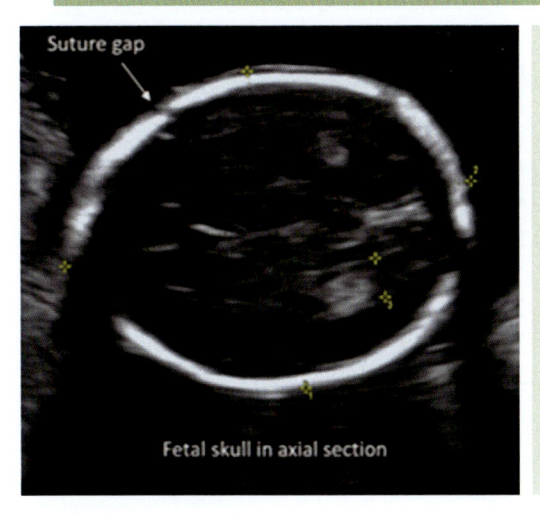

- Presence of the skull

- Normal contour of the skull usually checked in axial section

- Normal mineralisation of skull bones and presence of the "suture gaps"

Fig. 7.4 Normal fetal skull

Abnormalities of the fetal skull

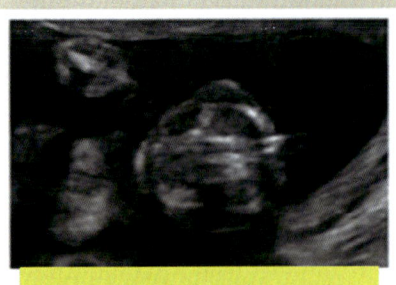

Absent cranial vault - acrania

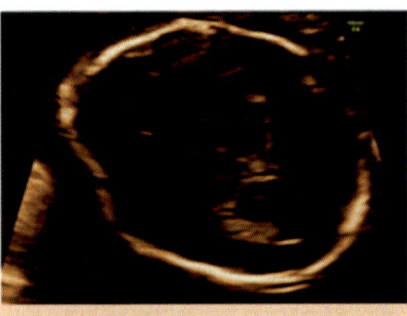

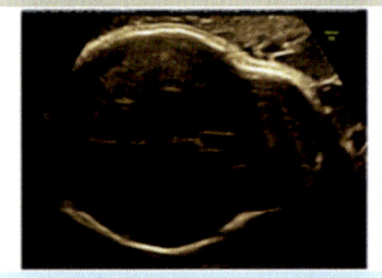

Clover leaf skull - craniosynostosis

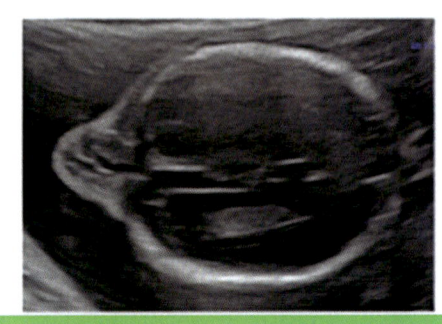

Frontal scalloping – lemon shaped skull

Defect in Occipital bone with encephalocele

Fig. 7.5 Abnormalities of the fetal skull

reasonable treatment available for the same. This often warrants termination of pregnancy and fortunately this diagnosis can be achieved in the first trimester scan, and thus obstetric decisions can be taken at a time safer for the woman.

7.4.2 Fetal Brain

The fetal brain is evaluated in the midtrimester scan based on the recommendations of the current practice guidelines by standard organizations. According to the ISUOG and the FMF guidelines, the expected standards of a routine anomaly scan should include evaluation of the fetal brain in three axial views (Fig. 7.6):

1. Transthalamic view
2. Transventricular view
3. Transcerebellar view

A checklist approach helps in establishing normal anatomical parameters for a given gestation, and in the midtrimester scan, it is recommended to check the following structures during fetal brain examination:

- Lateral ventricles
- Bilateral choroid plexi
- Cavum septi pellucidi
- The midline falx cerebri
- Thalami
- Cerebellum
- Cisterna magna

In case any abnormalities (Fig. 7.7) are detected during this basic brain evaluation, the fetus should be referred for a detailed "neurosonogram."

7.4 Fetal Anatomy Assessment

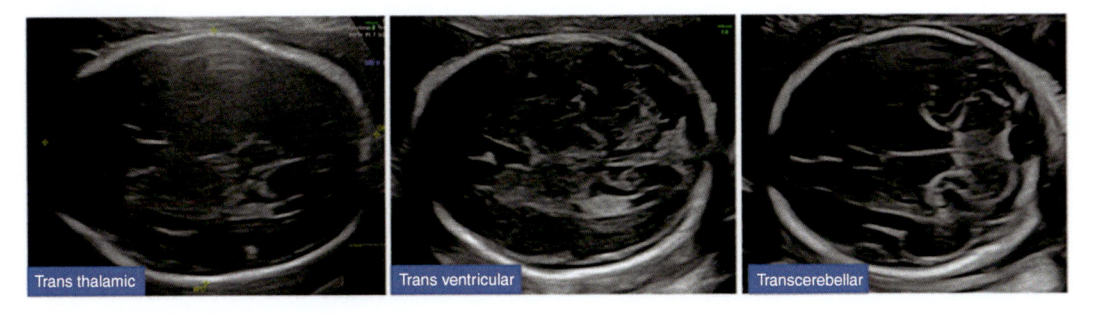

Fig. 7.6 Standard axial views of fetal brain

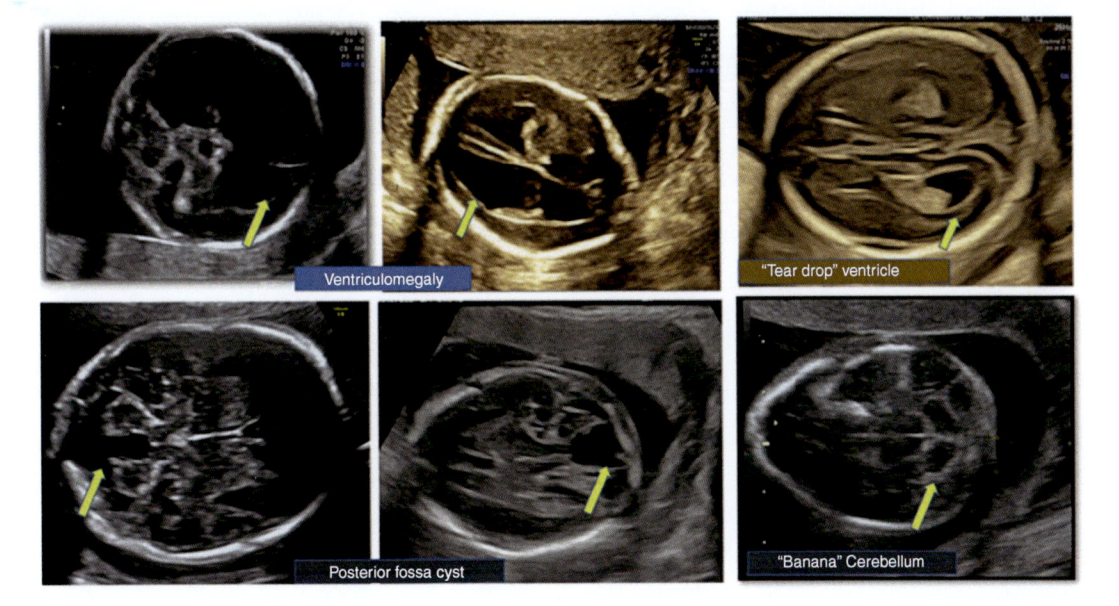

Fig. 7.7 Common fetal brain anomalies

It is also important to remember that the fetal brain is a developing structure, and even if all parameters appear normal at a certain gestation, it must be conveyed to the parents that some abnormalities may "evolve" over time and manifest during future scans.

7.4.3 Fetal Face

Fetal face is examined in the median sagittal plane and coronal views. The sagittal section helps to demonstrate the facial profile (Fig. 7.8) with the nasal protuberance, nasal bones, and upper and lower jaws. The frontal coronal view represents the intact upper lip and slight tilt can show the nostrils too. Another view to check fetal facial features is the axial view through the orbits and just below it, the fetal hard palate can be seen.

Common abnormalities of the fetal face are shown in Fig. 7.9 including cleft lip and palate, retro- or micrognathia, anophthalmia, hypo- or hypertelorism, or abnormal facial profile.

7.4.4 Fetal Neck

The normal fetal neck is (Fig. 7.10) seen as a cylindrical structure connecting the head and the body composed of the cervical vertebrae in the dorsal aspect and soft tissue anteriorly.

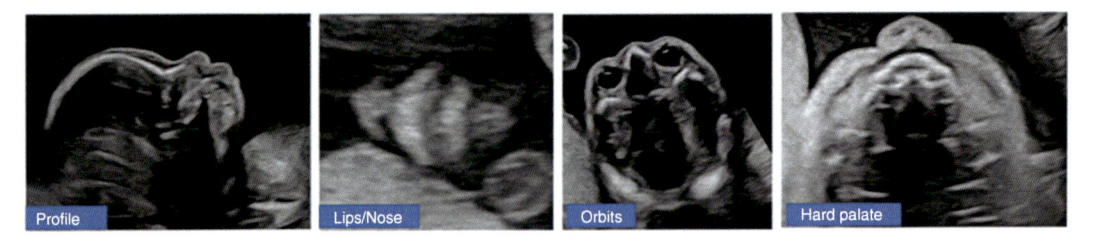

Fig. 7.8 Standard views of normal fetal face

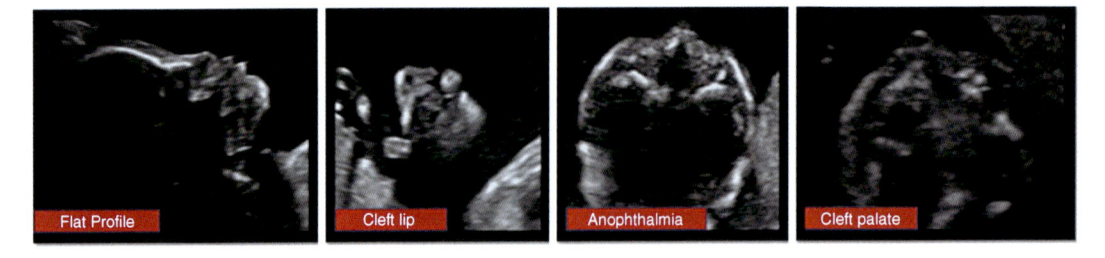

Fig. 7.9 Common abnormalities of the fetal face

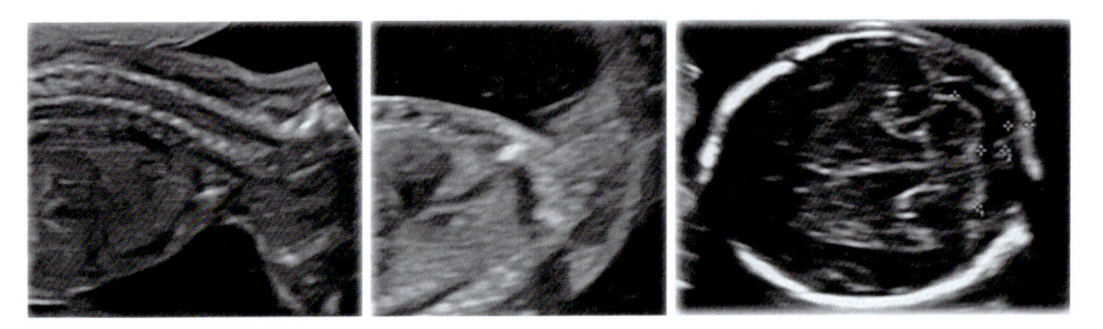

Fig. 7.10 Fetal neck in longitudinal section and axial view for nuchal fold assessment

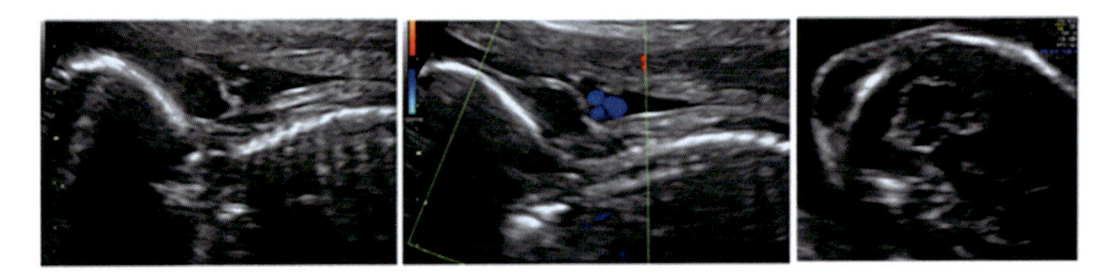

Fig. 7.11 Abnormal swelling in the dorsal aspect of fetal neck

No abnormal protrusions, masses, or cysts are expected in this area, and if any of these are seen, then it is deemed as an abnormality (Fig. 7.11).

Common neck masses include cystic hygromas, thyroid masses, hemangiomas, etc. The nuchal fold thickness is also measured in the fetus, and increased nuchal fold thickness is con-

7.4.5 Fetal Thorax

Evaluation of fetal thorax is done mostly on the axial views although the operator also evaluates a longitudinal view to assess the diaphragm, general appearance of the rib cage, and a smooth merging of the thoracic boundaries with the abdomen. In the axial section, the normal fetal thorax appears to have normal-shaped ribs outlining the cross section with the heart occupying the middle one third and flanked by two equal sized, similar appearing lungs on either side (Fig. 7.12).

In cases of abnormal contents or arrangement of thoracic organs (Fig. 7.13), there may be pressure effects on thoracic contents, and this usually has significant impact on fetal physiology as both heart and lungs are important organs.

7.4.6 Fetal Heart

Presence of fetal cardiac activity is one of the first steps in fetal assessment, but evaluating the fetal heart in the anomaly scan extends to a more structured evaluation of the cardiac chambers and outflow tracts. The basic cardiac examination (Fig. 7.14) includes demonstration of the normal four-chamber view with a normally placed heart defined by an orientation of the cardiac axis at $45 \pm 20°$ from the midline toward the left and beating rhythmically at a rate between 120 and 160 bpm.

An extended basic cardiac examination (Fig. 7.15) includes the evaluation of right and

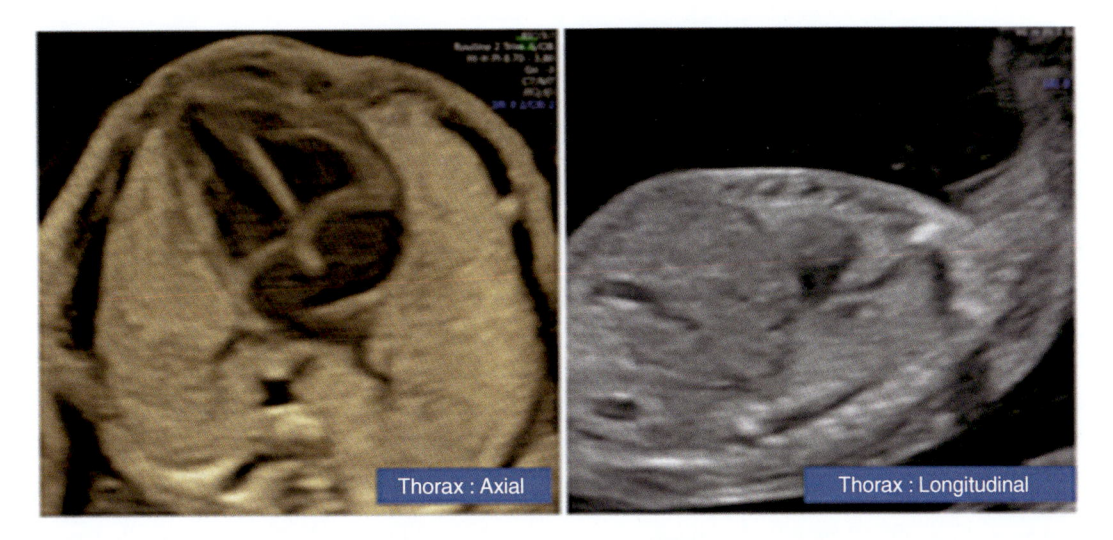

Fig. 7.12 Axial and longitudinal view of fetal thorax

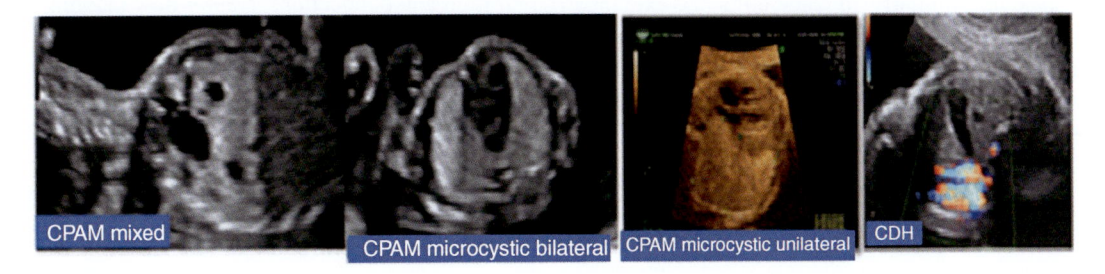

Fig. 7.13 Thoracic malformations

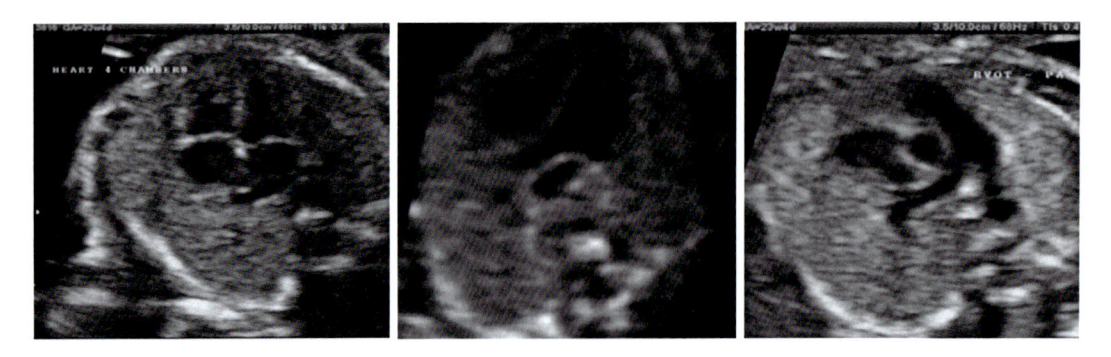

Fig. 7.14 Basic fetal cardiac views—normal

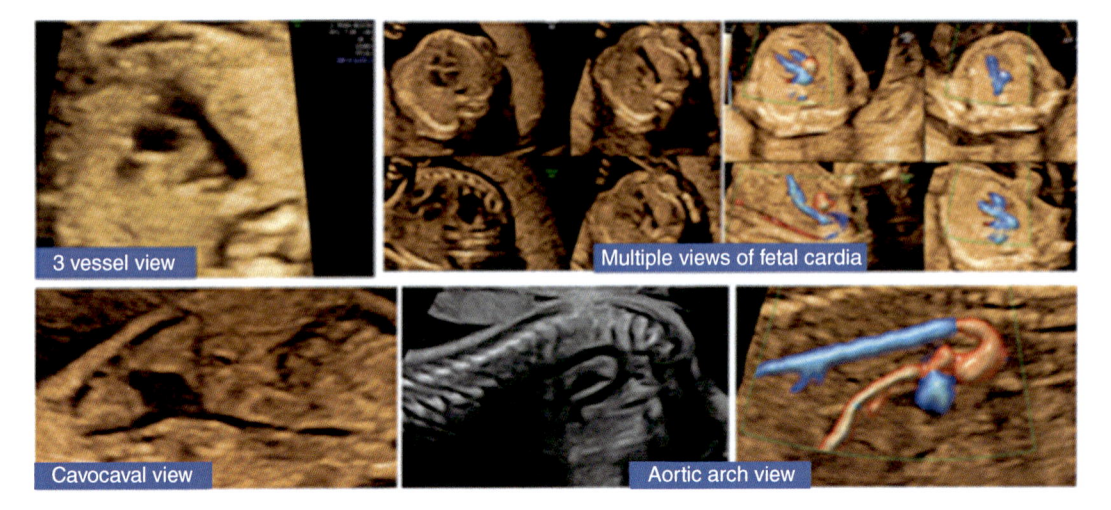

Fig. 7.15 Extended basic fetal cardiac views—normal

left ventricular outflow tracts which help excluding major cardiac anomalies like the conotruncal anomalies and transposition of great vessels. Addition of the "three-vessel view" is considered optional during a routine fetal anatomy scan as per guidelines. This view enhances the pickup of cardiac malformations' manifold as discrepancy of sizes and orientation of outflow tracts is easily picked up. Similarly, in some units, the extended protocol includes evaluation of the cavocaval views and the aortic arch views.

Considering that cardiovascular abnormalities are some of the commonest congenital malformations, a sturdy cardiac examination plan is a very useful part of the fetal anatomy assessment. It may be noted that most congenital cardiac malformations occur in the so-called "low-risk" pregnant women. A high index of suspicion and a disciplined evaluation protocol helps in detecting these problems. In case any deviation from normal is observed in the basic examination (Fig. 7.16), the fetus should be referred for a detailed "echocardiography."

Fetal echocardiography refers to a detailed evaluation of fetal cardiac anatomy and flow patterns. This includes a 2D evaluation of the configuration and connections, a color flow mapping of flow in the chambers and outflow tracts, and a Doppler spectral analysis of flow across the valves and in the outflow tracts. This can be supplemented by 3D and 4D studies. With the present-day machines and technology, it is possible to delineate structural anomalies and assess chamber capacity, contractility, and even pressure gradients so that optimum information can be provided to the cardiologist helping them

7.4 Fetal Anatomy Assessment

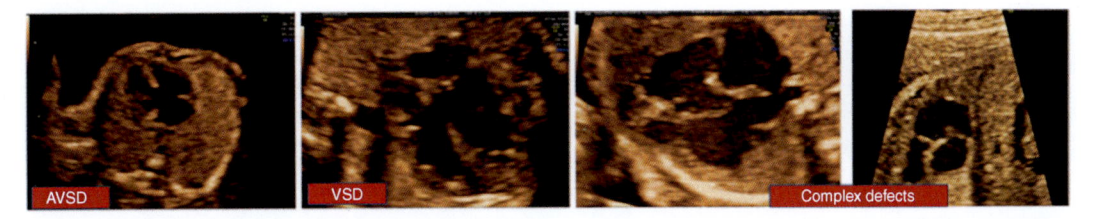

Fig. 7.16 Common congenital cardiac defects

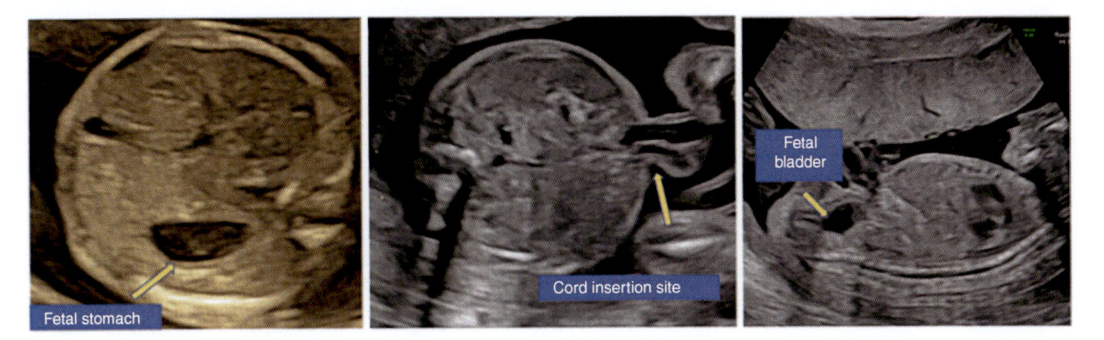

Fig. 7.17 Normal views of fetal stomach, abdominal wall, and urinary bladder

prognosticate the cardiac malformations while planning treatment.

7.4.7 Fetal Abdomen

The fetal abdomen is assessed in the axial and longitudinal views (Fig. 7.17) to examine the presence and position of the visceral organs along with evaluation of the abdominal wall and abdominothoracic diaphragm. Once fetal situs is established, presence of a normal-sized stomach "bubble" in the left hypochondrium is reassuring as it indicates patency of the upper GI tract and ability of the fetus to swallow amniotic fluid which fills in the stomach and makes it appear like an hypoechoic bubble. In case the stomach bubble is absent, it is important to wait for at least 40 min and recheck so that normal emptying and filling cycle of the fetal stomach is established. Absent stomach bubble is an important marker for fetal GI anomalies or neuromuscular conditions.

The fetal liver occupies the right hypochondrium, and in a transverse section, the umbilical vein is seen curving toward the liver, away from the stomach like a "hockey stick." The fetal "abdominal circumference" is measured at this level which is part of the routine biometry protocol.

Fetal bowel is seen filling the lower abdomen and the echogenicity of the bowel and liver is more or less similar although bowel shows intermittent peristalsis and is thus distinguishable. The lower abdomen shows a hypoechoic urinary bladder and the fetal kidneys are either in a transverse section of the lower abdomen or in coronal view from the back of the spine (Fig. 7.18).

The abdominal wall cord insertion can be documented either in a transverse section or in longitudinal view, and a normal insertion excludes any anterior abdominal wall defects. The differential diagnosis for any cystic structure seen around the umbilical cord and its insertion include pseudocyst, omphalomesenteric duct cyst, hemangioma, and omphalocele or anterior abdominal wall defects.

There is usually no free fluid seen in fetal abdomen and the bowel lumen also generally appears unremarkable. Unusual fluid collections like fetal ascites or abnormal bowel dilatation or

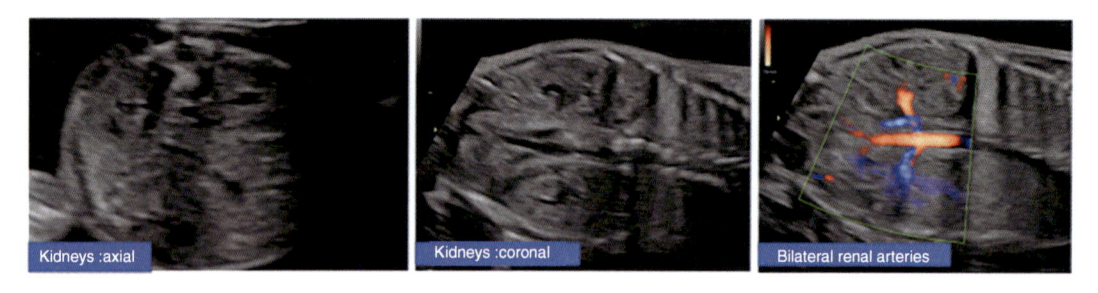

Fig. 7.18 Normal fetal kidneys

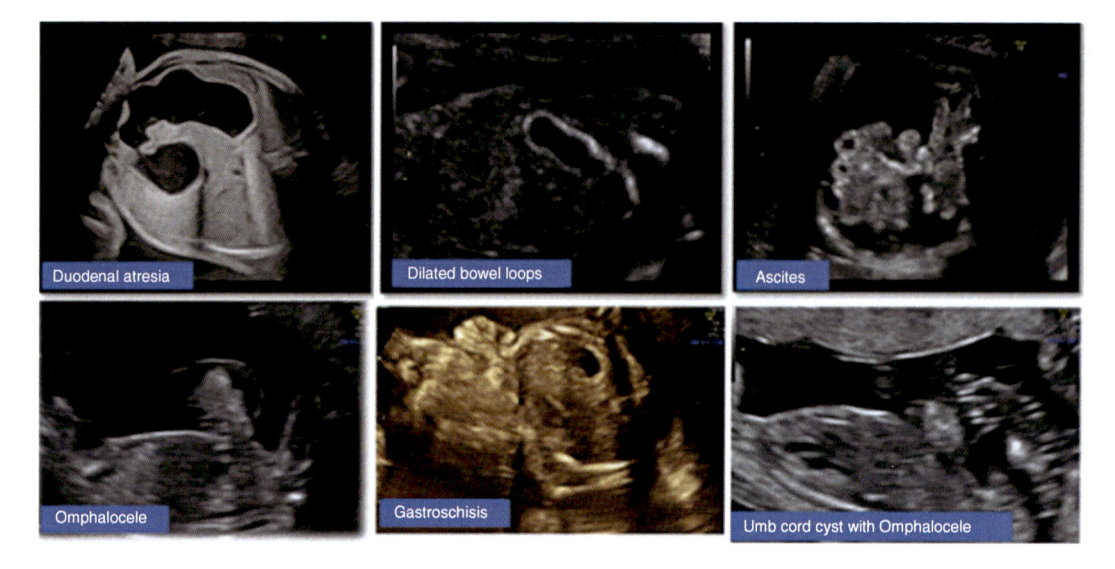

Fig. 7.19 Fetal GI anomalies

abdominal cysts should be noted and documented (Fig. 7.19).

7.4.8 Fetal Spine

Fetal spine is evaluated in the longitudinal, coronal, and axial views (Fig. 7.20). The best views are obtained when the fetus is dorsoanterior. It is imperative to visualize not only the normal skeletal elements of the vertebrae but also the intact skin above them so as to exclude possibility of any open spina bifida. Small meningoceles can be easily missed if the spine is not visualized in its entirety and with evidence of intact skin covering it. It is therefore useful to wait for such a position even if it demands an additional sitting for the scan.

It may be noted that many spinal defects (Fig. 7.21) can have intracranial manifestations, and hence any cranial abnormality like ventriculomegaly must warrant a detailed evaluation of the fetal spine.

Routine evaluation of the spine can be done on 2D grayscale imaging with remarkable clarity, and use of multiplanar imaging is not necessary as per standard guidelines of the fetal anomaly scan.

In cases where abnormalities are detected, multidimensional, multiplanar imaging (Fig. 7.22) helps in demonstrating the defect clearly and can be employed for better documentation.

7.4 Fetal Anatomy Assessment

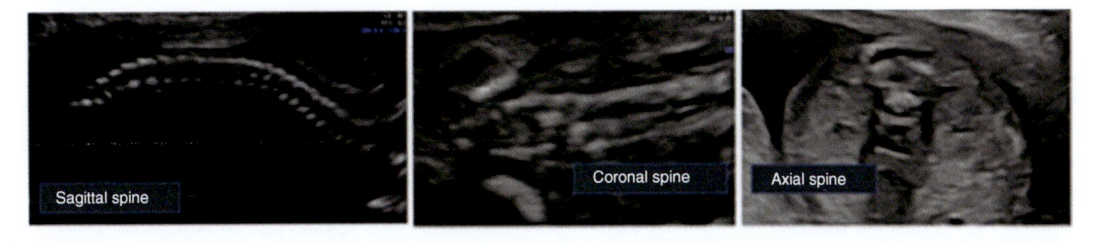

Fig. 7.20 Standard views of fetal spine

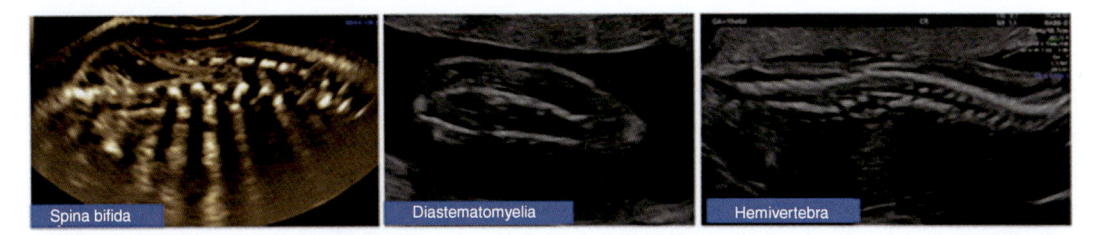

Fig. 7.21 Common fetal spine malformations

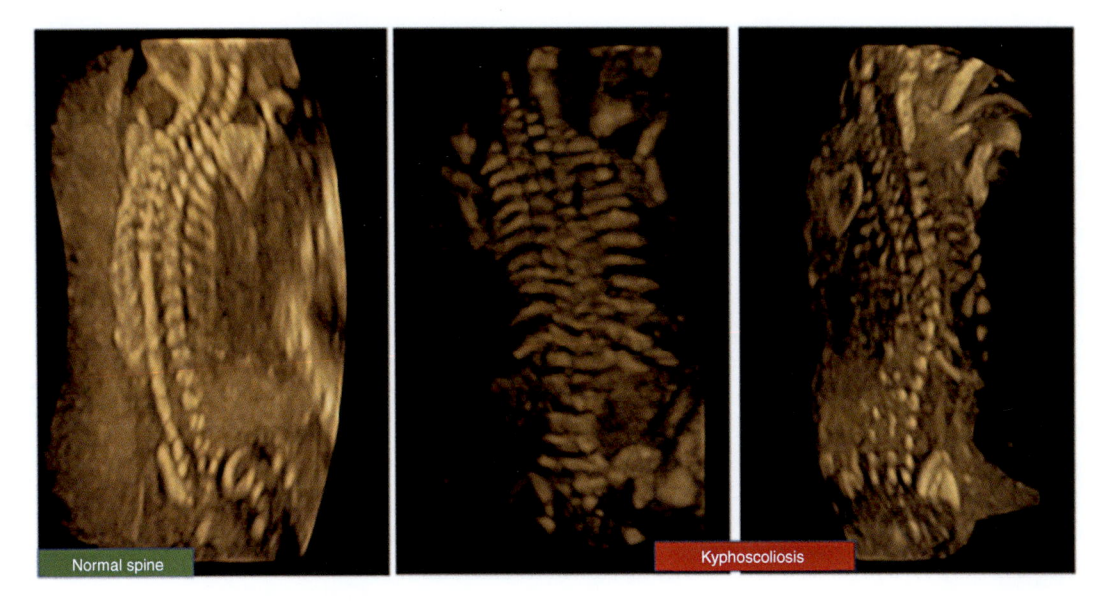

Fig. 7.22 3D rendering of fetal spine

7.4.9 Fetal Limbs

Evaluation of fetal limbs includes assessing all segments of both upper limbs and lower limbs. In each segment, the long bones are checked and the intersegmental joint mobility is assessed by noting unhindered movements of the limbs throughout the course of the scan (Fig. 7.23). While it is important to measure the femur length as part of the biometry protocol, all other long bones may be assessed as per unit protocol. Some units measure all long bones while others only follow a

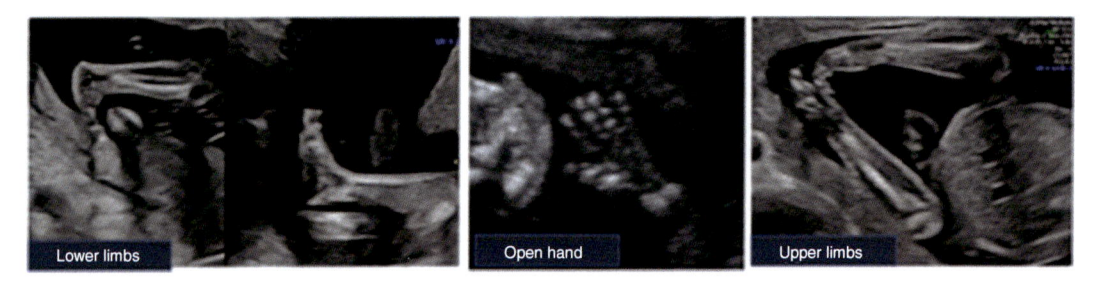

Fig. 7.23 Standard views of fetal limbs

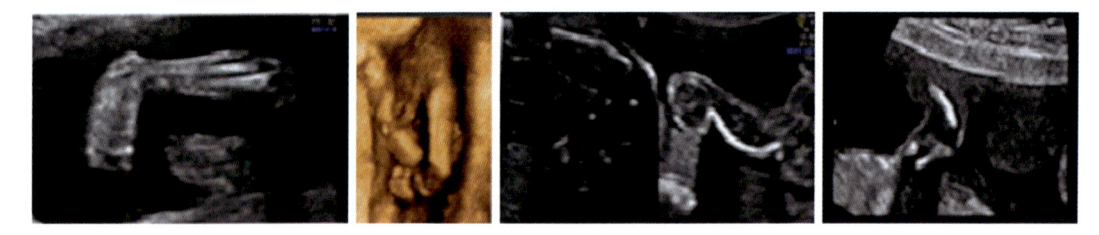

Fig. 7.24 Limb abnormalities

rule of "eyeballing" the long bones and limb movements. Each approach has its relevance depending on local requirements.

In case any abnormality is suspected or detected in any limb (Fig. 7.24), it is imperative to document the length of all long bones to make an objective assessment of limb anatomy. The hands and the feet must be checked to assess their presence and normal orientation along the wrist and ankle joints bilaterally.

However, counting of fingers and toes has not been specifically recommended in routine fetal anatomy assessment. This may need to be done in cases where specific anomalies are suspected or found.

7.4.10 Genitalia

The fetal genitalia "can" be assessed on the midtrimester anomaly scan as the basic external genitalia are distinctively formed by this time. However, whether they "should" be assessed and/or reported depends on the local legal guidelines. In some countries like India, the law prohibits routine evaluation of the genitalia but permits such examination only in situations allowed in the PCPNDT Act (Pre-Conception and Pre-Natal Diagnostic Techniques Act).

7.4.11 Other Parameters Assessed at the MTAS

Other important parameters assessed alongside fetal anatomy (Fig. 7.25) in the midtrimester anomaly scan include the evaluation of the placenta, umbilical cord, amniotic fluid, cervical length, and uterine artery Dopplers depending on the protocol of the unit in which the scan is being performed. Umbilical cord vessels may be counted as an optional component of the routine fetal anatomical survey. The technique to assess these parameters and their clinical relevance is discussed in specific chapters in this book. These parameters may not be directly listed under fetal anatomy evaluation, but they can affect the overall outcome of pregnancy and hence a midtrimester fetal evaluation will remain essentially incomplete unless such relevant information is also included in the report.

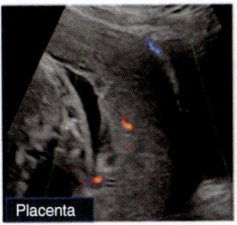

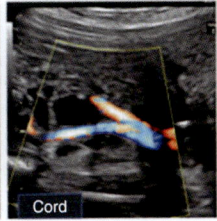

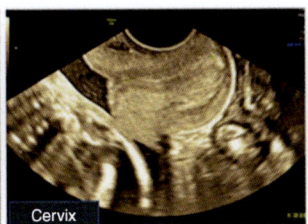

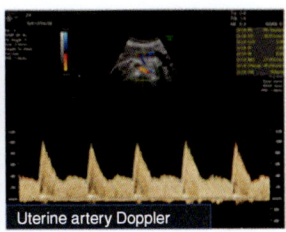

Fig. 7.25 Other parameters assessed at MTAS

7.5 Scope of the Midtrimester Anomaly Scan

Despite the fact that the second trimester anomaly scan is an important checkpoint for almost 90–95% of major structural anomalies, the fact remains that "all" fetal anomalies cannot be determined by ultrasound scan. We are used to inserting this sentence in our disclaimers, but more importantly, this information must be conveyed sensitively so as to allow them to have realistic expectations from the scan. Some fetal anomalies cannot be seen on ultrasound and some structural issues like late onset microcephaly, intestinal obstructive pathologies, nonlethal skeletal dysplasias, cerebral ventriculomegaly, congenital heart blocks, etc. may become apparent only later in pregnancy.

Detection of problems in the third trimester after an apparently normal second trimester evaluation causes of a lot of anguish to both parents and doctors. It is imperative, therefore, to include parents in an appropriate "pretest" counseling explaining to them that although a detailed anatomy check is undertaken, detection of structural anomalies will never be 100%. Detection rates will be different depending on the type of anomaly, the gestational age at scanning, the skill of the operator, the quality of the equipment used, and the time allocated for the scan. It is therefore also suggestive that all these parameters need to be optimized to obtain the best results from an anomaly scan.

It is important to explain the limitations of the scan to the parents. It may be useful to provide a "pretest" information leaflet to them so that they are well informed about the scope and limitations of the scan.

Every operator must make an attempt of obtaining the standard views and completing the checklist for fetal anatomy survey. If the standard views are unattainable despite correct position and machine settings, an anomaly is suspected. Based on the operator's knowledge of fetal anatomy, the anomaly is identified and defined. Presence of one anomaly must alert the operator to look for any other issue as isolated abnormalities and multisystem anomalies are different in terms of their cause, effect, and recurrence risk.

In case a fetal anomaly is detected on the second trimester anomaly scan, a detailed evaluation of the fetus must be done using advanced methods of evaluation available in contemporary medicine to firmly establish the anomaly and its severity. Fetal anomalies detected may be "lethal" or "nonlethal" but associated with significant postnatal morbidity and long-term disability. Some fetal conditions can be offered potential intrauterine therapy to prevent morbidity and mortality, while others will require postnatal investigation or treatment and lead to a reasonably good outcome. Thus, timely diagnosis of fetal anomalies allows for institution of a relevant multidisciplinary care team for counseling the parents, allowing them to clarify all their doubts and apprehensions summarily and planning further care.

7.6 Planning Further Care After Detecting Fetal Anomaly

Once a fetal anomaly is detected, the pathway of antenatal care changes direction in a manner to address the consequences of the specific anomaly that has been detected. After confirming the diagnosis and sensitively informing the parents about the anomaly, a decision for further testing and management is made. In case of correctable fetal anomalies, after ensuring that the given anomaly is isolated, its natural history and effect on antenatal fetal development need to be reviewed and a multidisciplinary team (MDT) is formed to provide further guidance. The MDT consists of the primary obstetrician, the fetal medicine specialist, a clinical geneticist, the neonatologist, and relevant pediatric subspecialist (e.g., the pediatric surgeon, neurosurgeon, or neurologist, pediatric cardiac surgeon or cardiologist, etc.).

Some anomalies may warrant specific prenatal intervention to mitigate the antenatal deterioration and help in postnatal repair. Few anomalies are amenable to primary antenatal repair in the appropriate settings, while most fetal anomalies are managed by postnatal correction. Details of some of these fetal "therapeutic" and "palliative" procedures are given in a separate chapter in this book.

Depending on the nature of the anomaly, a consultation with the relevant pediatric subspecialist and neonatologist can be arranged for the parents to get a better idea of the expected postnatal course. After the multidisciplinary consultation, the parents can now understand the anomaly better and have a clear perception of modifications in antenatal and postnatal course. They can make their personal arrangements accordingly to tackle the events that will follow. In many anomalies, the complete workup involves getting chromosomal/genetic tests done to exclude such associations. Prenatal testing like amniocentesis can be performed and the relevant genetic tests done. Details of prenatal testing and genetic tests are given in future chapters of this book.

Some anomalies may be lethal postnatally or may be such that the effect on the quality of life postnatally would be severely jeopardized and the parents may wish to discontinue the pregnancy. Within the legal limits applicable, such decisions may be duly supported by the medical staff as per the unit protocol. In case the etiology of the anomaly could involve chromosomal/genetic problems, an attempt to test for the same on the fetal sample should be made either by prenatal testing or on the postnatal sample. A discussion about the possibility of perinatal pathology examination may be made here so that parents are given the option of an autopsy of the fetus after termination. These issues may be difficult to discuss in cases where the parents are extremely distressed, but the onus lies on the fetal medicine specialist and obstetrician to help the parents understand the relevance of this workup which can help immensely in planning for future pregnancies.

Very often, given the delicate nature of the situation emotionally and even due to financial constraints, such discussions are ignored and valuable data is lost. Clinicians must understand the fact that if a pregnancy outcome is adverse, it is not the need of the story but the beginning of a puzzle that will need to be solved in the future. Vital clues can be obtained by effective perinatal workup, documentation, and counseling.

Suggested Reading

Bronshtein M, Gover A, Zimmer EZ. Sonographic definition of the fetal situs. Obstet Gynecol. 2002;99(6):1129–30.

Fetal Medicine. Fetal anomaly scan – FMF guidelines. London: Fetal Medicine. www.fetalmedicine.org.

Ratha C, Optimising Multidisciplinary Perinatal Care in Correctable Foetal Anomalies. In: Current Progress in Obstetrics & Gynaecology Volume-6. Studd J, Tan SL, Chervenak FA (eds). 2021.

Salomon LJ, Alfirevic Z, Berghella V, et al. Performance of the routine mid-trimester fetal ultrasound scan. Ultrasound Obstet Gynecol. 2011;37(1):116–26.

Basics of Doppler Imaging and Application in Fetal Medicine

8

The use of Doppler technology has revolutionized fetal evaluation in a very dynamic way not just literally because it deals with moving objects, but because this has enabled a real-time understanding of fetal hemodynamics opening up an opportunistic window for prediction, diagnosis, and prognostication of conditions affecting fetal health. The term "Doppler" in ultrasound is used to indicate information regarding blood flow in blood vessels. Technically, Doppler studies are based on the "Doppler effect" which enables echo-based delineation of moving objects. In a broader and simpler sense, "Doppler" imaging is based on interaction of the ultrasound beam to a "moving" target as opposed to a static one. It is based on the "Doppler" effect (Fig. 8.1) wherein the returning frequency of waves is altered by the relative movement of a source and a target. The classical example of the train siren appearing louder to the passenger standing on a platform as the train approaches and similarly appearing serially more feeble as the train departs indicates the "apparent change" in frequency of a sound due to the "relative motion" between the source and the receptor of the signal. The train blows the siren at a fixed frequency, but observers at two points perceive it differently depending on whether the train (source of sound) is moving toward them or away from them.

In fetal evaluation, blood flow patterns are studied using Doppler. The source and receptor of the signals are the ultrasound probe, and the moving target is a blood cell in the blood vessels in the region of interest. The returning signal is mapped in two ways—color or spectral. A map of the vessels can be obtained as "colors" which can be superimposed on the grayscale image. This is known as color flow mapping (Fig. 8.2). This indicates direction and velocity of flow.

The other method of mapping is known as the Doppler spectrum which consists of a graph showing flow characteristics as a waveform—spectral Doppler (Fig. 8.3). These can then be quantified as velocities, ratios, and indices. As shown in the figure, the "waveforms" are created by the phases of the cardiac cycle. The vessel shows a crest in blood flow during cardiac systole and a trough during diastole. If the vessel is compliant and the "resistance" of its walls is not very high, there is a smooth transition from systole to diastole, and there is some positive end-diastolic flow also through the lumen of the vessel being studied. If the peripheral resistance of the vessel wall is high, the transition from systole to diastole may be marked by a "notch," and sometimes the flows may be absent or reversed in diastole.

Visualizing the wave pattern gives a qualitative assessment of the blood flow but objectivity

© Springer Nature Singapore Pte Ltd. 2022
C. Ratha, A. Khurana, *Fetal Medicine*, https://doi.org/10.1007/978-981-19-6099-4_8

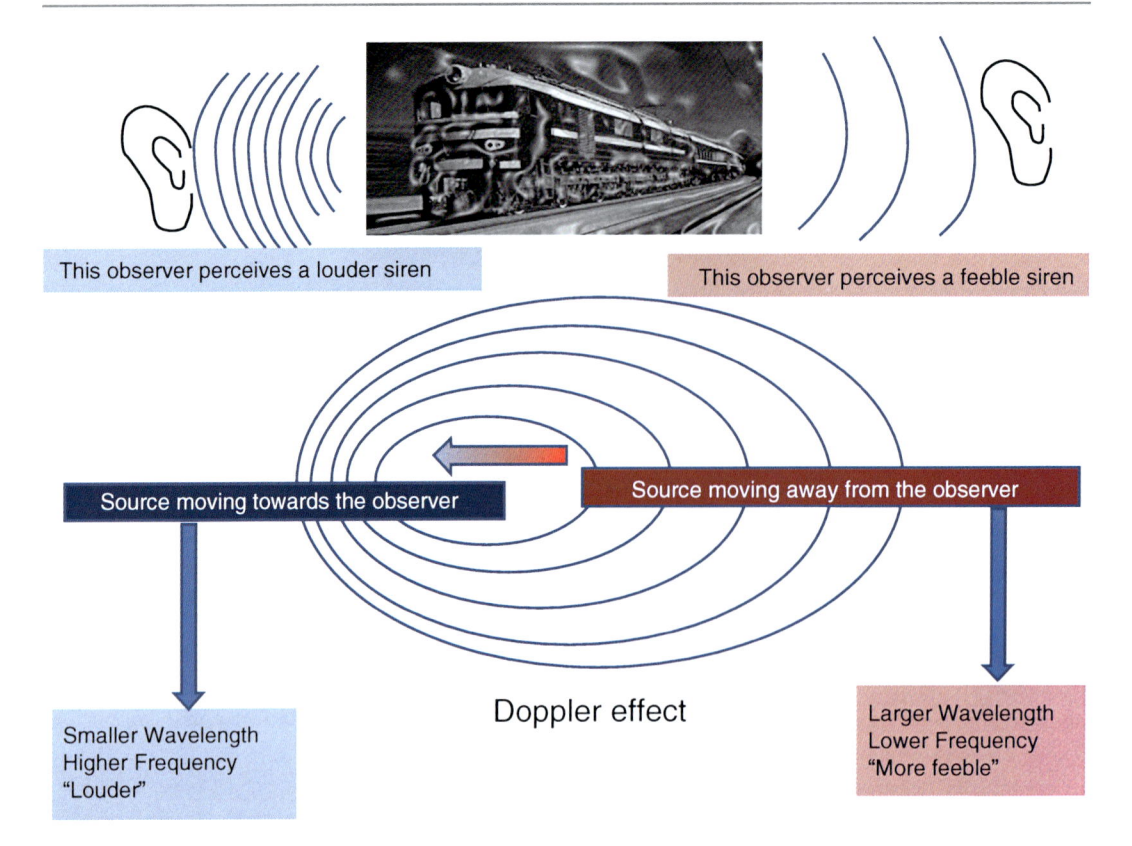

Fig. 8.1 Depiction of the "Doppler effect" when the source of sound is moving

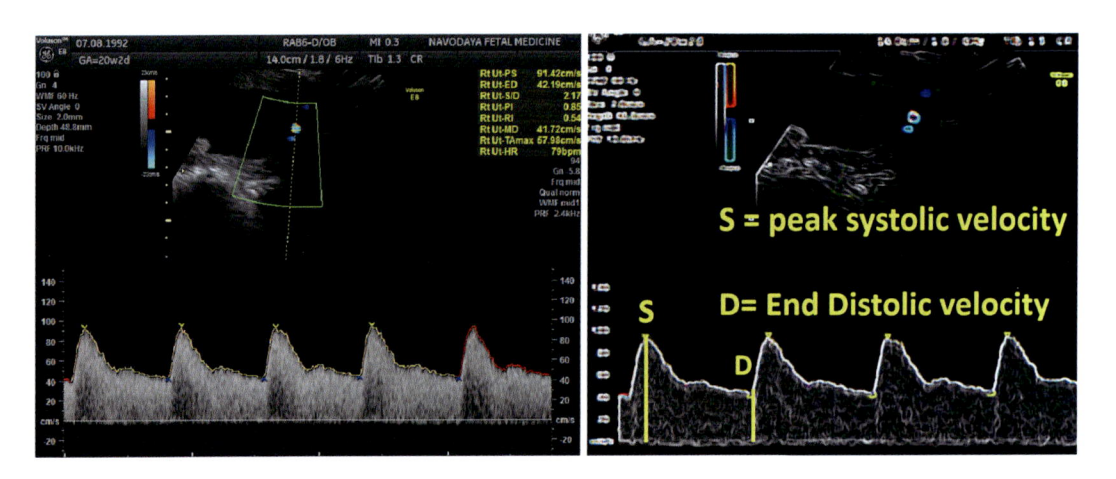

Fig. 8.2 Color flow mapping

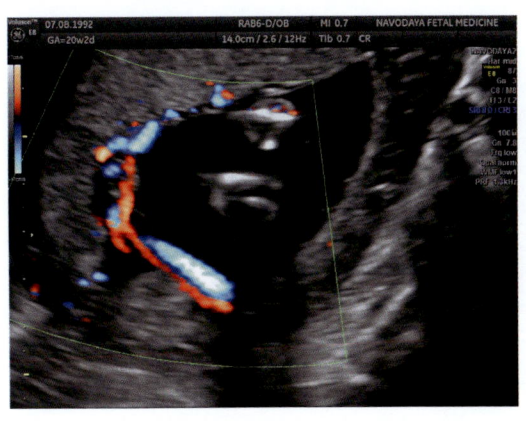

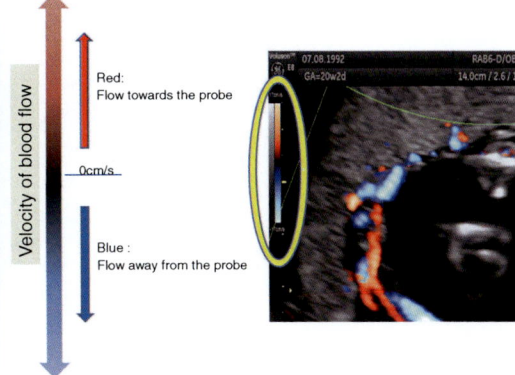

Fig. 8.3 Spectral flow

is best achieved by quantification. Hence, the need for measurable ratios and indices arises. The peak systolic velocity (S), the end-diastolic velocity (D), and the average velocity over one cycle (A) are determined.

Pulsatility index = $(S - D)/A$
Resistive index = $(S - D)/D$

It may be noted that while both are measures of vascular resistance, the pulsatility index functions better for statistical calculations as it will have a finite value even in absent diastolic flows. In fetal medicine, PI is the commonly used Doppler index. In assessing for fetal anemia, the peak systolic velocity (PSV) is used.

Color flow mapping gives information of blood flow over a large area of investigation, but the information is rather generic—presence or absence of flow and direction of flow. The colors are coded usually as red and blue with the code demonstrated on the screen such that one color denotes the movement of the target toward the probe and the other color denotes the same movement away from the probe. On closer evaluation of this "code," it is obvious that the shades within the color vary with the velocity of the blood flow in the area of investigation (Fig. 8.2). When there is no movement, there is obviously no signal and hence the color on the screen is "black." As movement starts, the colors become either red or blue depending on the direction of flow. A smooth, homogenous red or blue signal indicates smooth, laminar flow in the lumen. However, as the velocities increase, the color changes and red tends toward orange, while blue tends toward light blue as seen in the picture here. When there is "turbulence" in flow, then this smooth pattern turns into a riot of colors which is known in technical terms as "aliasing" (Fig. 8.4).

Power Doppler (Fig. 8.5) is another form of flow imaging. It uses amplitude of scatter rather than a frequency shift to make a map of tissue flow. It is by its inherent nature far more sensitive to slow flow and therefore proving to be useful in placental angiogenesis studies and in the vascular evaluation of some fetal malformations.

Based on real-time echoes from moving blood cells within the lumen of blood vessels, Dopplers help in establishing details of hemodynamics like velocity of blood flow during specific stages of the cardiac cycle. Fetal Doppler studies have

Fig. 8.4 Smooth and turbulent flows

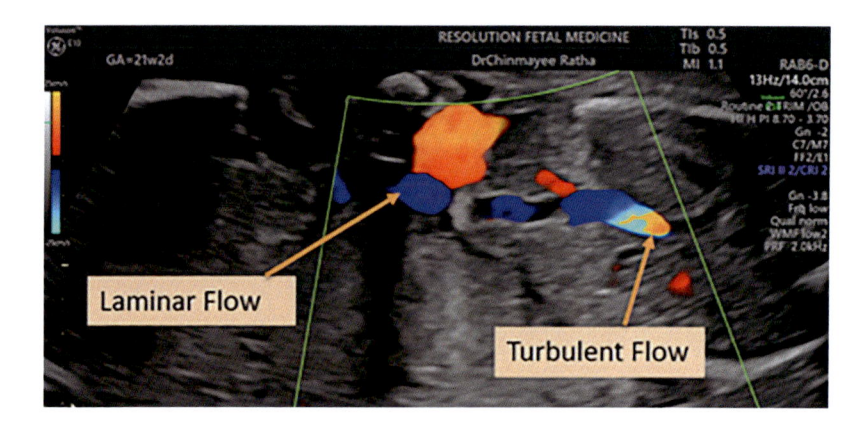

Fig. 8.5 Power Doppler

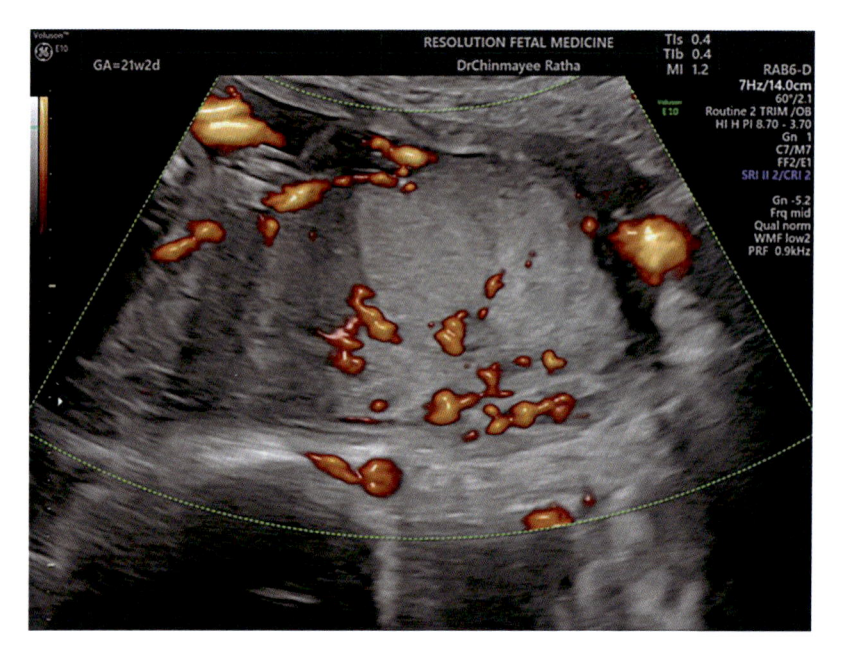

become crucial in planning management of growth-restricted fetuses in order to optimize perinatal outcome. With the emergence of more and more sophisticated ultrasound machines, we are able to define fetal hemodynamics really well, but the actual clinical significance of these studies depends on the extent of our comprehension of the fetal circulation. Understanding the pathways of fetal blood flow and the expected pattern of flow velocities and vessel resistance helps in defining the biophysical condition of the fetus. Color Doppler allows clear visualization of blood flow in the fetal circulation.

8.1 Fetal Circulation

Circulation of blood in the fetus is a dynamic circuit between the placenta and the fetal body. The fetus itself is not capable of respiratory function and thus relies on the maternal circulation to carry out gas, nutrient, and waste exchange. The fetal and maternal blood never mix; instead, they interface at the placenta which allows the exchange of gases and metabolites to help oxygenate, cleanse, and nourish the fetus. Consequently, the fetal lungs are nonfunctional, and a series of shunts exist in the fetal vascular

8.1 Fetal Circulation

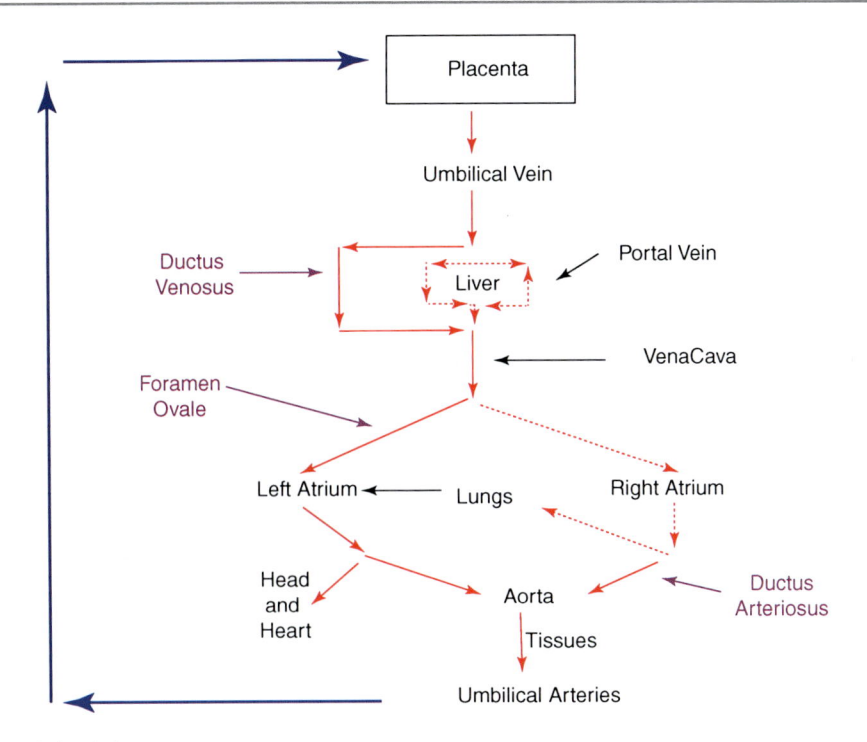

Fig. 8.6 Fetal circulation

pathways so that these organs are almost completely bypassed. Figure 8.6 is a systematic representation of the fetal circulation.

Oxygenated blood enters the fetus through the umbilical vein and through the ductus venosus in the liver, most of it bypassing the liver to enter the inferior vena cava. The ductus venosus links the umbilical vein to the caudal vena cava, and the flow of blood is controlled by a sphincter, enabling the proportion traveling to the heart via the liver to be altered.

In the fetal heart, oxygenated blood enters into the right atrium and the foramen ovale, which is an opening between the two atrial shunts' highly oxygenated blood from the right atrium to the left atrium enabling blood to be channeled directly into the systemic circulation, thereby bypassing the lungs. The septum secundum directs the majority of the blood entering the right atrium through the foramen ovale into the left atrium. Here it mixes with a small volume of blood returning from the nonfunctional lungs via the pulmonary veins.

The blood then goes to the left ventricle and gets pumped into the aorta and into the systemic circulation. The blood from the right ventricle is pumped to the pulmonary trunk where, due to the high resistance in the collapsed fetal lungs, a larger volume passes through the ductus arteriosus to the caudal aorta. The ductus arteriosus connects the pulmonary artery to the aorta and allows equivalent ventricular function in the fetus. The ductus arteriosus empties blood into the aorta after the artery to the head has branched off, thus ensuring that the brain receives well-oxygenated blood.

Most of the blood in the aorta is then returned to the placenta for oxygenation through the umbilical arteries. Once we have understood the basic fetal circulation, it is easy to understand the significance of the fetal vessels investigated to establish fetal well-being.

8.2 Umbilical Artery Doppler

The umbilical arteries are representative of the fetal peripheral circulation, and during normal fetal functioning, the umbilical artery Dopplers show a pattern with a good systolic and diastolic forward flow (Fig. 8.7). The umbilical Doppler is performed usually on a free loop of the umbilical artery using color Doppler to identify the vessel and then placing the pulse wave Doppler with a gate of 2–3 mm right in the middle of the vessel with the angle of the gate preferably aligned along the long axis of the vessel. There is a peak in cardiac systole and a trough in diastole with significant positive end diastolic flow seen in all cycles.

When the fetus is under stress, the umbilical artery resistance to flow increased which is reflected in increase in the height of the peaks and progressive diminution of diastolic flow leading to "absent end-diastolic flow" (AEDF) as the first sign of a physiological decompensation mechanism. When fetal distress persists, there is a hemodynamic reversal with "reversed end-diastolic flow" (REDF) in the umbilical arteries as shown in the figure below.

8.3 Fetal Middle Cerebral Artery Doppler

The other important blood vessel investigated during fetal evaluation is the fetal middle cerebral artery (MCA). The MCA arises from the internal carotid and supplies blood to many parts of the lateral cerebral cortex, the anterior temporal lobes, and the insular cortices. This vessel carries about 80% of the flow volume received by the cerebral hemisphere. This vessel is interrogated at the junction of the proximal one-third and the distal two-thirds of its length. The Doppler gate is 2–3 mm and the angle of insonation should be as close to zero as possible such that the velocity measurements are reliable. The normal flow pattern in the fetal MCA is one with tall peaks in systole (Fig. 8.8). During fetal hypoxemia, there is cerebral vasodilatation and the blood flow pattern in MCA changes so that the diastolic flow increases and the phenomenon is called the "brain sparing" effect. This is a sign of physiological compensation in the fetal circulation to maintain perfusion to the vital organ—the fetal brain.

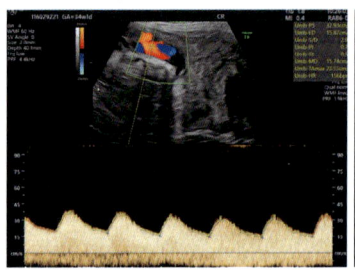

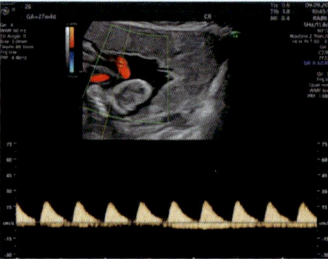

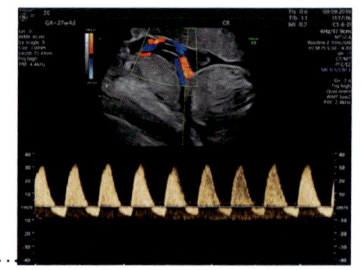

Fig. 8.7 Umbilical artery flow patterns (normal, absent EDF, reversed EDF)

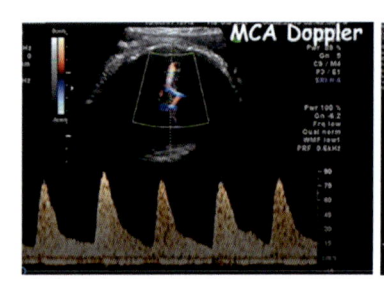

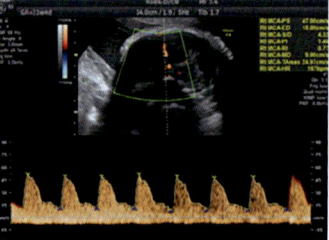

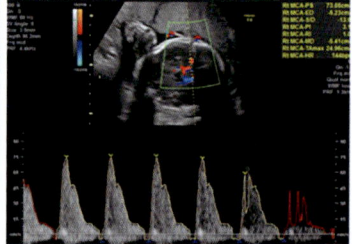

Fig. 8.8 MCA flows

The fetal middle cerebral artery blood flow pattern helps in diagnosing another important condition which affects fetal hemodynamics—fetal anemia. When the fetus becomes anemic, the peak systolic velocity of the fetal MCA rises above 1.5 times the multiple of median for that stage of gestation. The charts of nomograms for MCA-PSV at different stages of gestation are available, and it is useful to plot the MCA-PSV on a serial nomogram while monitoring fetuses at suspicion for developing anemia. As a ballpark figure, the 1.5 MoM at any gestation is roughly twice the gestational age in weeks, e.g., at 32 weeks of gestation, a PSV in the fetal MCA greater than 64 cm/s would be likely suggestive of fetal anemia. It is recommended however that standard charts be followed and the graphs plotted accordingly.

The sensitivity of fetal MCA-PSV in detecting fetal anemia is so accurate (>99%) that in a setting of clinical suspicion, raised MCA-PSV is enough to diagnose anemia, and there are methods of quantifying it to warrant a fetal blood transfusion. The details of this evaluation and management are given in the Chap. 16.

8.4 Fetal Ductus Venosus Doppler

The fetal ductus venosus is a conduit between the umbilical vein and the inferior vena cava. The umbilical vein brings in oxygenated blood from the placenta to the fetus, and hence the DV carries this oxygenated blood into the IVC into which shunts in order for this to reach the fetal cardiac right atrium. The flow pattern in the ductus venosus reflects the portocaval pressure gradient and the pressure on the right side of the heart (Fig. 8.9).

Normal flow in the fetal ductus venosus represents blood flow velocities during ventricular and atrial contraction phases. Abnormal venous waveforms are characterized by a decrease of diastolic peak forward and increase of peak reverse velocities with atrial contraction in the inferior vena cava and right hepatic vein. The DV is one of the last vessels to be compromised in fetal growth restriction due to fetal compensatory mechanisms as it is critical to the supply of oxygenated blood to the fetus. Abnormal DV Doppler is the single most important indicator of risk of fetal demise as it indicates a breakdown of fetal hemodynamic compensatory mechanisms in the face of hypoxia.

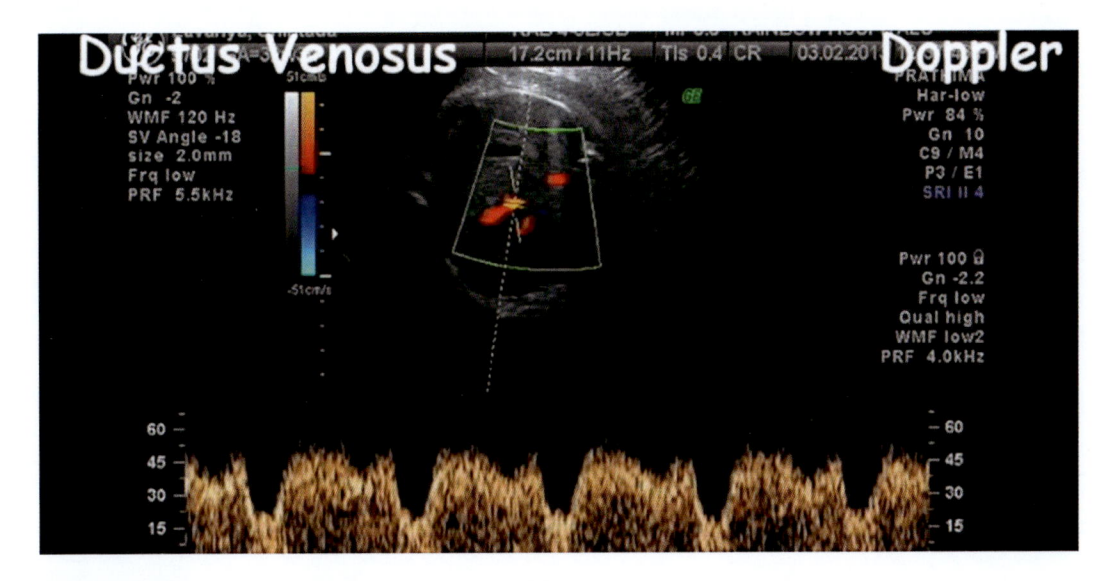

Fig. 8.9 DV flow

Another Doppler studied in the fetus is that of the aortic isthmus. The aortic isthmus is the region in the fetal aorta between the origin of the left subclavian artery and the junction of the ductus arteriosus. This isthmus represents an interface between highly oxygenated blood that flows toward the upper part of the body and the partly deoxygenated blood going toward the lower parts of the body in the fetal circulatory outflow. Under normal circulatory patterns, there is forward flow in the ductus arteriosus in all stages of the cardiac cycle. The isthmus is a narrow zone and shows a sharp peak flow in systole with a forward flow in diastole that follows a narrow incisura post systole. However, reversal of diastolic flow in the aortic isthmus is considered abnormal and indicates reduced oxygen supply to the fetal brain. These changes in aortic isthmus occur almost a week before the changes in ductus venosus flow, so it has become a potential marker for prognosticating "intact survival" rather than only "survival." However, the technical difficulty in assessing the aortic isthmus flow and the interobserver variability and lack of robust data has limited its wide application in clinical practice as of now (Fig. 8.10).

In the cascade of events leading to fetal compromise in fetal growth restriction, the umbilical artery changes occur first. The early changes like increased resistance with positive diastolic flow are followed by late changes like absent or reversed end-diastolic flow. The late changes are representative of fetal decompensatory mechanisms, and unless the gestational age is the limiting factor, the fetus may be delivered to avoid further intrauterine compromise. Progressive fetal compromise is associated with changes in middle cerebral artery, aortic isthmus, and then the venous flow changes which are indicative of severe fetal decompensation. The challenge in managing these fetuses in distress is to strike the right balance between in utero maturation at the cost of further compromise and ex utero survival at the cost of prematurity. The interpretation of

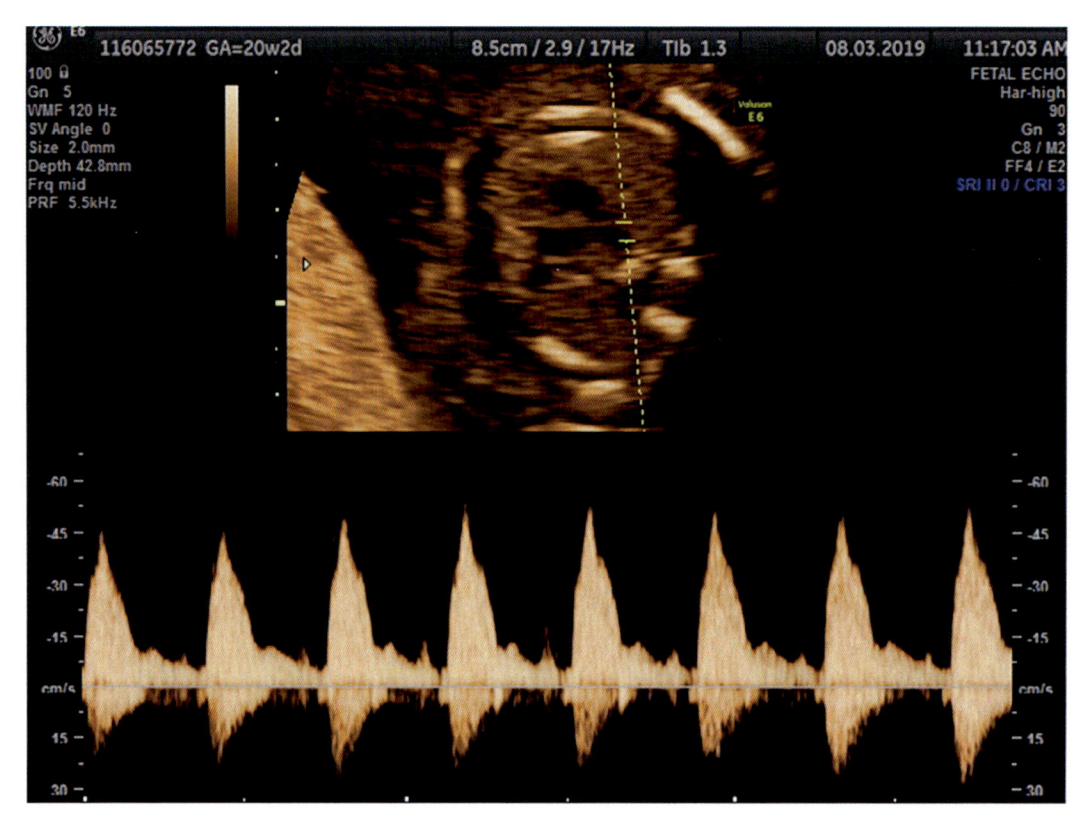

Fig. 8.10 Aortic isthmus Doppler

these Doppler changes is thus of paramount importance in understanding the level of fetal stress and optimizing the timing of delivery. This is the most important decision in a case of fetal growth restriction, but many factors are taken into account prior to finalizing this decision—fetal evaluation, maternal comorbid conditions, neonatology facilities available, and also parental wishes.

The significance of interpreting the fetal Dopplers is getting a clarity about the fetal circulation along with its unique shunt mechanisms, namely, the ductus venosus, foramen ovale, and ductus arteriosus.

The fetal circulation maintains fetal physiological functions through exchange of oxygen, nutrients, and metabolites through the placenta throughout pregnancy. At birth, with the disconnection of the placental pathway, there are significant circulatory changes that occur in the newborn baby due to the replacement of the placenta by the lungs as the organ of respiratory exchange. When a newborn baby takes its first breath, the lungs and pulmonary vessels expand, thereby significantly lowering the resistance to blood flow. This subsequently lowers the pressure in the pulmonary artery and the right side of the heart. On the other hand, the removal of the placenta causes an increase in the resistance of the systemic circulation and hence an increase in the pressure of the left side of the heart—these changes cause the closure of the foramen ovale which was patent throughout pregnancy.

The birth of the baby also triggers the closure of the other fetal circulatory shunts. The ductus venosus is weakly responsive to prostaglandin E2 (PGE2) and prostacyclin (PGI2) which behave as vasodilators. With improved pulmonary clearance resulting from the absence of an umbilical blood supply, these prostaglandin effects are diminished. This loss of blood supply also causes the sphincter in the ductus venosus to constrict, thereby diverting blood to the liver. Closure of the ductus venosus becomes permanent after 2–3 weeks of birth, and the remnant of the ductus venosus forms the ligamentum venosum.

The ductus arteriosus is a muscular artery and immediately after birth, increased oxygen content of the blood passing through it and the production of bradykinin, which causes smooth muscle contraction which closes the shunt. This physiological closure causes blood to be directed from the pulmonary arteries to the lungs which now have expanded and are functioning. Although functional closure occurs first, the actual anatomical closure takes about 2 months and occurs by infolding of the endothelium and proliferation of the subintimal connective tissue layer resulting in a residual ligament called the ligamentum arteriosum. The closure of these unique shunt mechanisms marks the transition of fetal circulation to postnatal circulatory adaptations, and the fetal dependence on placenta for oxygen shifts to the neonatal dependence on its lungs.

8.5 Uterine Artery Doppler

The uterine artery is a maternal blood vessel that is studied for predicting the risk of maternal pre-eclampsia and fetal growth restriction in pregnancy. Uterine artery arises from the anterior division of the internal iliac artery and can be evaluated close to the cervix in the first trimester and at the crossover across the external iliac vessels in the second trimester. Both uterine arteries are evaluated and the mean PI is determined. This can be used for risk assessment of abovementioned issues in an extended screening protocol which is discussed in detail in the Chap. 11.

In addition to assessing stages of fetal hypoxia and its associated compensatory events, specific Doppler findings can be used to correlate risk factors for fetal aneuploidies, to diagnose and prognosticate fetal anomalies, and to define unique problems of multiple pregnancies. The individual conditions will be dealt with in detail in their respective chapters in the book, but here is a comprehensive table (Table 8.1) summarizing the application of fetal Doppler in various clinical situations.

Clearly, the technology of Dopplers has revolutionized the assessment of the anatomy and physiology of the fetus and can be implemented in diagnosing, prognosticating, and even treating problems in fetal health. It is therefore imperative that every obstetrician acquires a reasonable understanding of the basics of the use of Dopplers in obstetrics.

Table 8.1 Application of fetal Doppler in specific clinical conditions

	Doppler examination	Clinical condition	Interpretation
1.	Spectral Doppler across cardiac valves	To assess fetal heart rate	The fetal heart rate and rhythm can be assessed to establish viability, normal patterns, or abnormalities like arrhythmias or heart blocks
2.	First trimester fetal ductus venosus	Risk assessment for fetal aneuploidies	Raised resistance to DV flows is correlated with high risk of fetal aneuploidies
3.	First trimester fetal tricuspid regurgitation	Risk assessment for fetal aneuploidies and cardiac anomalies	Tricuspid regurgitation raises the risk of fetal aneuploidies and cardiac anomalies
4.	Midtrimester perivesical umbilical vessels	Color flow is used to ascertain two patent umbilical arteries	Normal cord vasculature can be demonstrated and anomalies like two-vessel cord can be detected
5.	Midtrimester cardiac chambers and outflow tracts	Color flow is used to check chamber patency and flow patterns	Abnormal flow patterns can reveal septal defects, valvular dysfunctions, or abnormal connections
6.	Assessment of fetal anomalies	Color flow is used to identify several conditions, e.g., vascular malformations and presence of certain blood vessels or altered course of the same can be checked to prognosticate anomalies	Presence of renal arteries rules out renal agenesis, abnormal course of superior mesenteric artery helps in identifying bowel herniation through fetal diaphragm, etc.
7.	Assessment of problems in multiple pregnancies	Color flow assessment for blood flow discordance in monochorionic twin complications	Abnormal Doppler flows help in classifying TTTS, TAPS, and TRAP in MC twins
8.	Assessment of fetal hemodynamic compensation in physiological disturbances	Spectral flows across critical vessels help in diagnosing fetal anemia and prognosticating fetal growth restriction	High PSV in MCA is indicative of fetal anemia. High resistance flows in umbilical arteries, DV, and aortic isthmus indicate worsening compensatory efforts on fetal growth restriction just as low resistance flow in MCA is a marker for fetal hypoxia

8.6 Safety Issues with Fetal Doppler

Doppler involves exposure of the fetus to high-frequency signals and thus there are safety concerns, so the principle of ALARA (as low as reasonably achievable) must be adhered to while using this technology. The safety issues are discussed in the chapter on "basics of fetal imaging" too. As with any technology, the best results of using Dopplers in fetal medicine can be obtained only by optimal use, proper case selection, and adherence to the correct protocols of practice.

> **Key Learning Points in Doppler Imaging**
> 1. Doppler technology provides a very useful method to assess feto-maternal hemodynamics.
> 2. Appropriate use of Doppler studies provides very important information regarding physiological and pathological processes in the feto-maternal-placental unit.
> 3. A thorough understanding of fetal circulation is of paramount importance in interpreting fetal Doppler results.

4. Blood vessels have definite flow patterns which can be studied quantitatively by Doppler indices and used for correlating clinical outcomes.
5. Use of fetal Doppler can help provide a very reliable method to prognosticate fetal outcome in conditions like fetal growth restriction, anemia, MC twin complications, and other fetal anomalies such that rational decisions to deliver can be made.
6. Doppler studies have emerged as the technology providing the basis to support most crucial clinical decisions in current perinatal practice.

Suggested Reading

ISUOG. Practice guidelines: use of Doppler ultrasonography in obstetrics. Ultrasound Obstet Gynecol. 2013;41(2):233–9.

Fetal Growth Disorders

Fetal "growth" is a continuous process that starts at conception and continues till birth in a regulated manner depending on its inherent genetic potential. "Growth" is considered to be a basic characteristic of human life and is defined as an increase in physical size. Here it is important to recall that "size" and "growth," although closely related, have a basic difference. Size can be defined by current biometric parameters and this may or may not be within normal ranges, but "growth" is a serial process—so even if "size" may be within normal limits, growth may be suboptimal, while even if size is small, interval growth may be normally maintained.

We have explained in the Chap. 6 that fetal parts can be measured, and these composite measurements provide a statement of fetal "size." At every stage of gestation, there are specific fetal growth parameters that can be measured and expressed as a percentile for that stage of gestation. Whenever we want to quantify fetal growth and label it in comparison to expected parameters at that gestational age, it is a good practice to plot the actual growth into charts representing the 5th, 50th, and 95th centiles of that parameter as expected in that period of gestation. Most ultrasound machines used today for obstetric scans have these charts inbuilt in their reporting format. There are also specific obstetric ultrasound reporting software which enable the user to plot the fetal biometry at each evaluation date and obtain trends of fetal growth.

A normal growth process involves attaining these parameters in a certain time frame. A deviation from the expected growth trajectory is classified as a growth disorder—growth may either be less or more than expected. The figure below (Fig. 9.1) shows an example of a growth chart and the expected trend of fetal growth alongside the actual observed trend thus showing the difference.

In Fig. 9.1, it is seen that the observed growth parameters were below the expected levels and hence this is an example of "slowing" of growth velocity. The three reference curves indicate the 10th, 50th, and 90th centiles of fetal growth which is represented by the fetal weight in grams along the vertical axis (Y-axis on the graph) for that stage of gestation in weeks (X-axis on the graph). Fetal biometry is considered appropriate for gestational age if individual measurements are falling within the 10th to 90th centile for that stage of gestation. Fetal growth disorders are diagnosed when there is significant deviation from the expected growth pattern. The accepted definition of "crossing centiles" is a slowing by more than 2 quartiles as compared to an earlier growth estimate. "Normal fetal growth" is

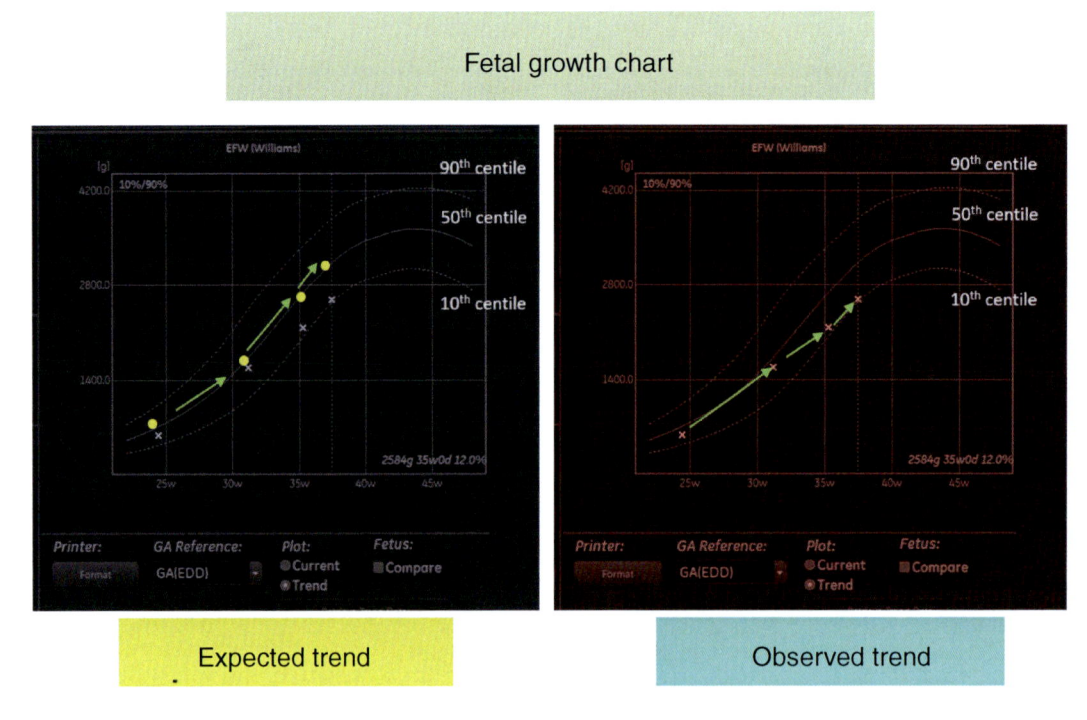

Fig. 9.1 Observed and expected fetal growth pattern plotted on a growth chart

expected to follow a "growth curve" maintaining a trajectory of similar centiles upon serial biometry, as gestation advances.

In any case, where fetal biometry parameters are not "appropriate for gestational age," we have to consider the possibilities of:
1. Mistaken dates
2. Fetal growth disorders—small or large for dates

Once again, this brings us to the revision of the concept of dating a pregnancy which has been discussed in earlier chapters. No fetal evaluation should be started without first confirming the actual dates of the pregnancy. An early pregnancy ultrasound with an appropriately measured CRL is by far the most appropriate method of dating a pregnancy. The criteria of correct measurement of CRL are given in the earlier chapter on "fetal biometry."

Once an early pregnancy ultrasound is performed, the dates allocated by the CRL at that stage should correspond to the dates based on the woman's recollection of her last menstrual period, with an allowance of disparity within 7 days. If the disparity exceeds 7 days, then it is better to redate the pregnancy based on the early pregnancy CRL. Once the dates are confirmed, each pregnancy can be allocated an "EDD" (expected date of delivery) which corresponds to 40 weeks of gestation. Henceforth, in this pregnancy, the EDD should be used for dating to avoid any confusion whatsoever.

Despite correction of dates if the fetal growth curve varies from the expected trend, then we diagnose fetal growth disorders. The more common growth disorder encountered in clinical fetal medicine is fetal growth restriction and we shall discuss this first.

9.1 Fetal Growth Restriction

Inability of a fetus to achieve its genetically determined potential for growth is called fetal growth restriction. This is a very important clinical condition and has tremendous impact on perinatal health; hence, it is imperative that all doctors involved in fetal and neonatal care understand this concept very clearly. Over the decades, we have witnessed massive amount of research in this area, and although macroscopically, it seems that concepts are changing in reality, it is just that we are understanding the core issues better and redefining the "cause-effect" relationship of various biophysical, biochemical, and ultrasound parameters. We are now able to correlate the clinical events in utero to their logical sequelae ex utero by prognosticating the disease in a stage-based manner.

The time tested Barker's hypothesis of "fetal origin of adult disease" finds numerous examples in the pathophysiology of fetal growth restriction where the in utero stress on various organs and systems has the capacity to present as organic malfunctions in later life. With further understanding of the origin of these stressors and better ability to monitor these fetuses along with refinement of neonatal care, today meaningful management of fetal growth restriction involves greatest emphasis on ensuring not just ex utero survival but also "intact survival" for the neonate and future adult.

9.1.1 Etiology and Classification of Fetal Growth Restriction

Fetal growth is affected by the inherent genetic growth potential of the fetus along with external factors which could be maternal conditions, placental support issues, and finally inherent fetal problems like malformations. Figure 9.2 highlights the major factors that could be causing fetal growth restriction.

As is evident from the figure (Fig. 9.2), many of these factors are interdependent, and hence fetal growth is a result of a complex interplay of forces which finely balance themselves to facilitate the process of fetal growth and development. If any of the adverse forces become predominant, then fetal growth is "restricted."

Fetal growth restriction was classified earlier as "symmetric" or "asymmetric". In symmetric FGR, all fetal parts lagged behind in biometry proportionally to each other, while in "asymmetric" the fetal head biometry was less affected than fetal abdominal biometry parameters. This classification aimed to distinguish the etiology of FGR with the presumption that symmetric FGR could result from problems like inherently poor genetic potential to grow. On the other hand, asymmetric FGR represented a "restriction" to growth due to extraneous factors like placental insufficiency which would start after some degree of "normal growth" that would have happened earlier on in pregnancy. As a natural adaptive mechanism, there would be a "redistribution" of resources to try and preserve fetal brain growth while compromising on the peripheral organs. Thus, fetal head biometry (BPD or HC) may still be within normal limits, while the fetal abdominal circumference (AC) is at lower centiles–the ratio of BPD/AC and HC/AC therefore gets altered in asymmetric FGR. There is also lesser blood flow to kidneys leading to less amniotic fluid and with serial progression classical Doppler changes ensue.

Symmetrical FGR is usually due to inherent fetal problems like aneuploidies and genetic syndromes where the potential to grow is lesser than normal, but instead of "constitutional," it is classified as "growth restriction" because there is serial fall in growth velocity indicating a worsening growth potential due to "restriction" related to the pathology.

The more recent classification of fetal growth restriction has been into "early" and "late" FGR depending on the time of onset of growth restriction in pregnancy. An arbitrary cutoff has been set at 32 weeks of gestation such that if FGR is identified before 32 weeks, then it is called early FGR, while typically late FGR is expected to set in only after 32 weeks. Here it is important to realize that just because a case of FGR is diagnosed at 35 weeks, it cannot automatically be labeled as "late onset" unless there is evidence to show that till 32 weeks the growth was following normal centiles. Serial monitoring of fetal growth will help reduce this confusion as "late onset FGR" and late identification of "early onset IUGR" will have different prognoses as they represent different pathophysiological processes.

Factors causing Fetal Growth Restriction

PLACENTAL FACTORS

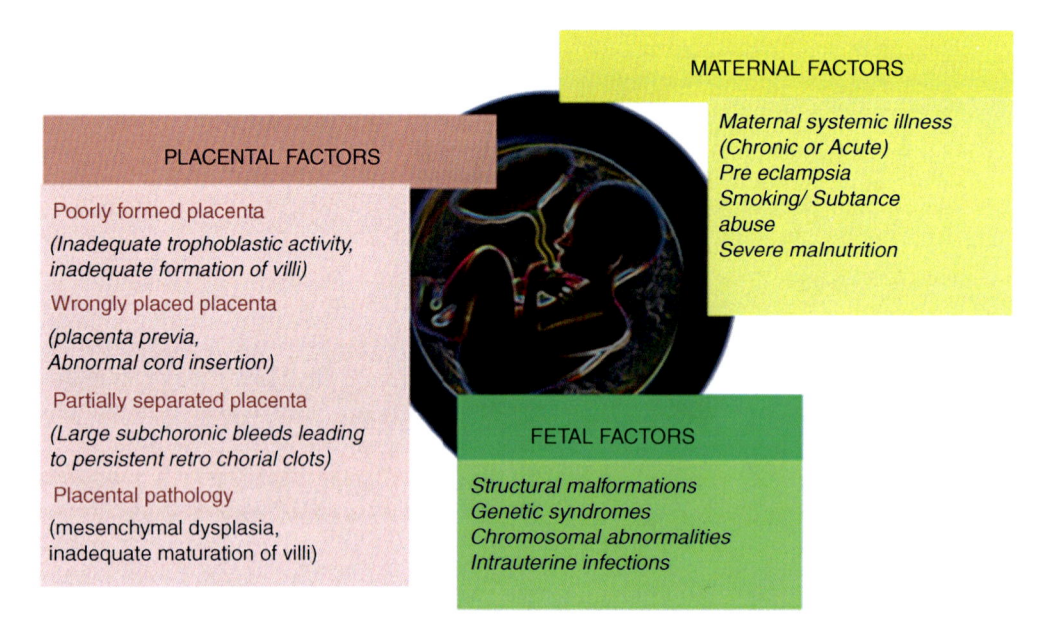

Poorly formed placenta
(Inadequate trophoblastic activity, inadequate formation of villi)

Wrongly placed placenta
(placenta previa, Abnormal cord insertion)

Partially separated placenta
(Large subchoronic bleeds leading to persistent retro chorial clots)

Placental pathology
(mesenchymal dysplasia, inadequate maturation of villi)

MATERNAL FACTORS

Maternal systemic illness (Chronic or Acute)
Pre eclampsia
Smoking/ Substance abuse
Severe malnutrition

FETAL FACTORS

Structural malformations
Genetic syndromes
Chromosomal abnormalities
Intrauterine infections

Fig. 9.2 Factors causing fetal growth restriction

This classification of "early" and "late" FGR involves looking at the placenta playing a pivotal role in facilitating fetal growth. If the placenta malfunctions, then one or the other type of growth restriction ensues depending on the timing of placental dysfunction. In early FGR, it has been shown that the placentae generally are smaller and have a smaller number of villi per unit surface area. This results in poor exchange of nutrients as well as a high vascular "resistance" in the placental bed. This resistance may be reflected by high resistance flows in the umbilical arteries of the fetus and uterine arteries of the mother. The details of fetal circulation and Doppler flows are given in the chapter on "fetal Dopplers."

9.1.2 Diagnosis and Evaluation of Fetal Growth Restriction

The fact that "growth restriction" and "smallness" are not always synonymous has been clarified in the preceding sections. Therefore, the diagnosis of fetal growth restriction involves methods beyond simple biometry. Appropriate dating and serial biometry remain the most important clues for suspecting fetal growth restriction, but fetal Doppler studies help in establishing the diagnosis and segregating the group of "constitutionally" small fetuses. Figure 9.3 depicts an algorithm to establish the diagnosis of fetal growth restriction.

Fig. 9.3 Algorithm to diagnose fetal growth restriction

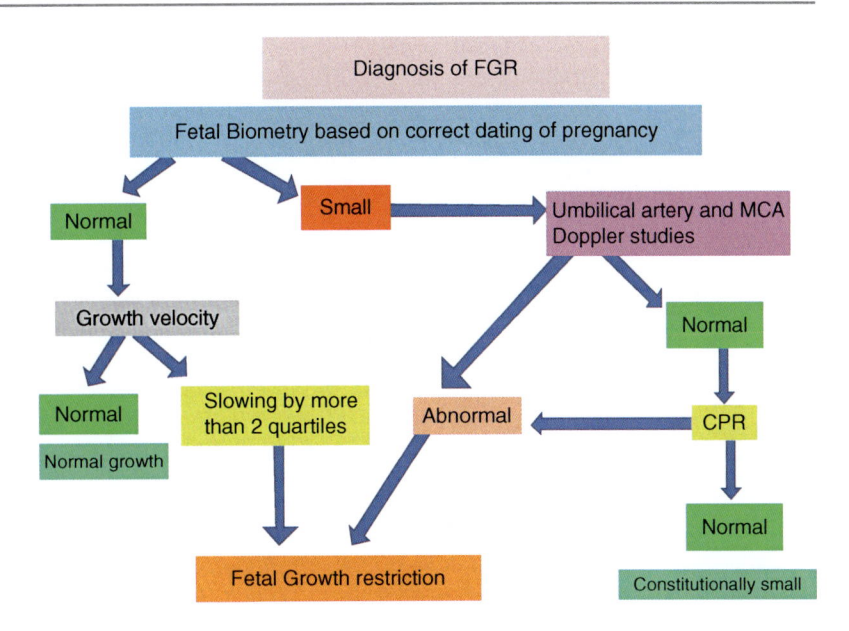

Umbilical artery Doppler changes are evident once at least 30% of the placental function is compromised. In "early onset FGR," the placental villi are deficient and hence the placental function is suboptimal, so it will be expected that umbilical artery Doppler changes start early. The cascade of umbilical artery Doppler deterioration starts with increased resistance followed by absent end-diastolic flow and finally reversed end-diastolic flow. This aggravated placental resistance then exerts stress on the entire fetal hemodynamic system which then responds by "redistributing" the fetal circulation in a manner to favor vital organs while reducing the perfusion of peripheral structures like the intestines, kidneys, and limbs. This redistribution is a compensatory mechanism and as it gets severe, it has adverse effects on fetal organs.

In "late onset FGR," the placental villi lack maturity and start to dysfunction later in pregnancy such that the manifestations are usually seen as suboptimal fetal growth after 32 weeks. The Doppler changes are rather subtle in late FGR such that there may be reduction in the MCA PI with little change in the umbilical flows. In this situation, sometimes the ratio of MCA PI and umbilical artery PI—the cerebroplacental ratio or CPR—shows perceptible changes even when the individual parameters may not be significantly altered. Therefore, in late FGR, the MCA Doppler and CPR are good indicators of fetal compromise unlike early FGR where umbilical artery changes precede the others and are far more obvious in severity. Table 9.1 summarizes the various differences between early onset and late onset FGR.

Once the diagnosis of fetal growth restriction is established, fetal Dopplers play an important role in evaluation and have a very important prognostic role. Most management decisions will be guided by the Doppler abnormalities as these closely correlate with the severity of the fetal physiological changes due to FGR. Figure 9.4 shows the clinical significance of Doppler abnormalities in fetal growth restriction.

Table 9.1 Differences between early and late onset FGR

	Early onset FGR	Late onset FGR
Gestation at "onset"	Less than 32 weeks	Onset after 32 weeks GA
Prevalence	Approx. 1%	3–5%
Fetal biometry	The EFW is usually below the 10th or even 5th centile	The EFW may or may not be below 10th centile always but growth restriction is noticed due to significant drop in centiles from preceding trend
Doppler changes	Umbilical Doppler is altered first followed by MCA and DV changes	The MCA alteration is more apparent, while umbilical changes may be subtle and DV may remain normal. CPR changes are obvious
Placental pathology	The placenta is expected to have less number of villi with significantly lower villous vascular area	The placental villi are not reduced in number but have inadequate maturation
Clinical challenges for the fetus	Severe prematurity in addition to smallness and morbidity due to hemodynamic redistribution	Risks of hypoxia in a "near-term" fetus with less reserve and possibility of severe compromise due to inability to detect the clinically "subtle" signs
Clinical challenges for the mother	Usually associated with maternal comorbidity like preeclampsia	Maternal comorbidity is uncommon but increased risk of operative delivery
Challenge to clinician	Optimizing the timing of delivery by balancing the odds of severe prematurity with the risk of in utero compromise	Identifying the problem and optimizing the timing of delivery to avoid risk of fetal hypoxic injury

Clinical significance of Abnormal Dopplers in FGR

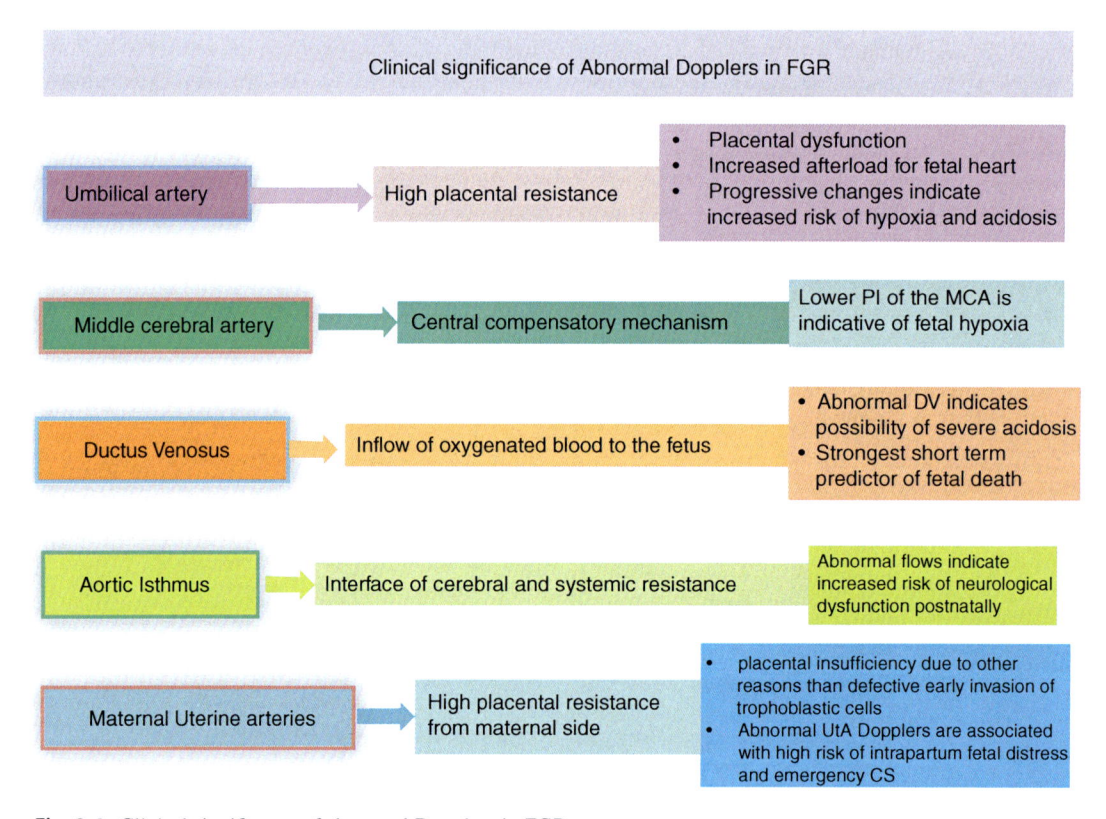

- **Umbilical artery** → High placental resistance
  - Placental dysfunction
  - Increased afterload for fetal heart
  - Progressive changes indicate increased risk of hypoxia and acidosis

- **Middle cerebral artery** → Central compensatory mechanism
  - Lower PI of the MCA is indicative of fetal hypoxia

- **Ductus Venosus** → Inflow of oxygenated blood to the fetus
  - Abnormal DV indicates possibility of severe acidosis
  - Strongest short term predictor of fetal death

- **Aortic Isthmus** → Interface of cerebral and systemic resistance
  - Abnormal flows indicate increased risk of neurological dysfunction postnatally

- **Maternal Uterine arteries** → High placental resistance from maternal side
  - placental insufficiency due to other reasons than defective early invasion of trophoblastic cells
  - Abnormal UtA Dopplers are associated with high risk of intrapartum fetal distress and emergency CS

Fig. 9.4 Clinical significance of abnormal Dopplers in FGR

9.1.3 Management of Fetal Growth Restriction

The problem in fetal growth restriction is that the fetus in utero is not being able to grow despite having the capacity to do so otherwise. This translates into the fact that intrauterine environment is not conducive for fetal growth and the solution would involve an intervention such that either that environment is modified or the fetus is removed from that environment and allowed growth ex utero. Both these strategies may sound logical but have inherent challenges. Modification of in utero environment in advanced gestation has extremely limited possibilities, e.g., treating maternal malnutrition and preventing smoking or substance abuse, and as is evident, these are issues pertinent to a very small fraction of cases with fetal growth restriction. Improving maternal diet seems to be a reasonable empirical "intervention," but unless the mother has definite malnutrition, this is unlikely to be of palpable benefit based on the evidence provided by studies. There are no proven medications as yet that can be started in the second half of pregnancy to improve uteroplacental circulation. It is safe to say that till date, there is no proven "treatment" of fetal growth restriction. It therefore remains a fact that finally the goal of management is to monitor a fetus in utero till it becomes reasonable to deliver and "relieve" the fetus of the "intrauterine" growth restriction. This is the crux of the principle of management of FGR.

The growth-restricted fetus in utero copes with the stresses on its system by developing compensatory mechanisms. The severity of compensatory mechanisms correlate with neonatal morbidity, and decompensation finally results in intrauterine fetal demise. The challenge in managing fetal growth restriction is to optimize the timing of delivery as the perfect balance between not allowing nonreversible fetal damage due to the stress of nutritional and hemodynamic compensation while ensuring optimal maturity for an intact postnatal survival and avoiding the risk of intrauterine fetal demise.

The target of fetal monitoring is to achieve a reasonable maturity and hence at 37 weeks offering delivery would be a prudent decision. Continuing these pregnancies beyond 37 weeks does not show any benefit, and if the Dopplers are not severely compromised, even induction of labor is acceptable at term. However, at earlier gestation, decision to deliver is derived by multifactorial assessment, and the mode of delivery is abdominal as these fetuses cannot be further subjected to the stress of labor. Figure 9.5 summarizes the challenges in managing FGR at different gestational ages and the factors based on which decisions to deliver may be taken.

As is evident from the preceding discussion, the decision to deliver a growth-restricted fetus is taken while considering many factors, and in reality, every clinical scenario will be different. The wishes of the parents, the NICU facilities, and the maternal condition are all confounding variables in real life. In case there is a coexisting maternal medical condition, then the perinatal decisions are skewed in favor of maternal health. It is therefore not possible to have one blanket algorithm covering management of fetal growth restriction. At best, one can follow the basic principles of healthcare of beneficence and nonmaleficence and weigh the pros and cons of every case before taking a final decision to deliver. Managing fetal growth restriction remains one of the toughest challenges of present-day healthcare.

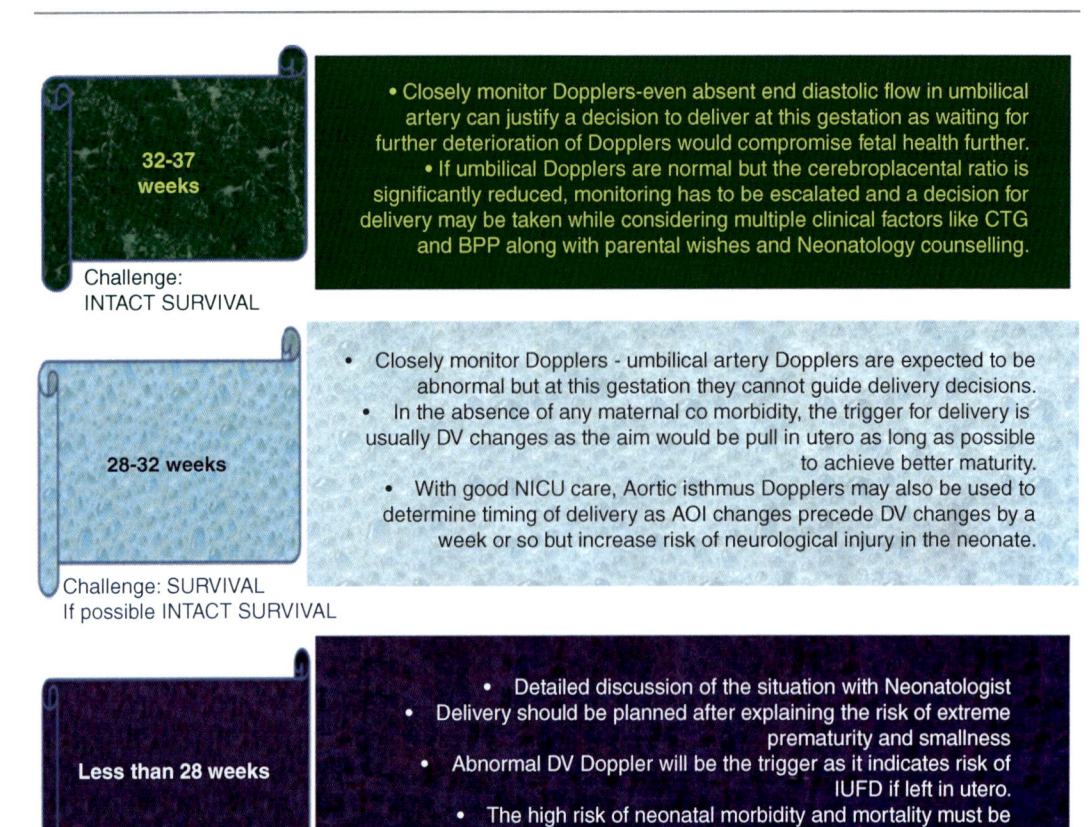

32-37 weeks
Challenge: INTACT SURVIVAL
- Closely monitor Dopplers-even absent end diastolic flow in umbilical artery can justify a decision to deliver at this gestation as waiting for further deterioration of Dopplers would compromise fetal health further.
- If umbilical Dopplers are normal but the cerebroplacental ratio is significantly reduced, monitoring has to be escalated and a decision for delivery may be taken while considering multiple clinical factors like CTG and BPP along with parental wishes and Neonatology counselling.

28-32 weeks
Challenge: SURVIVAL
If possible INTACT SURVIVAL
- Closely monitor Dopplers - umbilical artery Dopplers are expected to be abnormal but at this gestation they cannot guide delivery decisions.
- In the absence of any maternal co morbidity, the trigger for delivery is usually DV changes as the aim would be pull in utero as long as possible to achieve better maturity.
- With good NICU care, Aortic isthmus Dopplers may also be used to determine timing of delivery as AOI changes precede DV changes by a week or so but increase risk of neurological injury in the neonate.

Less than 28 weeks
Challenge: SURVIVAL
- Detailed discussion of the situation with Neonatologist
- Delivery should be planned after explaining the risk of extreme prematurity and smallness
- Abnormal DV Doppler will be the trigger as it indicates risk of IUFD if left in utero.
- The high risk of neonatal morbidity and mortality must be discussed

Fig. 9.5 Decisions to deliver in FGR based on gestational age

9.2 Fetal Overgrowth Conditions

When the fetal biometry exceeds the expected centiles and is above the 90th centile for that stage for gestation, it is called "large for dates" or LGA (large for gestational age). It is reiterated here that in any suspicion of fetal growth disorder, the first and foremost point to be checked is dating of the pregnancy. In case of mistaken dates, fetal growth may be misinterpreted and a false diagnosis may be added. To avoid any such confusion, the pregnancy dates must be reconfirmed.

If despite correction of dates the fetus appears LGA, then the two important points to be checked are maternal sugars and fetal anatomy. Maternal hyperglycemia increases the chances of fetal macrosomia, and with the rising trend of maternal diabetes, this is becoming increasingly common. If maternal diabetes is detected, then treating the same and achieving euglycemia can help in stabilizing the fetal growth velocity. In some cases, there may be associated fetal anomalies with an LGA fetus and some known genetic fetal overgrowth syndromes must be ruled out. Figure 9.6 shows an algorithm for workup for fetal macrosomia.

In case the fetal overgrowth syndromes are suspected, a genetic opinion may be sought, and specific genetic diagnosis can be obtained which helps in counseling the couple regarding the prognosis and recurrence in future pregnancies.

In case no specific cause is found and the fetus is structurally normal, the condition may represent a constitutional or familial trait. In such cases, the fetal prognosis is good.

Unless maternal diabetes is confirmed, elective induction of labor due to suspected macrosomia is still not recommended by current guidelines. Every case of fetal macrosomia presents a tremendous challenge to the obstetrician as macrosomia

9.2 Fetal Overgrowth Conditions

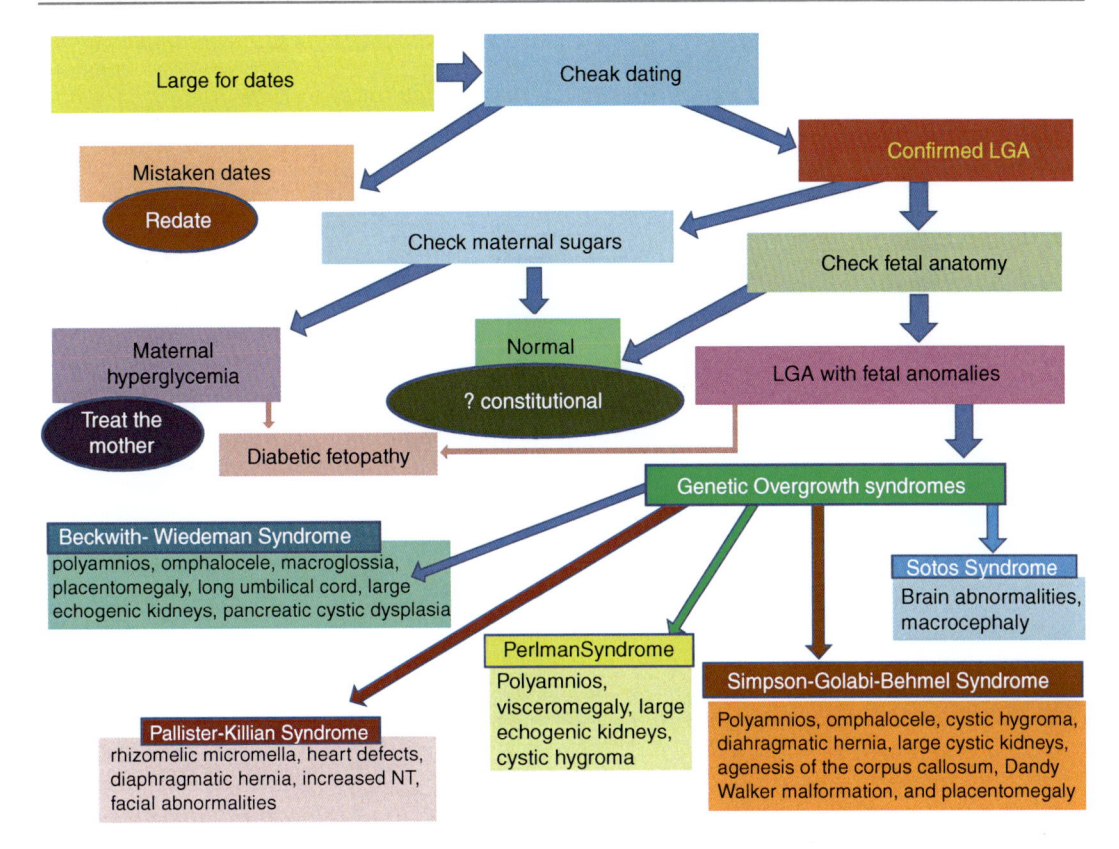

Fig. 9.6 Algorithm for workup for an LGA fetus

is associated with increased risk of birth trauma (e.g., shoulder dystocia, brachial plexus injuries), operative delivery, and also sudden stillbirth. It is therefore imperative to identify the cases of LGA fetuses accurately and conduct a thorough antenatal workup to facilitate a good plan of perinatal care by anticipating the challenges thereof.

Key Learning Points in Fetal Growth Disorders

1. Fetal growth is a steady process that starts at conception and continues throughout life.
2. There is an established "expected" pattern of growth which is defined as "physiological" at different stages of life. Any deviations from this expected pattern can lead to growth disorders.
3. Accurate dating of a pregnancy is vital in assessing fetal growth.
4. Serial biometry with use of charts depicting biometry centiles can help assess growth patterns.
5. Fetal growth restriction is more common than fetal overgrowth conditions.
6. Fetal growth restriction (FGR) can occur due to various etiologies, and the currently classification of early versus late FGR along with an understanding of evolution of the condition provides guidelines for management of FGR. Doppler studies are of paramount importance in FGR surveillance.
7. Fetal overgrowth can occur due to maternal metabolic disorders or fetal genetic conditions, and prognosis depends on inherent etiology.

Suggested Reading

Alfirevic Z, Stampalija T, Dowswell T. Fetal and umbilical Doppler ultrasound in high-risk pregnancies. Cochrane Database Syst Rev. 2017;6(6): CD007529.

American College of Obstetricians and Gynecologists. Practice Bulletin No. 173: Fetal Macrosomia. American College of Obstetricians and Gynecologists' Committee on practice bulletins—obstetrics. Obstet Gynecol. 2016;128(5):e195–209.

Figueras F, Gratacos E. An integrated approach to fetal growth restriction. Best Pract Res Clin Obstet Gynaecol. 2017;38:48–58.

Gordijn SJ, Beune IM, Thilaganathan B, Papageorghiou A, Baschat AA, Baker PN, Silver RM, Wynia K, Ganzevoort W. Consensus definition of fetal growth restriction: a Delphi procedure. Ultrasound Obstet Gynecol. 2016;48:333–9.

ISUOG. Practice guidelines: diagnosis and management of small-for-gestational age fetus and fetal growth restriction. Ultrasound Obstet Gynecol. 2020;56:298–312.

The "First Trimester (11–14 Weeks) Scan"

10

The first trimester of pregnancy is a very important phase where fetal formation begins into a definitive form and maternal adaptations to pregnancy start. We are all traditionally aware of the role of the first trimester ultrasound in defining fetal viability and dating in early pregnancy. Today, the first trimester scan has transcended its potential and can be optimized to define fetal structure so well such that many fetal anomalies can not only be detected so early but those requiring prognosticating tests can be worked up early. The lethal fetal anomalies are definitively defined and those requiring pregnancy termination can be addressed in the first trimester which makes the procedure safer— medically and socioethically. With the advancing maternal age in the general population and prevalence of consanguinity in some regions, the first trimester scan markers for aneuploidies and genetic syndromes have a potent role in screening for the same. Such screening facilitates decisions for definitive prenatal testing.

Prediction of preterm births, fetal growth restriction, and maternal complications like preeclampsia is possible with the ability to provide objective risk assessment in the first trimester by use of ultrasound. Such prediction will help triaging women requiring special care and adequate preventive measures can be initiated early. This optimization of the first trimester scan has a practical advantage which is definitely cost-effective and can be adopted in most clinical settings. It is thus imperative to invest in skill enhancement for first trimester ultrasound in all obstetric settings today.

The first trimester 11–14 weeks' scan has now become a benchmark for a comprehensive fetal evaluation and has the following potential uses:

1. Reconfirmation of fetal viability and dating
2. Detailed structural assessment to diagnose major anomalies, e.g., anencephaly, limb agenesis, etc.
3. Screening for some anomalies that may become apparent later, e.g., intracranial translucency for spina bifida
4. Screening for fetal aneuploidies by measuring fetal nuchal translucency and other markers like nasal bone, tricuspid valve blood flows, and ductus venosus flows
5. Basic workup of multifetal pregnancy like confirmation of chorionicity and amnionicity, viability, and dating issues along with establishing any condition like early discordance in fetal growth or anatomy among the multiple fetuses
6. Evaluation of maternal uterine artery Doppler as a screening tool for preeclampsia or fetal growth restriction in current pregnancy
7. Evaluation of maternal cervix to assess risk of preterm birth

10.1 Reconfirmation of Fetal Viability and Dating

Fetal viability is assessed by detecting a rhythmic pulsation in the region of fetal cardia in early pregnancy. By the 11–14 weeks' scan, the fetal heart is a well-defined structure and the fetal heart beat is a convincing activity signifying fetal viability. As soon as the fetus is visualized on the scan, one of the most important observations by the operator is to establish a definite fetal cardiac activity. Once this is noticed, the rate can be measured by placing either an M-mode Doppler (Fig. 10.1) or a pulse wave Doppler (Fig. 10.2) across this region of activity, and the reading is taken across one or two cycles depending on the machine settings and reported as "number of beats per minute," e.g., "148 bpm."

It is a real-time assessment but a documentation of the same by a convincing picture with the measurement of the fetal heart rate should be part of every scan report at 11–14 weeks.

Dating of a pregnancy is best done by the crown-rump length (CRL) of the fetus in early pregnancy, and again this is better done at 11–14 weeks as compared to very early scans simply because the fetus is a much better defined structure now and the possibility of error in measurement is very low if standard guidelines are followed.

Several professional bodies have recommended guidelines to measure the fetal CRL correctly as it is such an important parameter and the dating of a pregnancy finally rests on this measurement. A few important common points to all are as follows:

1. The fetal CRL should be measured from the top of the crown to the bottom of the rump in the midsagittal section without including

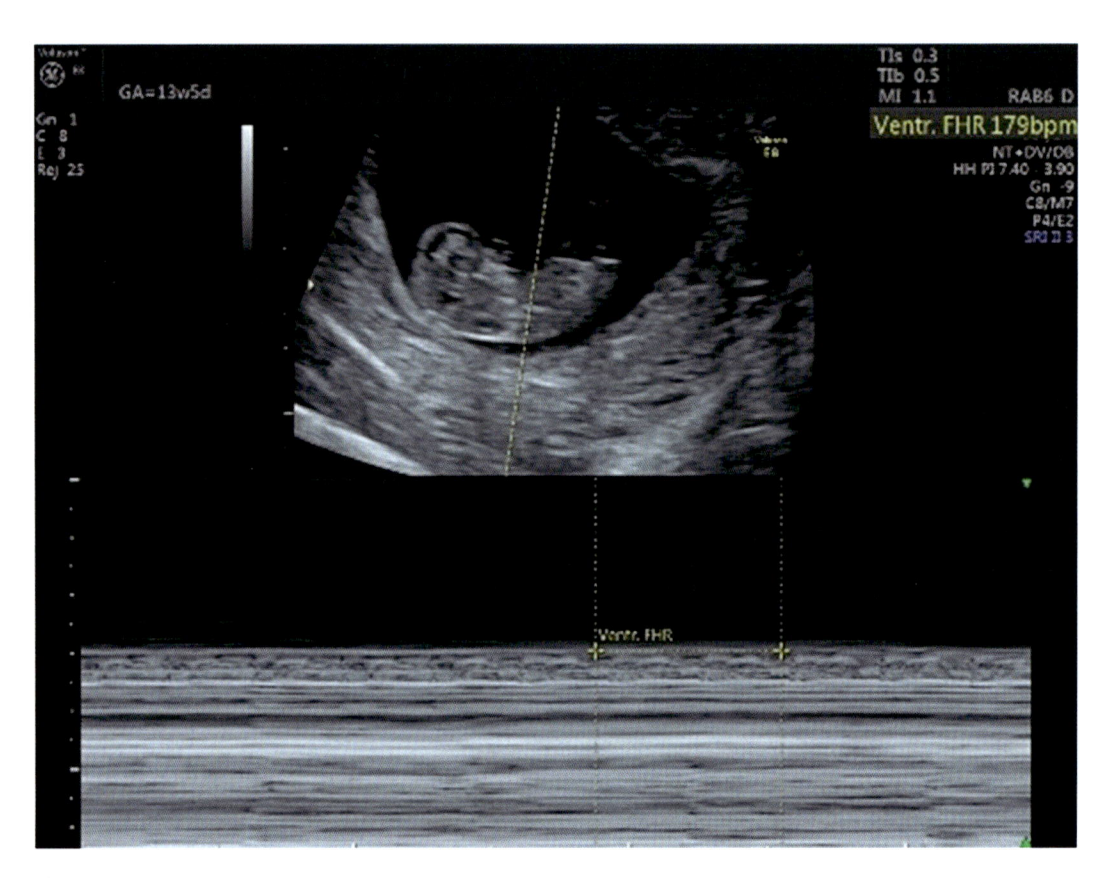

Fig. 10.1 FHR M-mode

10.1 Reconfirmation of Fetal Viability and Dating

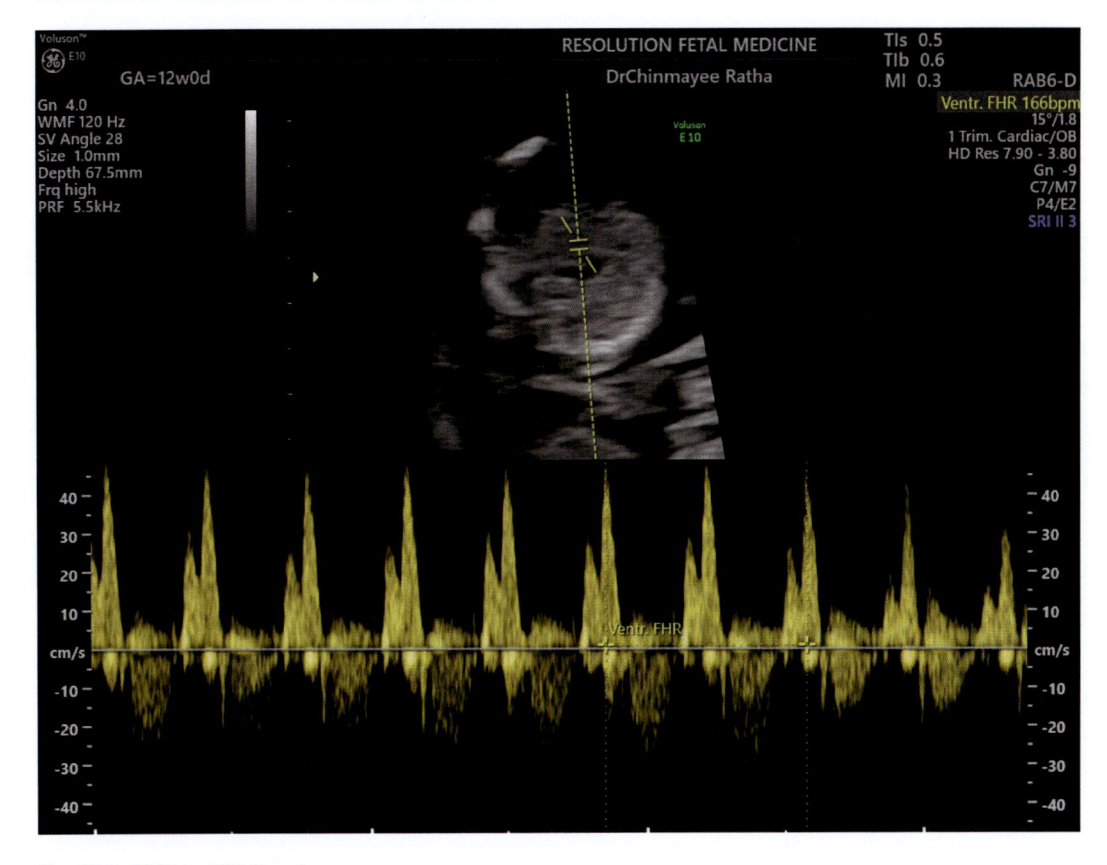

Fig. 10.2 FHR by PW Doppler

limbs or yolk sac in the measurements (Fig. 10.3).
2. The fetal attitude should be neutral and too much flexion underestimates the length, while a highly extended fetus might appear to have a longer CRL as opposed to one in neutral position which is ideal (Fig. 10.4).
3. As the fetus is not stationary and would be constantly moving through the examination, it is advisable to take several measurements of the CRL and finally take an average of the three best images to report the final CRL at that stage of gestation.

As it is evident that fetal appearance is better defined at the 11–14 weeks' scan, in some cases, there may be a disparity as compared to very early pregnancy scans like 5–6 weeks. If there is a convincing picture of a CRL measurement at those scans, then one has to refer the case to a specialize fetal care unit for detailed evaluation and assessment of the reason for disparity. However, in most cases, the error may be due to suboptimal positioning of calipers in early pregnancy scans as the fetus is rather small, and unless one is very particular, it is possible to get a rather oblique view of the fetus or a bit of "end-on" appearance such that there is a scope of over–/underestimation. In most cases, for all practical purposes, the CRL defined at the 11–14 weeks' scan is taken for dating the pregnancy.

An important rule in fetal care is to establish the dating firmly by the 11–14 weeks' scan and NOT to change it repeatedly thereafter. The purpose of dating a pregnancy is to establish the limits of gestational age, and it is neither wise nor correct to keep changing the same later on. Sometimes, a woman is not sure of her dates or is sure but the dates are not matching the fetal age after we have redated her at 11–14 weeks' scan—in such cases, it is imperative to explain

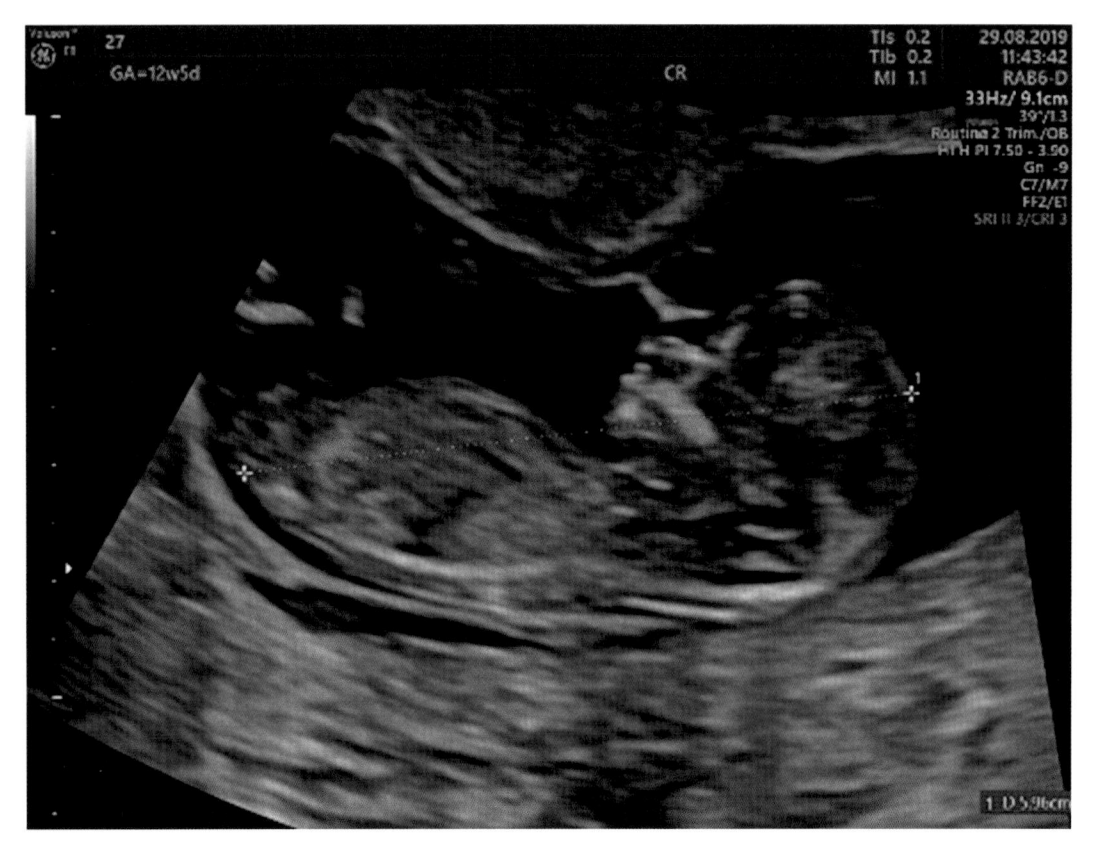

Fig. 10.3 Correct measurement of CRL at 11–14 weeks' scan

the situation to the woman and tell her the projected "EDD" which signifies the date when her pregnancy will complete 40 weeks. It is very useful to clarify this aspect to her now and even advise her that during all future consultations, she can make sure that these corrected dates are used in her evaluation. In all subsequent fetal scans, it is a good practice point to start the report by stating the final EDD as allocated in the first trimester so that future growth is corroborated to this correct dating. This prevents confusion lingering over such an important issue in pregnancy.

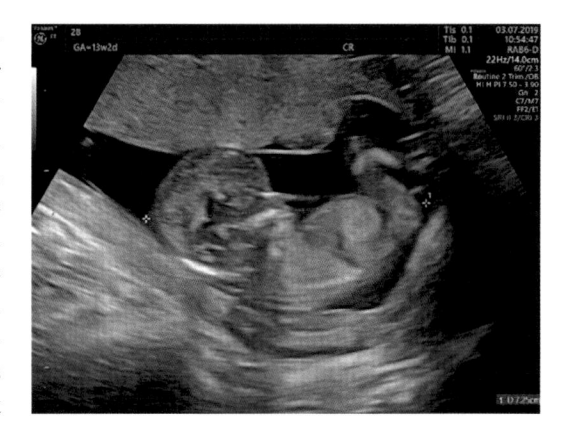

Fig. 10.4 Extreme flexion affecting CRL measurement

10.2 Detailed Fetal Structural Assessment at the 11–14 Weeks' Scan

The fetus can be examined from "head to toe" to complete a detailed structural evaluation at 11–14 weeks' scan.

Head The fetal head is evaluated in the transverse section and a smooth bony outline of the skull is seen along with a midline falx and choroid plexuses that seem to be filling the lateral ventricles and give a characteristic "butterfly" appearance when the falx cerebri is seen as a midline division (Fig. 10.5).

In cases where such a well-defined fetal head is either not seen or has some unusual appearance, one is alerted to the possibility of major CNS anomalies. Some major anomalies can be unequivocally diagnosed at the time of the first trimester scan such as absence of the cranial vault—anencephaly (Fig. 10.6)—improper cleavage of the forebrain leading to holoprosencephaly (Fig. 10.7) or outpouching of the brain, and meninges through defects in the cranial bones, encephaloceles (Fig. 10.8). Many of these problems have an adverse prognosis which are either lethal or carry risk of severe neurodevelopmental delay. An early diagnosis of such problems helps in taking

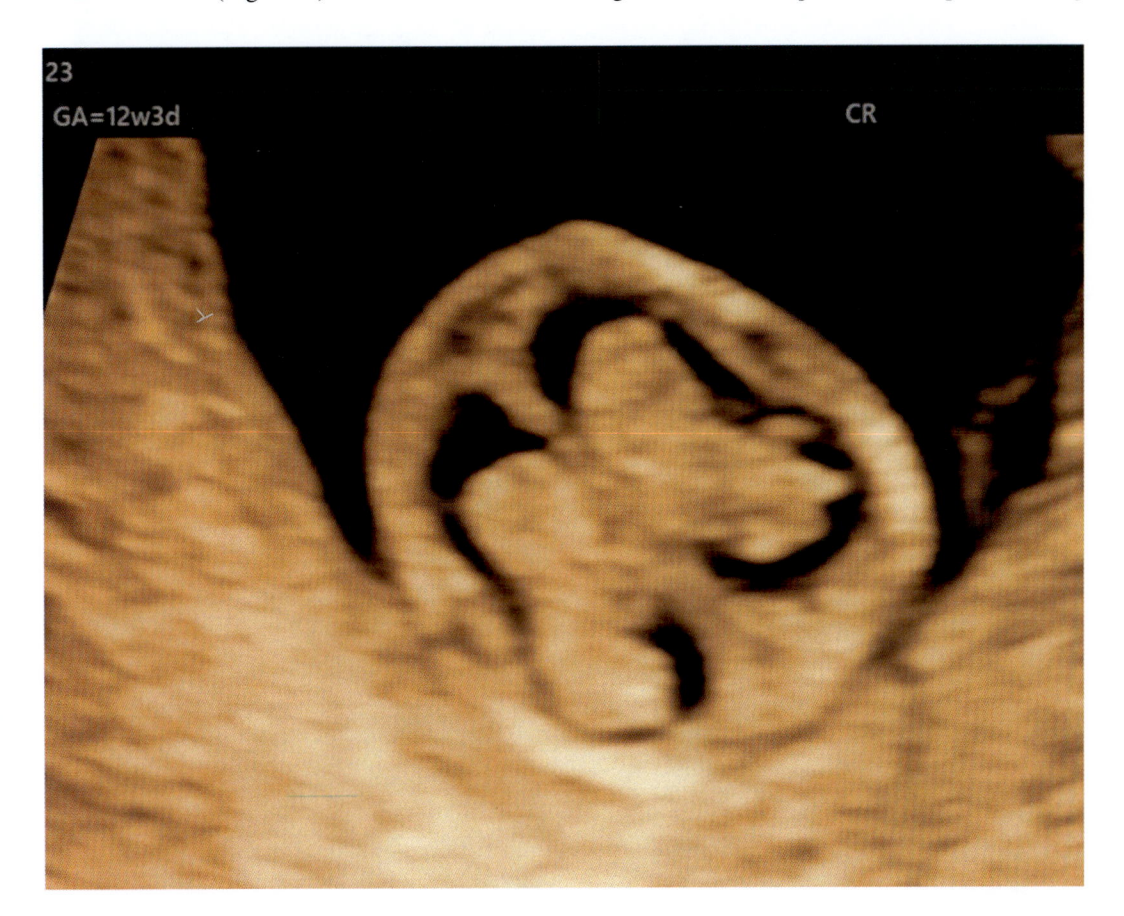

Fig. 10.5 Normal fetal head at the 11–14 weeks' scan

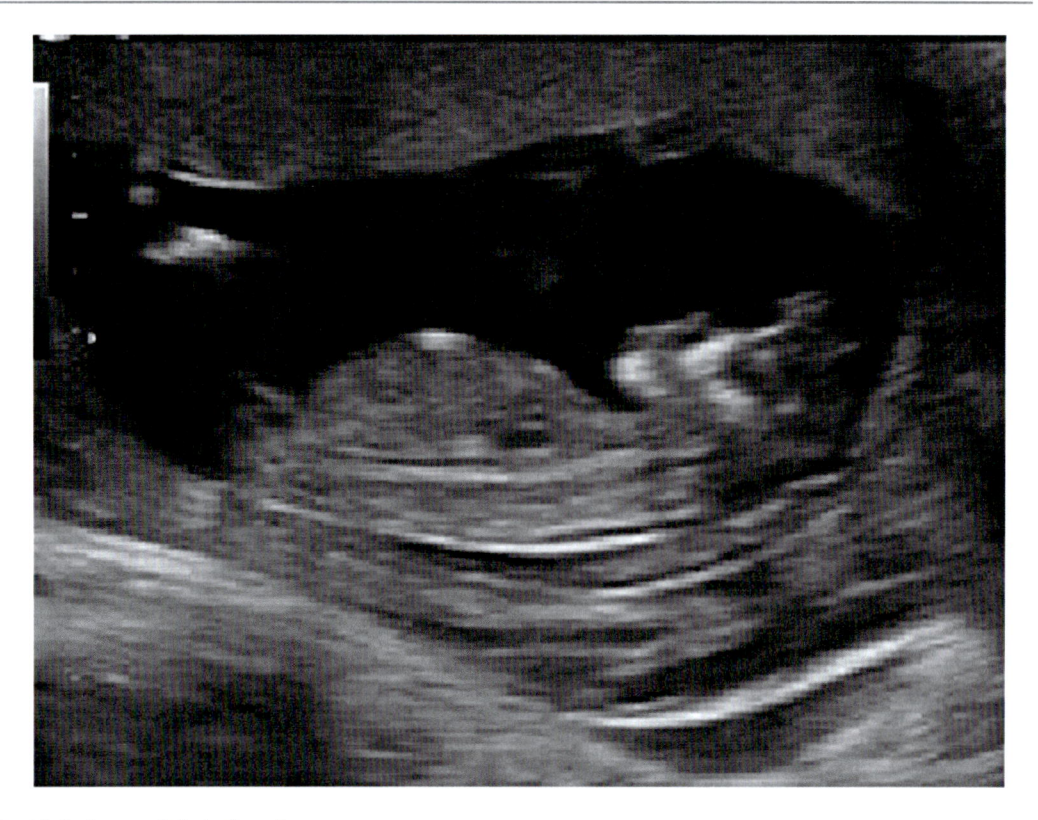

Fig. 10.6 Anencephaly in first trimester scan

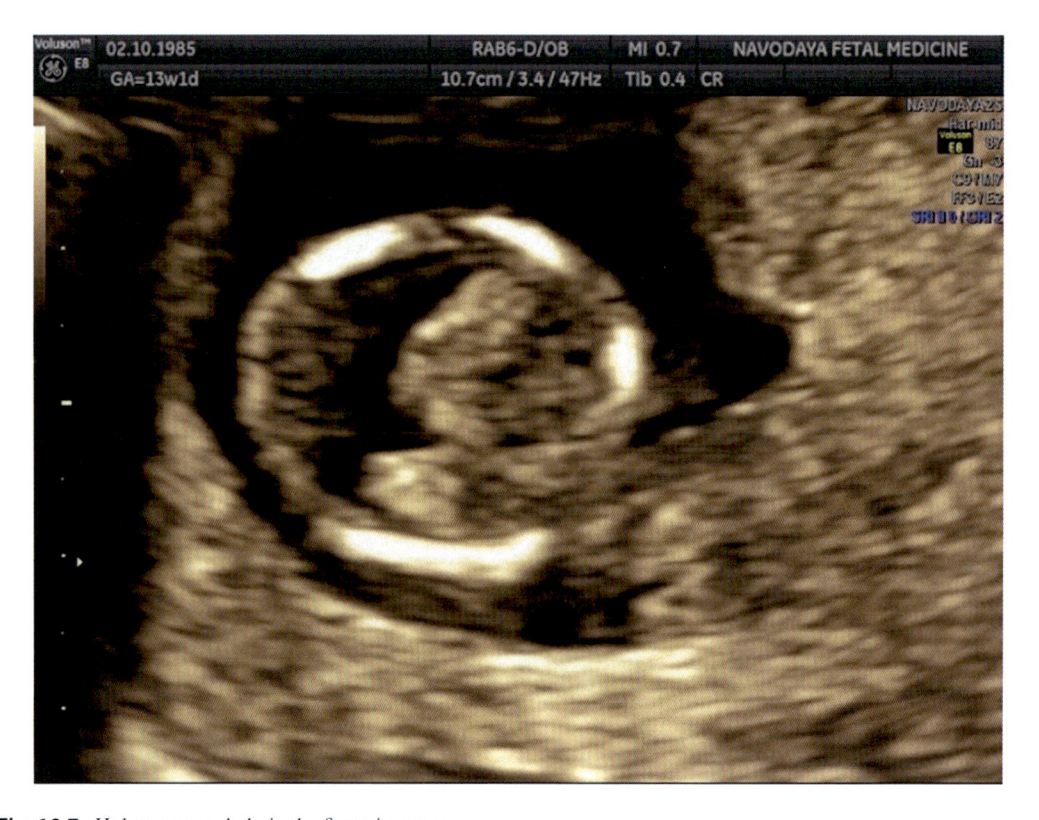

Fig. 10.7 Holoprosencephaly in the first trimester

10.2 Detailed Fetal Structural Assessment at the 11–14 Weeks' Scan 87

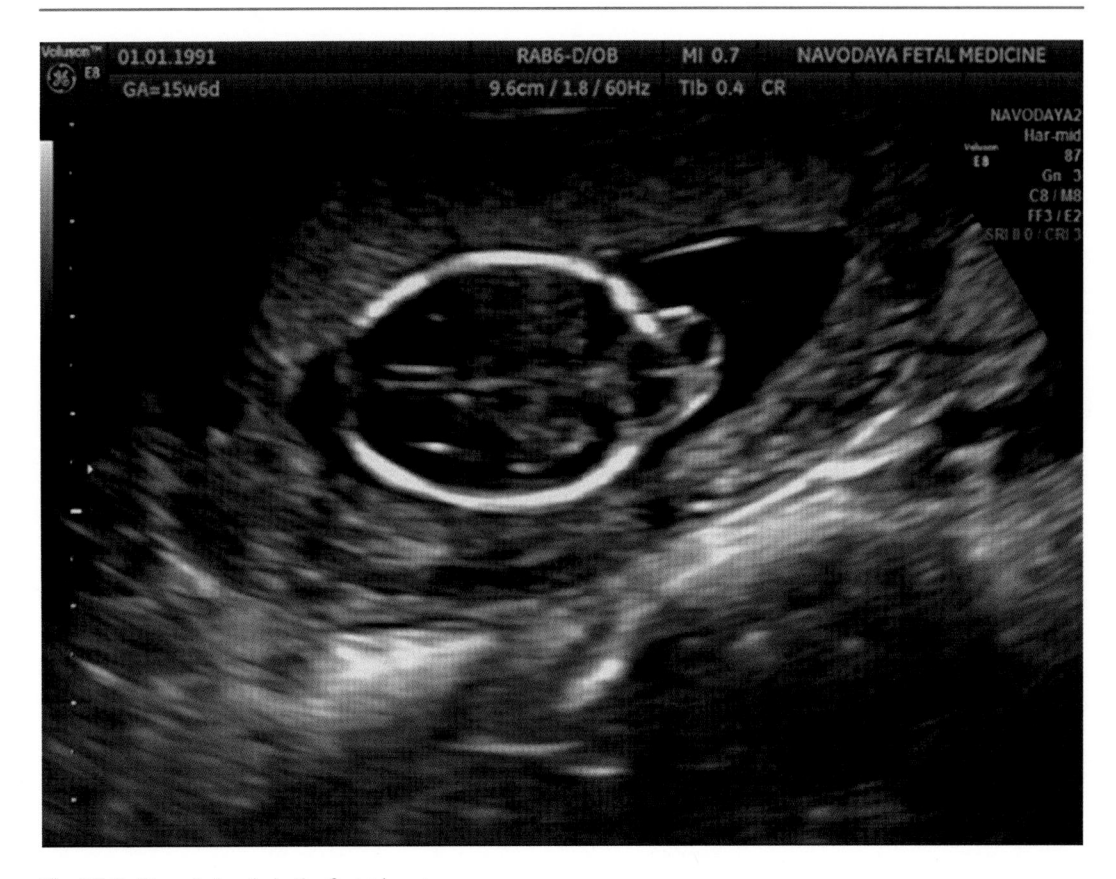

Fig. 10.8 Encephalocele in the first trimester

appropriate decisions in pregnancy at an early stage.

Neck The fetal neck is evaluated in the midsagittal section in the first trimester of pregnancy. The presence of any neck swelling or masses is noted. The "nuchal translucency" or "NT" is the collection of fluid posteriorly under the skin of the fetal neck in the first trimester and is an important feature to be evaluated at the 11–14 weeks' scan as a marker for fetal aneuploidies and structural anomalies.

A normal appearance of the fetal neck region is very reassuring not only in terms of structural assessment but also as a factor reducing the risk for fetal aneuploidies if the measurement is taken according to a standard protocol as suggested by the Fetal Medicine Foundation, UK, and if that measurement is then applied to the first trimester risk assessment protocol (Fig. 10.9).

In contrast, abnormal appearance of the fetal neck which can range from mild increase in the "nuchal translucency" to appearance of large cystic dilatations and even swelling enveloping the entire fetus are features which increase the risk of structural and chromosomal abnormalities in the fetus. The different manifestations of abnormal appearance of the fetal neck in the first trimester is shown in Fig. 10.10a–i.

Thorax The fetal thorax is evaluated in the axial section in the first trimester (Fig. 10.11), and it usually shows the fetal heart occupying the mediastinum and roughly one-third of the total area of the thoracic section flanked by two equal appearing

88　　10　The "First Trimester (11–14 Weeks) Scan"

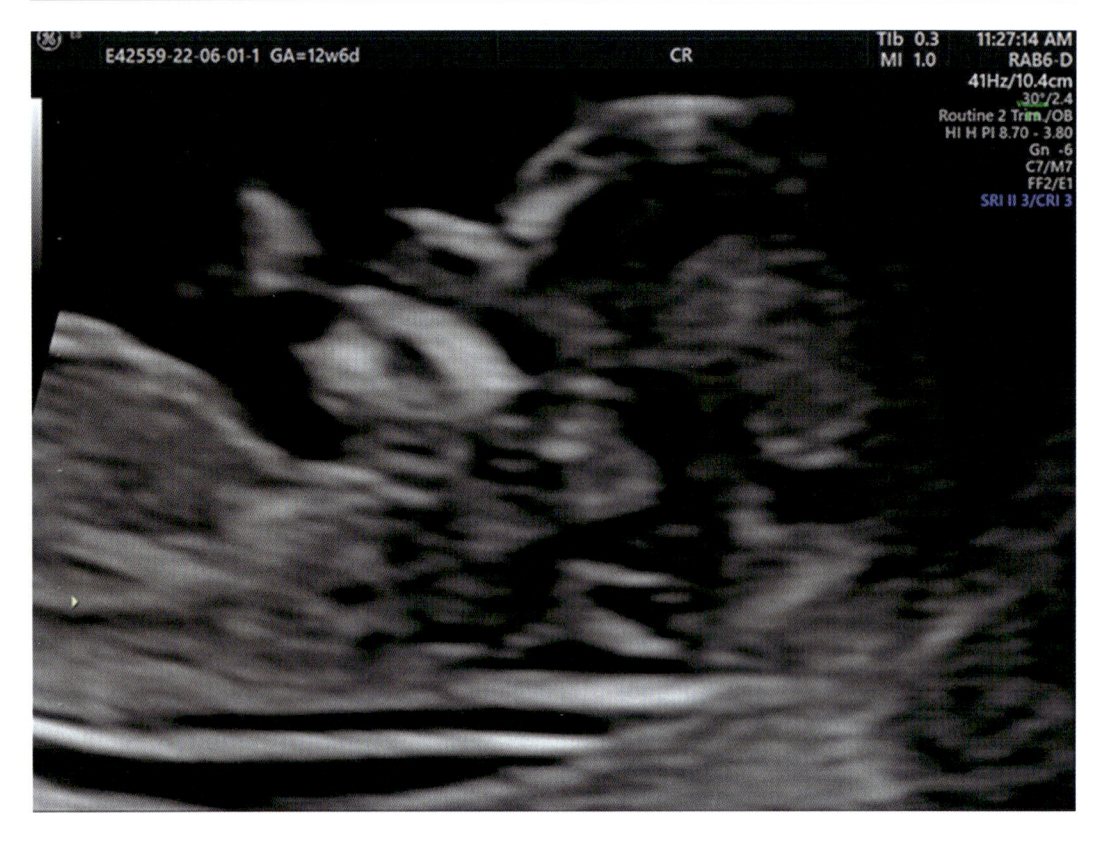

Fig. 10.9 Normal appearance of fetal neck in the first trimester

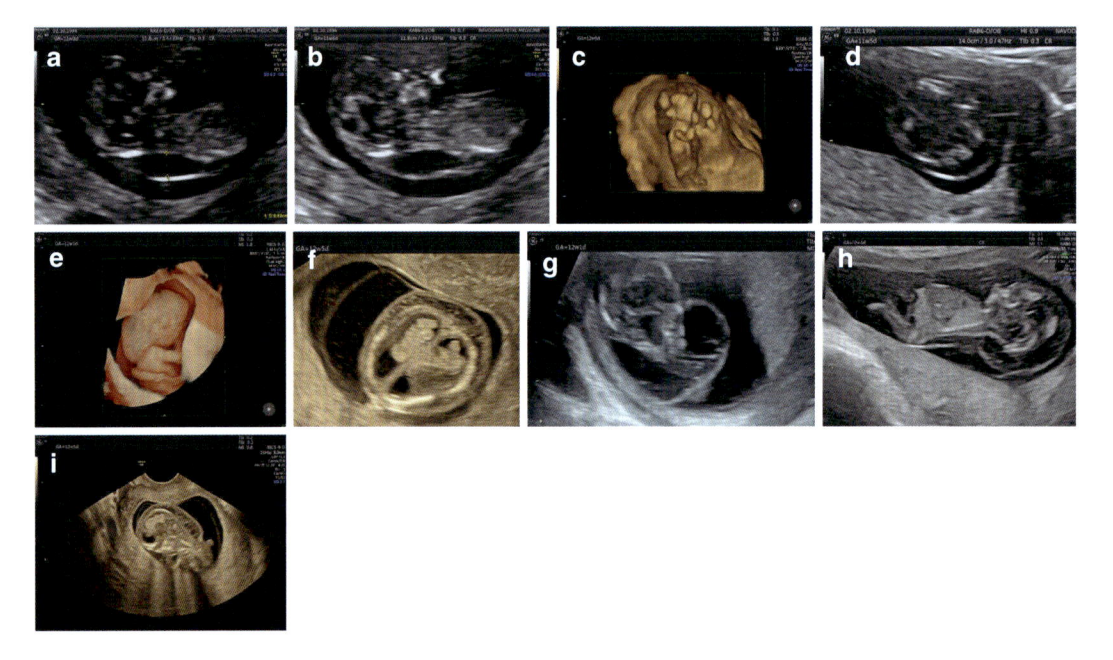

Fig. 10.10 (a–i) Increased NT or cystic hygroma in first trimester

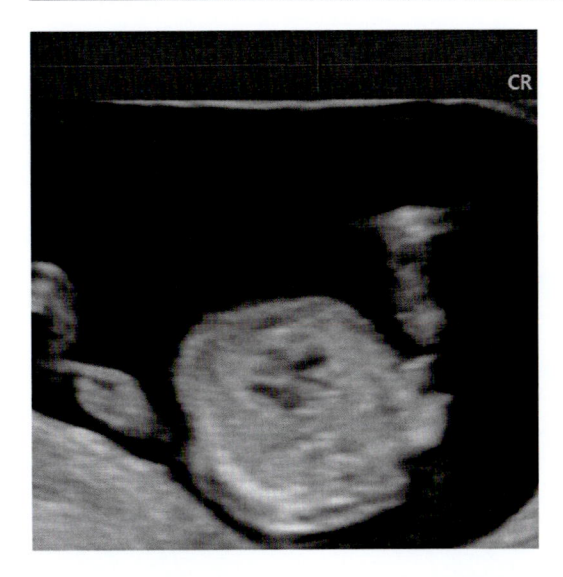

10.2 Detailed Fetal Structural Assessment at the 11–14 Weeks' Scan

Fig. 10.11 Normal appearance of normal fetal thorax in the first trimester

lungs on either side. Presence of any lung masses or pleural effusion is noted as signs of abnormalities (Fig. 10.12) that warrant further workup.

Heart The first trimester is a good window for a preliminary evaluation of the fetal heart. With the advent of high-resolution machines and better understanding of the anatomy of the fetal heart, the possibilities of detailed imaging of the fetal heart in the first trimester are increasing by leaps and bounds such that first trimester fetal echocardiography is a definite reality in specialized fetal medicine units. However, in general fetal medicine practice, at least a four-chamber view of the fetal heart along with a basic outflow tract evaluation would suffice for a good practice protocol that is practical, efficient, and easily reproducible with reasonable skill sets.

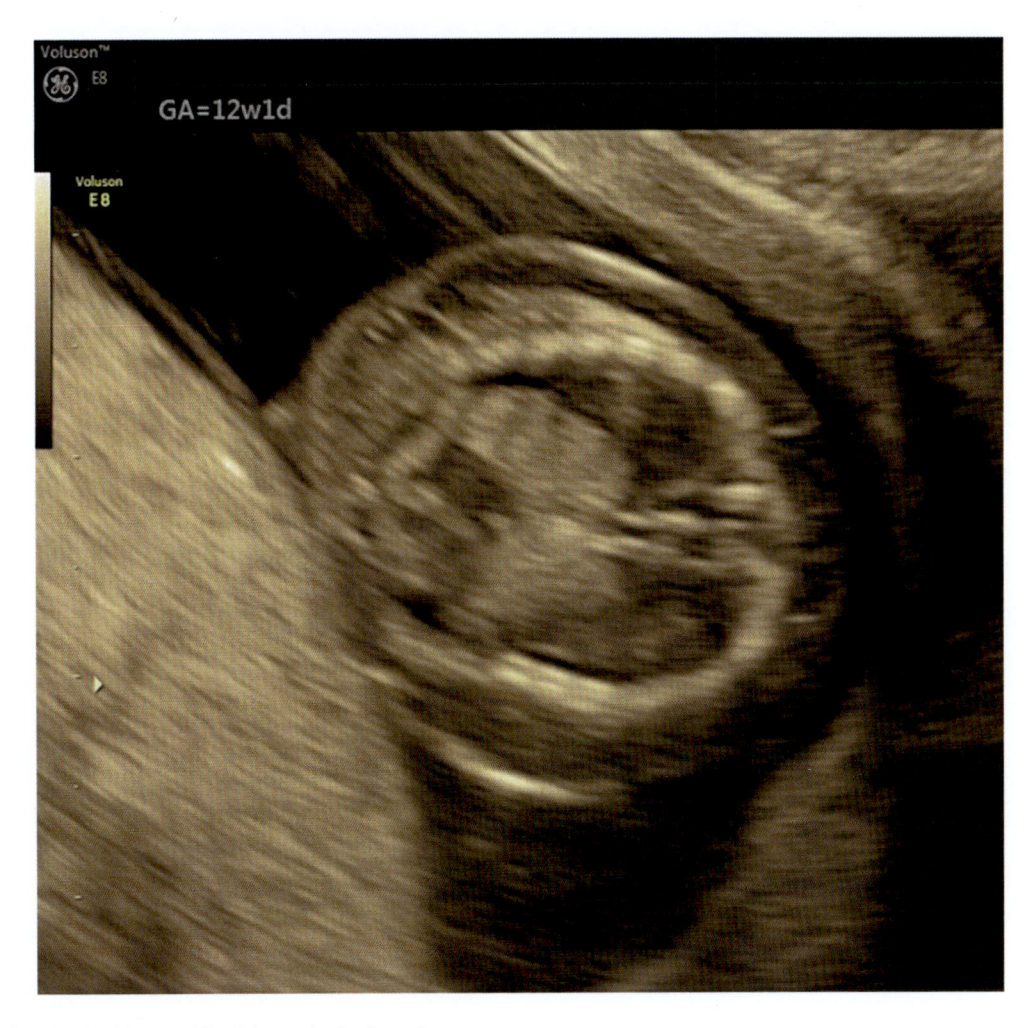

Fig. 10.12 Abnormal fetal thorax in the first trimester

Application of color flow to generate the "X" sign to represent the normal crossover of outflow tracts and the "Y" sign for the normal three-vessel trachea view further enhances the detection rate for major cardiac anomalies in the first trimester. Normal appearances of the fetal heart in the first trimester are seen in Fig. 10.13a–b. Any deviation from the normal appearance such as disproportionate chambers or obvious outflow abnormalities can be picked up at this stage of pregnancy (Fig. 10.14a–d).

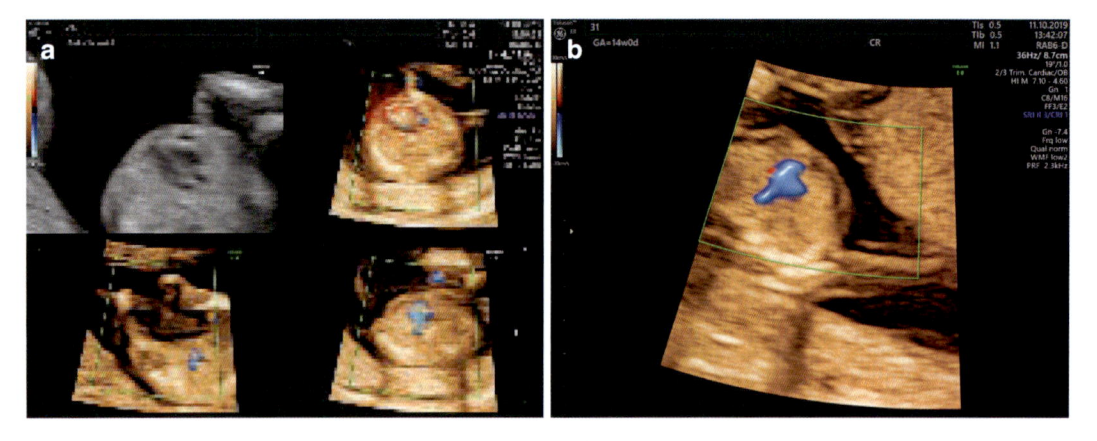

Fig. 10.13 (a, b) Normal views of the fetal heart in the first trimester

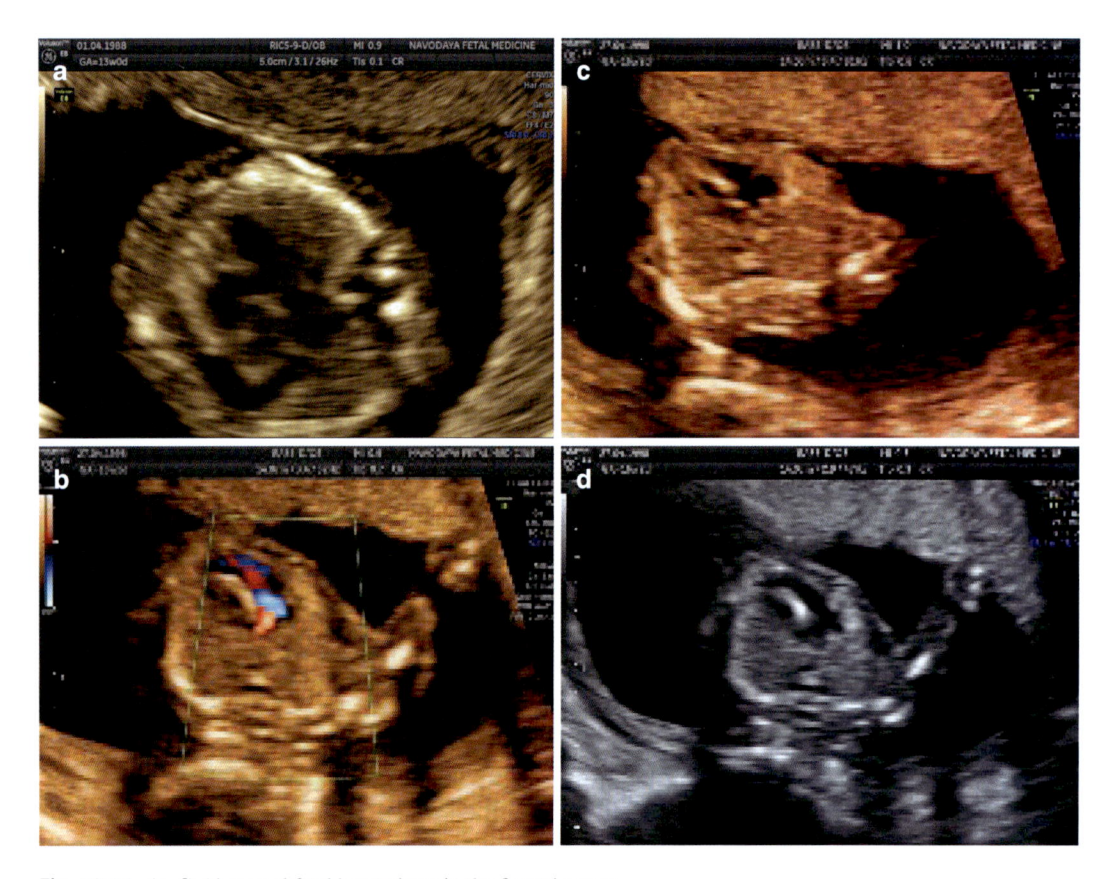

Fig. 10.14 (a–d) Abnormal fetal heart views in the first trimester

10.2 Detailed Fetal Structural Assessment at the 11–14 Weeks' Scan

Abdomen The evaluation of the fetal abdomen includes an upper abdomen axial view at the level of the stomach to demonstrate a normal-sized fetal stomach bubble which essentially indicates a patent upper GI tract such that amniotic fluid is being swallowed by the fetus and reaches the stomach to create the appearance of a "bubble" on ultrasound. A very small or persistently absent stomach bubble in the first trimester scan indicates the possibility of an upper GI tract obstruction or a poor swallowing effort by the fetus due to neuromuscular problems. It may be noted here that sometimes an absent stomach bubble may be a transient finding and hence it should be evaluated repeatedly over a period of time to establish definite, persistence absence of the same before labeling it in the diagnosis (Fig. 10.15).

Another plane to evaluate the fetal abdomen is at the level of the umbilical cord insertion to show a normal anterior abdominal wall contour at this site and thus rule out any anterior abdominal wall defects like exomphalos or gastroschisis (Fig. 10.16).

The physiological exomphalos of early pregnancy is expected to have regressed by 11 weeks of gestation, and hence if the anterior abdominal wall defect is seen after the completion of 12 weeks, it is definitely pathological. These defects may be associated with other defects or fetal aneuploidies, and thus appropriate testing and modification of care can be planned after this condition is diagnosed early in pregnancy (Fig. 10.17).

In the lower abdomen, another hypoechoic area representing the fetal urinary bladder is also noted in the first trimester. In case of doubt, demonstration of the umbilical arteries flanking this cystic area is confirmation of this being the fetal urinary bladder. The direct visualization of the fetal kidneys is possible around 12–13 weeks but may not be very clear in earlier first trimester

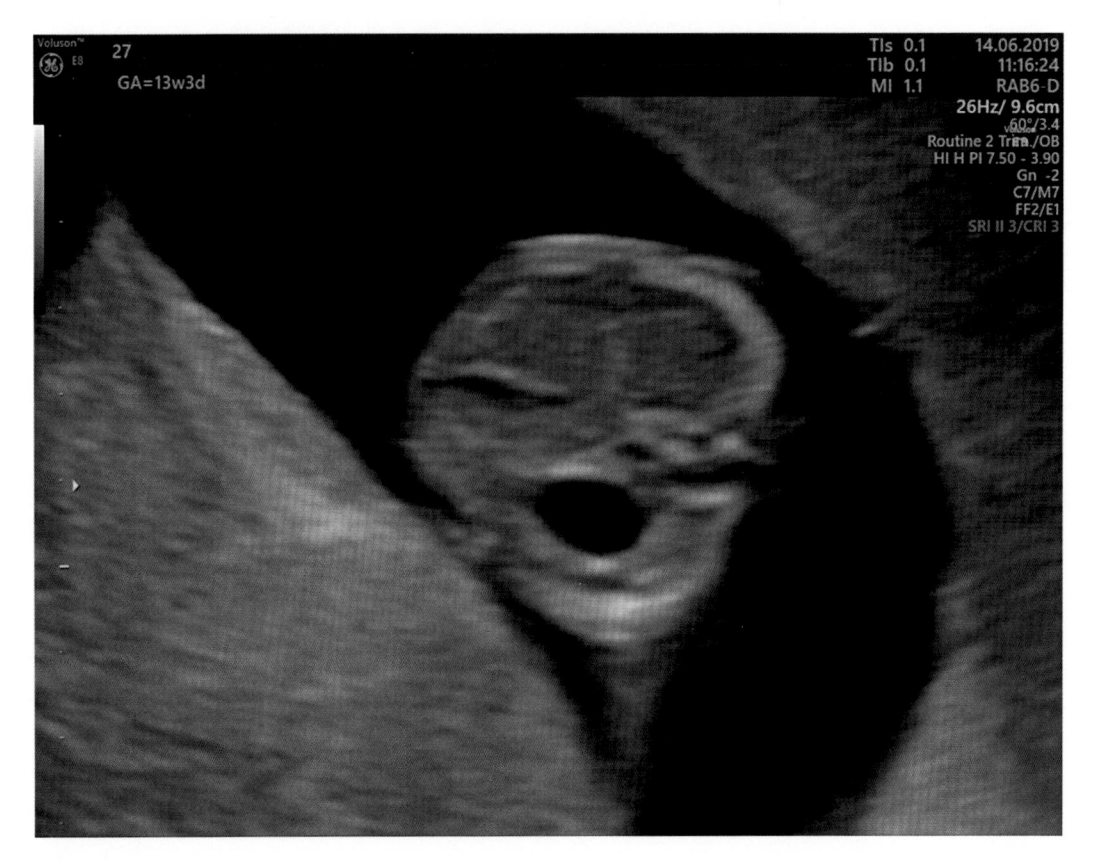

Fig. 10.15 Fetal stomach bubble in the first trimester

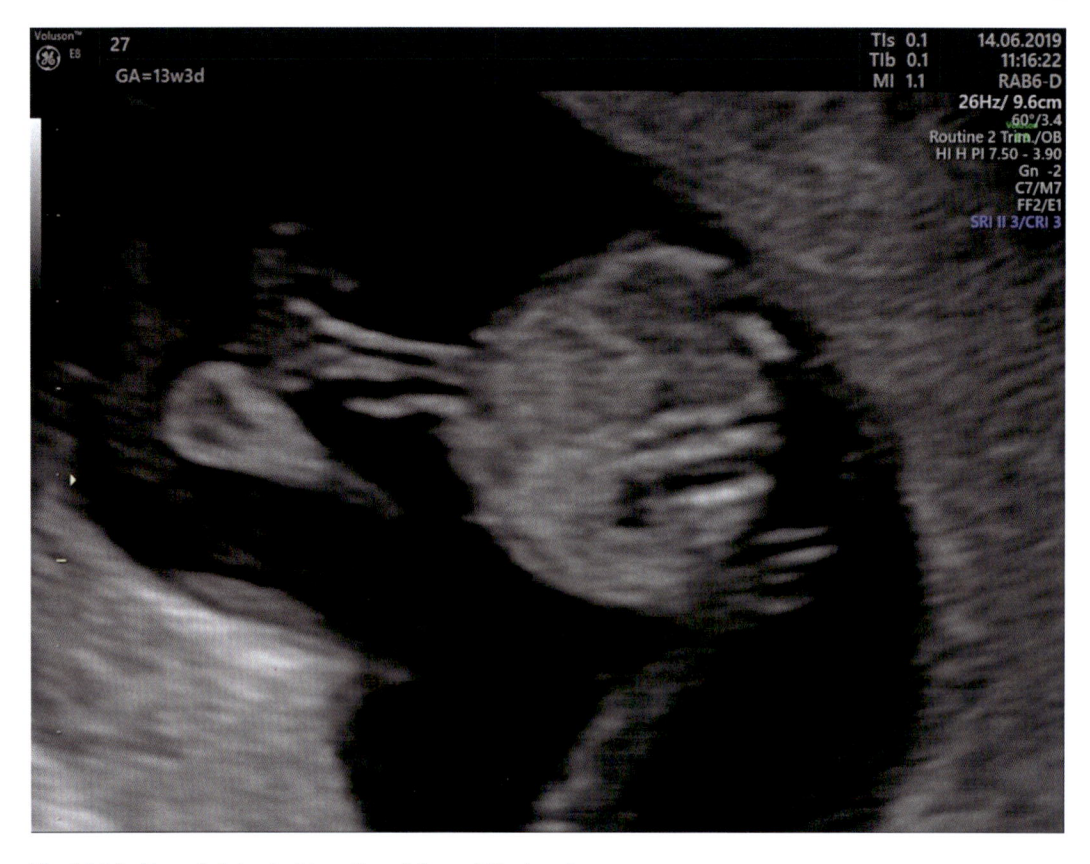

Fig. 10.16 Normal abdominal insertion of the umbilical cord

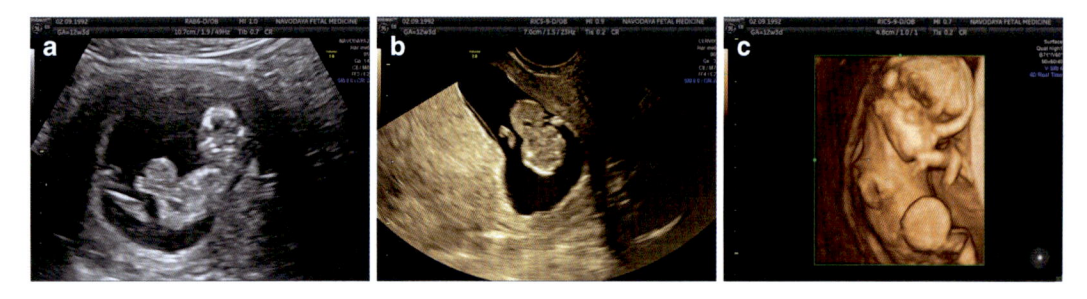

Fig. 10.17 (a–c) Exomphalos seen at the 11–14 weeks' scan

scans. Presence of a normal-sized fetal urinary bladder is an indirect indicator of functioning fetal kidneys which are producing urine that is filling the bladder (Fig. 10.18a–b).

The longitudinal diameter of the fetal urinary bladder is less than 7 mm in the first trimester, and when it exceeds 7 mm, it is labeled as "megacystis" (Fig. 10.19a, b). Megacystis below 14 mm is a marker for fetal aneuploidies, while more than 14 mm is more likely to be caused by bladder outflow obstruction.

Persistent nonvisualization of the fetal bladder in the first trimester scan may be indicative of bilateral renal agenesis or nonfunctioning kidneys. The liquor amnii in the first trimester is also produced by the placenta and fetal membranes so

10.2 Detailed Fetal Structural Assessment at the 11–14 Weeks' Scan

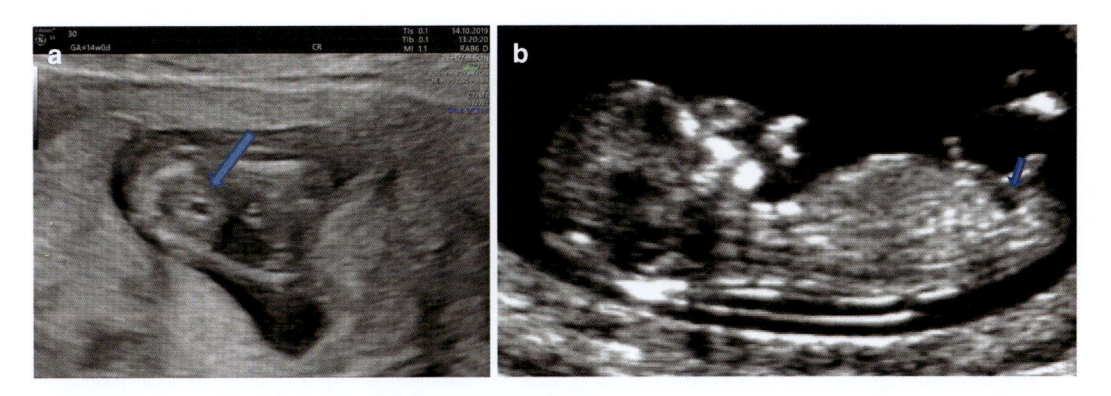

Fig. 10.18 (a–c) Normal fetal urinary bladder in the first trimester

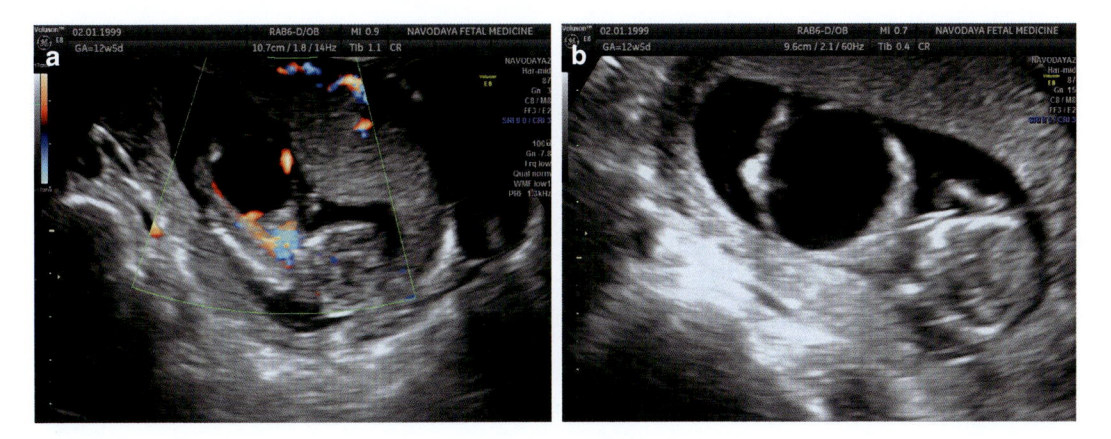

Fig. 10.19 (a, b) Megacystis in the first trimester

it is not a good indicator of renal function. In cases where the fetal bladder is not seen in the first trimester scans, it is useful to recall the mother at 16 weeks for a detailed reassessment of fetal kidneys.

Limbs The first trimester scan provides an optimal opportunity to evaluate the fetal limbs—all three segments of all four limbs can be clearly demonstrated at this stage. Simultaneous visualization of both upper limbs and both lower limbs is possible in the first trimester scan so this is actually a better time to detect major anomalies of the fetal limbs like agenesis or hypoplasia of limb segments. Both upper limbs are seen arising from the fetal trunk in the axial section of the body, and all the three segments—arms, forearms, and hands—are well visualized as shown in Fig. 10.20.

Both fetal lower limbs are also similarly seen (Fig. 10.21a–d), and it is a good practice to document an image of both legs simultaneously in the report. Such documentation is very reassuring and helps establish the presence of limbs at this stage of fetal evaluation in cases of rare evolving anomalies arising due to transverse limb amputation by amniotic bands, etc.

Spine The fetal spine is evaluated in the sagittal or coronal section (Fig. 10.22a, b) in the first trimester where a normal contour along with a complete overlying skin cover is highly reassuring.

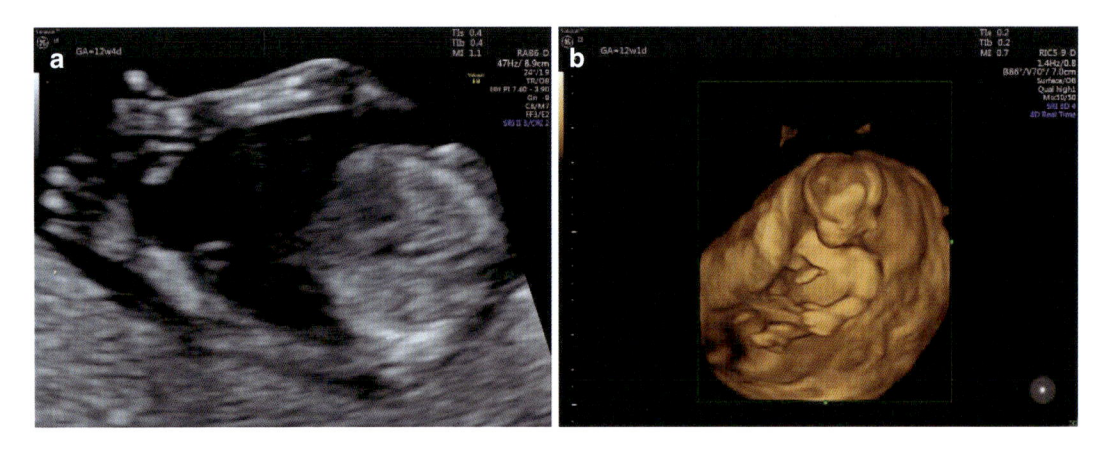

Fig. 10.20 Normal upper limbs in the first trimester

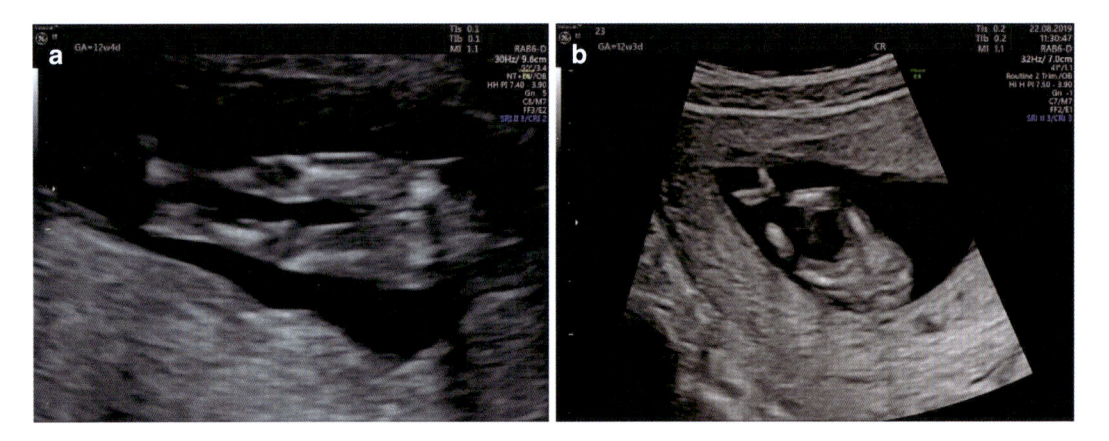

Fig. 10.21 (a, b) Normal lower limbs in the first trimester

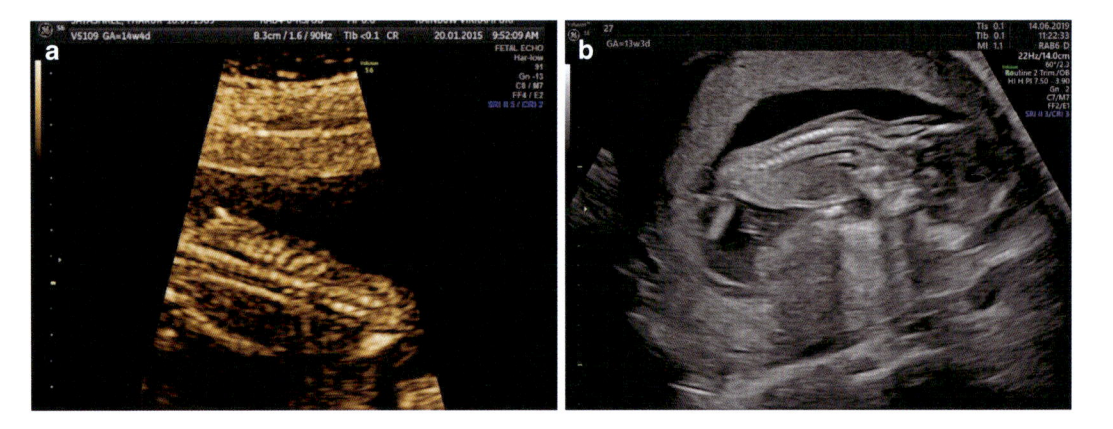

Fig. 10.22 (a, b) Normal fetal spine in the first trimester

Abnormal contours with major bends along the longitudinal axes may represent kyphoscoliosis or even open spina bifida (Fig. 10.23a–c). The abnormalities in spinal contour that present very obviously even in the first trimester are likely to have significant clinical impact on the fetal well-being, and such early diagnosis allows to explain the prognosis to the parents and get relevant workup done.

Open spina bifida may or may not be directly seen in the first trimester, but there is a screening

10.3 Screening for Spina Bifida by IT (Intracranial Translucency)

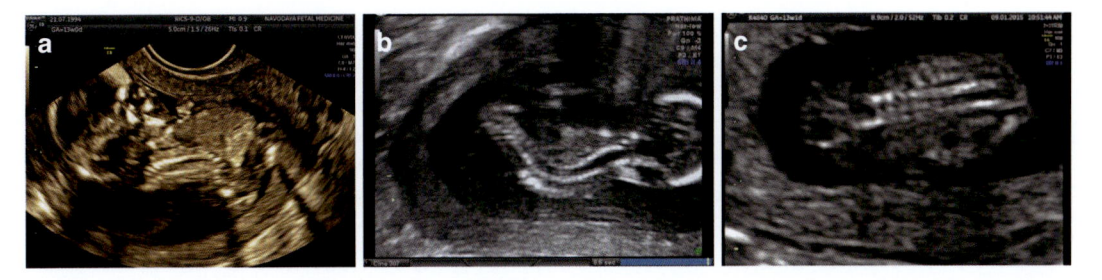

Fig. 10.23 (a–c) Abnormal fetal spine in the first trimester

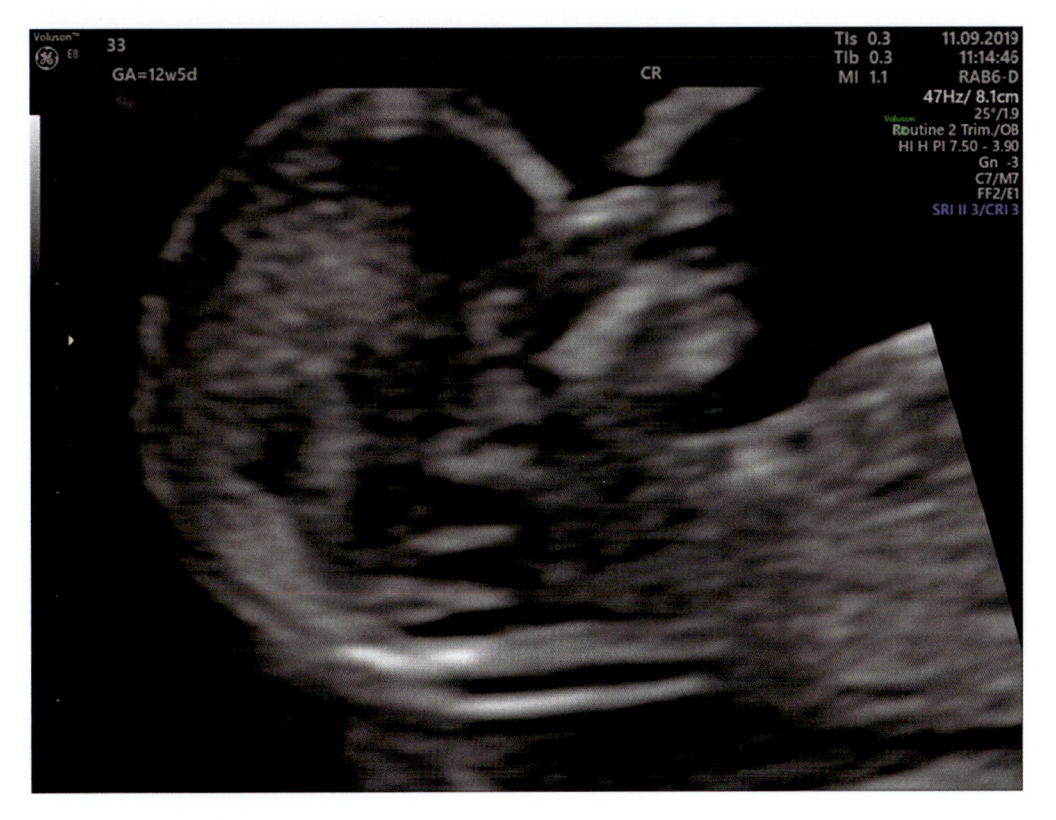

Fig. 10.24 Intracranial translucency

marker for these abnormalities called intracranial translucency or "IT" which has emerged as a useful marker in triaging fetuses who need recall for an early anatomy assessment at 16 weeks.

10.3 Screening for Spina Bifida by IT (Intracranial Translucency)

The "intracranial translucency" (IT) actually represents the appearance of the fourth ventricle in a midsagittal view of the fetal head and neck in the first trimester of pregnancy. In the same section that is used to evaluate the fetal NT, the fetal brain stem, fourth ventricle, and the cisterna magna are seen as almost parallel spaces. The IT appears as a hypoechoic area and represents the fourth ventricle of the fetal brain at the 11–14 weeks of gestation. A normal appearing IT (Fig. 10.24) is reassuring, while a collapsed IT represents compression of the fourth ventricle due to caudal displacement of the brain stem in open neural tube defects. The actual defect may not be big enough to be clearly seen on the first trimester scan, but an abnormal IT raises the index of suspicion for such problems and facilitates an earlier detection with better follow-up.

10.4 Markers for Fetal Aneuploidy Screening in the 11–14 Weeks' Scan

The 11–14 weeks' scan is a landmark for screening for fetal aneuploidies. The various markers assessed at this scan with the background of maternal age can provide a screening test for trisomy 21 with a sensitivity of up to 85–90% for a false-positive rate of less than 5%.

The details of fetal aneuploidy screening and risk assessment protocol issues are given in Chap. 4 ("Principles of Screening for Fetal Aneuploidies"). In this chapter, we will emphasize upon the correct imaging for these markers during the conduct of the first trimester scan.

10.4.1 Fetal NT

As per the guidelines given in by the Fetal Medicine Foundation (FMF UK), it is expected that the image would be magnified to an extent that the ultrasound screen is occupied almost entirely by the head and the neck of the fetus in "midsagittal" view. The attitude of the fetus should be such that the neck is aligned in line with the head. The fluid between the chin and the chest of the fetus indicates that the neck is not too flexed and it should not be too extended but rather in a "neutral position." The image should have adequate contrast which is attained by reducing the "gain" settings, and the sharp margins of the lines behind the neck should be seen. The fetal NT is then measured placing "plus-shaped" calipers in a manner that the horizontal line of the caliper merges with the inner borders of the area representing the nuchal fluid. If the gain settings are not optimal, this sharp margin will not be delineated and the measurement will be erroneous. The calipers have to be adjusted such that each movement changes the measurement by 0.1 mm.

For purposes of risk allocation for fetal aneuploidies, it is mandatory that fetal CRL is between 45 and 84 mm and the NT is measured according to the criteria defined by the FMF. Since the exact measurement of the NT is vital to get a correct risk assessment for fetal aneuploidies, it is imperative upon all operators to learn this technique perfectly. The Fetal Medicine Foundation website which has been referenced in the "suggested reading" section at the end of this chapter has clear description of the technique and a certification process for this scan.

This process has been one of the most successful self-learning strategies in which the operator can follow instructions and improvise his/her own images and once a satisfactory level of confidence is gained, one can send images for an online assessment by an FMF expert. This evaluation provides feedback regarding the quality of the images, and if the images are satisfactory, the operator is certified to conduct the NT measurement for risk assessment by the FMF UK. The process comes highly recommended for all operators who want to conduct a meaningful NT scan as this certification helps in standardizing image procurement and reduces interoperator variability (Fig. 10.25).

10.4.2 Fetal Nasal Bone

The fetal nasal bone can be assessed in the same view as the NT and the magnification, attitude, and gain criteria are similar as described above. To demarcate the nasal bone, it is useful to hold the scan probe in the direction of the nose, and with very fine lateral tilts, one can observe a second line parallel to the skin of the nose. This parallel line arrangement, also called the "equal" sign, has the skin as the upper line and the lower line representing the nasal bone, seen normally brighter than the skin as seen in Fig. 10.26.

If the lower line is not seen or is not brighter than the skin, then the nasal bone is deemed as absent or hypoplastic, respectively. It has been clearly stated in literature that for purposes of risk calculation, "absent" or "hypoplastic" nasal bone is deemed as a common entity.

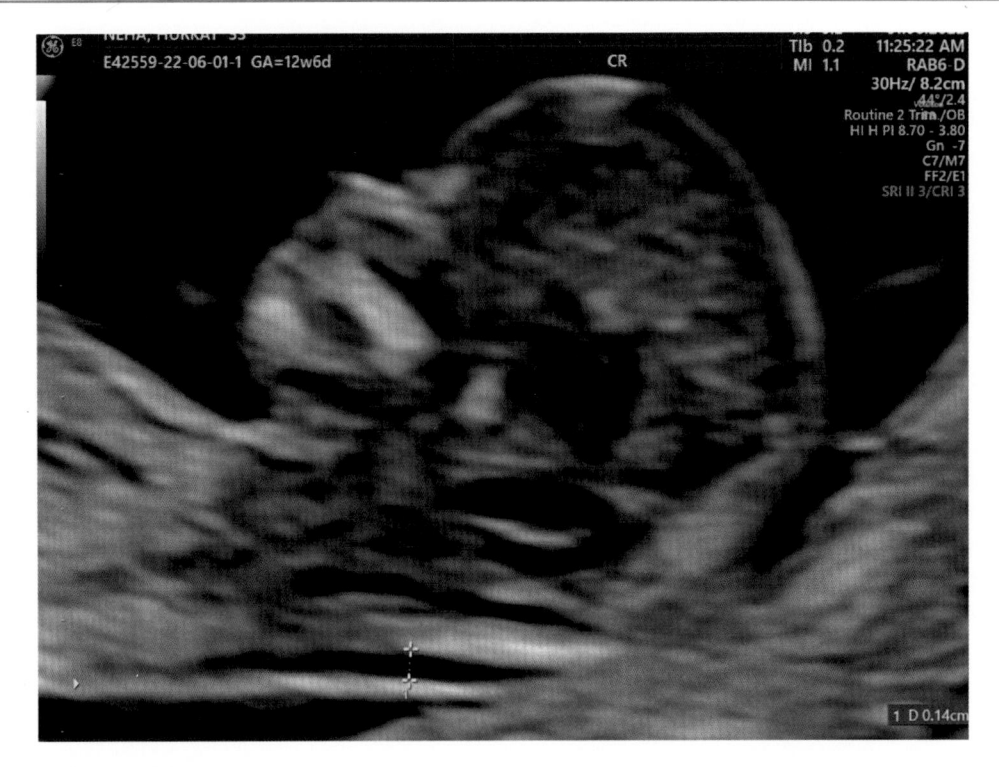

10.4 Markers for Fetal Aneuploidy Screening in the 11–14 Weeks' Scan

Fig. 10.25 Fetal NT

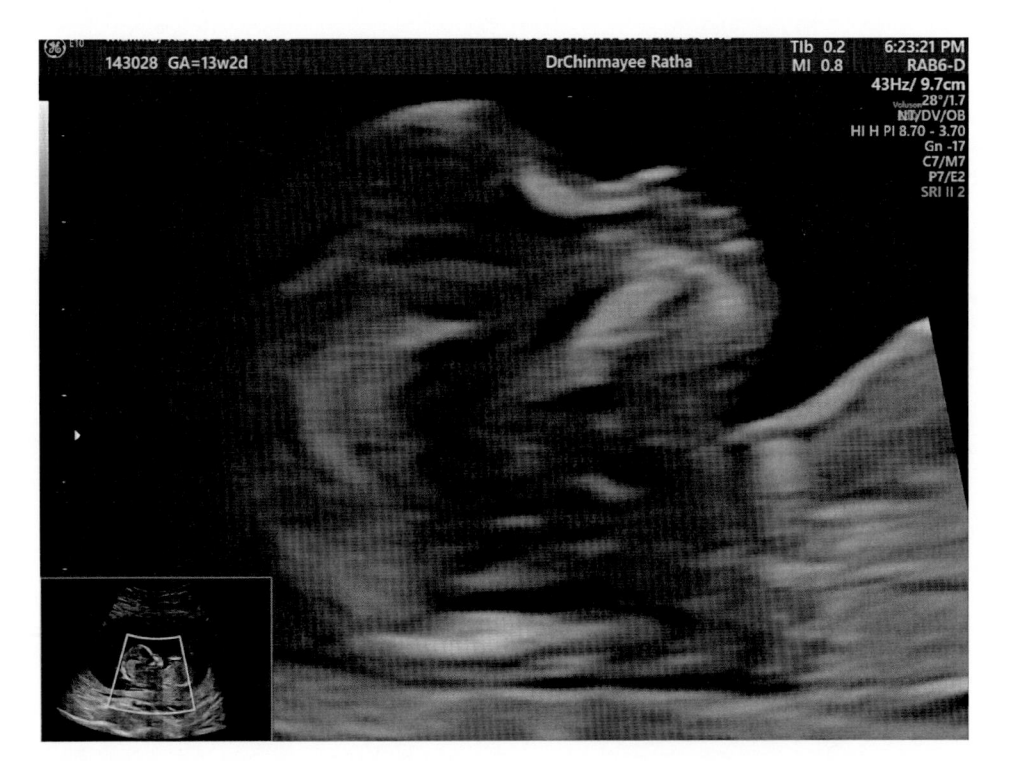

Fig. 10.26 Fetal NB

10.4.3 Tricuspid Blood Flow

The blood flow across the tricuspid valve is expected to be unidirectional and a normal flow pattern is seen in Fig. 10.27.

The presence of tricuspid regurgitation is considered as a minor marker for fetal aneuploidies and is also associated with a higher risk of fetal cardiac anomalies.

The correct method of evaluation of tricuspid blood flow according to the FMF criteria is on the axial section of the fetal thorax with the apical four-chamber cardiac view occupying 75–80% of the screen. The pulse wave Doppler with a gate size of 2–3 mm is placed across the tricuspid valve with the angle aligned ideally along the direction of blood flow but never more than 30° away. The sweep speed is adjusted to 2–3 cm/s and flow pattern is noted. During ventricular systole, no backflow is expected but sometimes there may be small physiological jets. In case the regurgitant jet speed is 60 cm/s or more and if this jet occupies more than half of systole, then it is considered as tricuspid regurgitation as seen in Fig. 10.28.

10.4.4 Ductus Venosus Blood Flow

The fetal ductus venosus (DV) is a continuation of the umbilical vein and forms a narrow conduit before joining the IVC. Due to the narrow caliber, the blood flow through the DV shows "aliasing" upon application of color Doppler and is thus identified. It is better to measure the DV blood flow when the fetus is not moving and with a smaller sample gate of 0.5–1 mm in size owing to the small size of this vessel (Fig. 10.29).

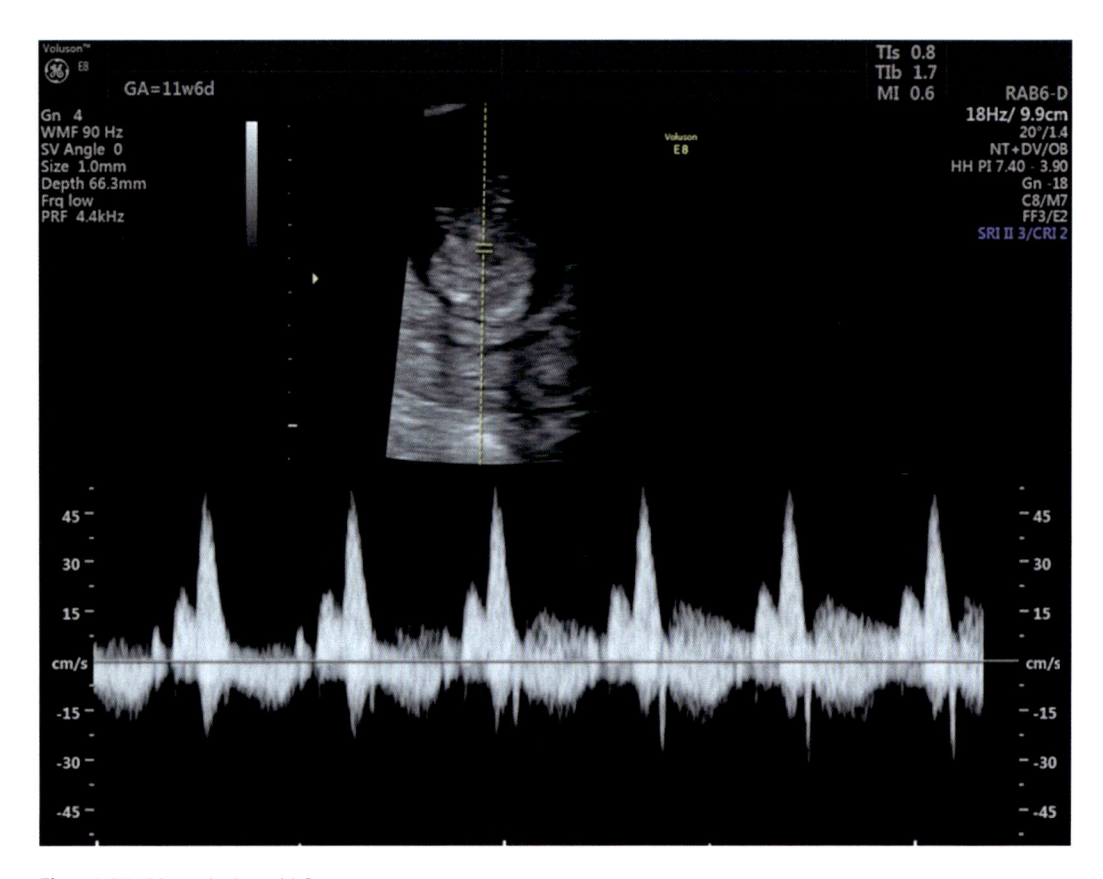

Fig. 10.27 Normal tricuspid flow

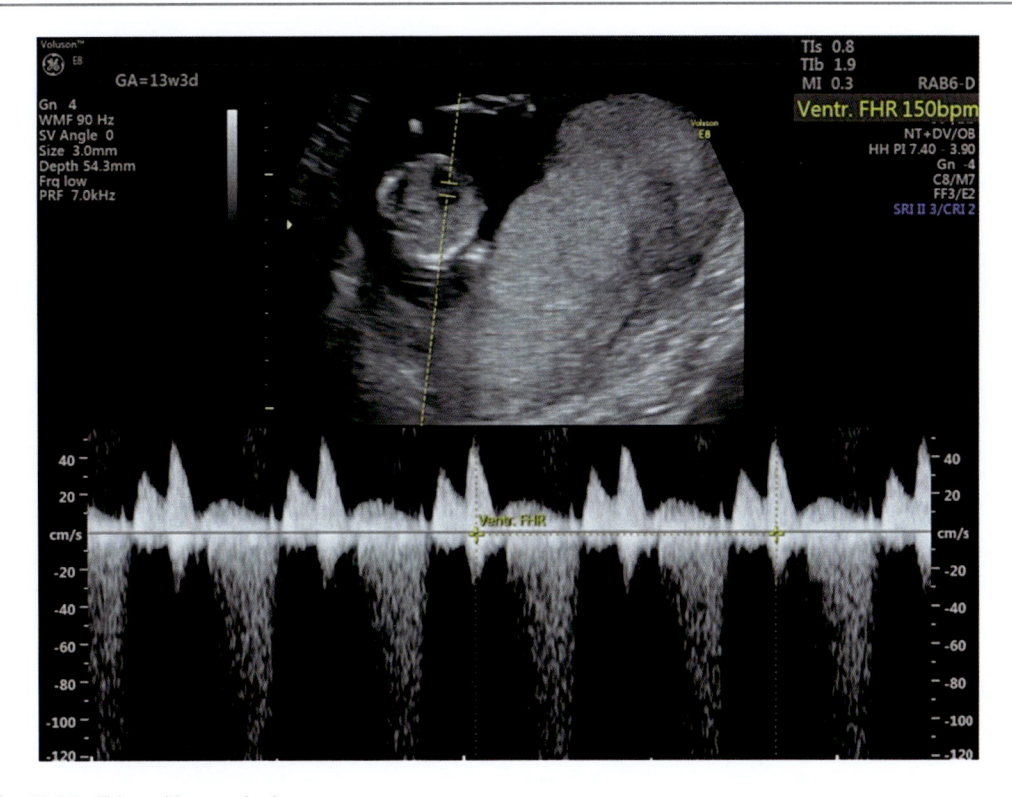

10.4 Markers for Fetal Aneuploidy Screening in the 11–14 Weeks' Scan

Fig. 10.28 Tricuspid regurgitation

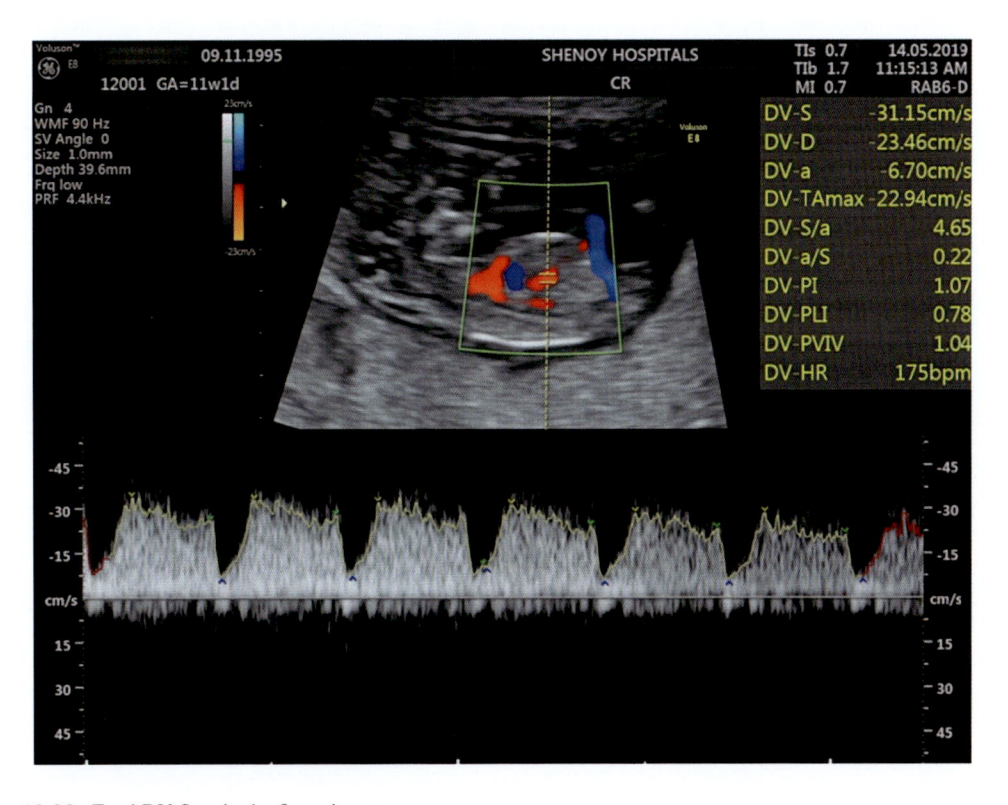

Fig. 10.29 Fetal DV flow in the first trimester

The fetal DV can be identified in the midsagittal section of the fetal abdomen with color Doppler as a small area of aliasing between the umbilical vein and IVC. A low-frequency wall motion filter (50–70 Hz) helps in getting the triphasic wave of this vessel which is affected by the right atrial activity.

The DV pulsatility index is used as a parameter for risk calculation in the scan-based fetal aneuploidy risk assessment protocol. Abnormal DV flow indices are associated with higher risk of aneuploidies, fetal cardiac anomalies, and even risk of fetal demise.

10.5 Basic Workup of Multifetal Pregnancy at the 11–14-Week Scan

The most important aspect of multifetal pregnancy assessment in the first trimester remains the assessment of number of fetuses and establishment of chorionicity unequivocally. If both placentae in twins are seen distinctly separate, then the assignment of "dichorionicity" is easy. However, if the placentae are close by, the "lambda" sign (Fig. 10.30a, b) denotes dichorionicity, while the "T" sign represents monochorionicity (Fig. 10.31). Individual fetal evaluation will be similar to that in singletons, and specific protocols for multiple pregnancy evaluation in general are described in Chap. 11 ("Multiple Pregnancy Evaluation").

In cases of triplets, the "Benz" sign denotes triamnionicity (Fig. 10.32). Chorionicity will be determined by assessment of the "lambda sign" or "T sign" at the interface of the different placentae. Triamniotic triplets can therefore be trichorionic, dichorionic, or monochorionic.

Chorionicity is the most important prognostic factor for multifetal pregnancy and this is optimally achieved at the 11–14 weeks' scan. Not allocating chorionicity in a first trimester scan for multiple pregnancy should be considered a suboptimal evaluation.

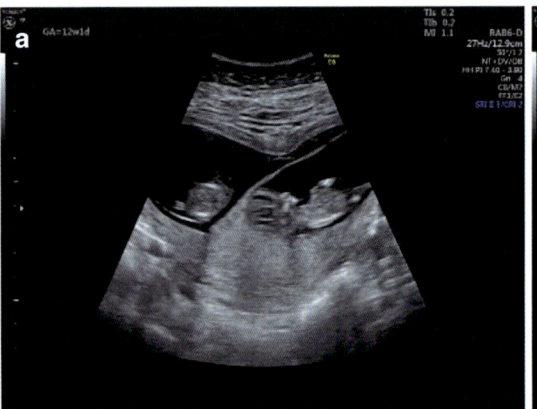

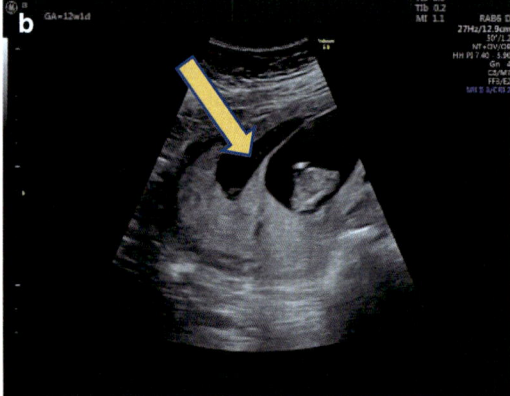

Fig. 10.30 (a, b) Dichorionic twins—lambda sign

10.5 Basic Workup of Multifetal Pregnancy at the 11–14-Week Scan

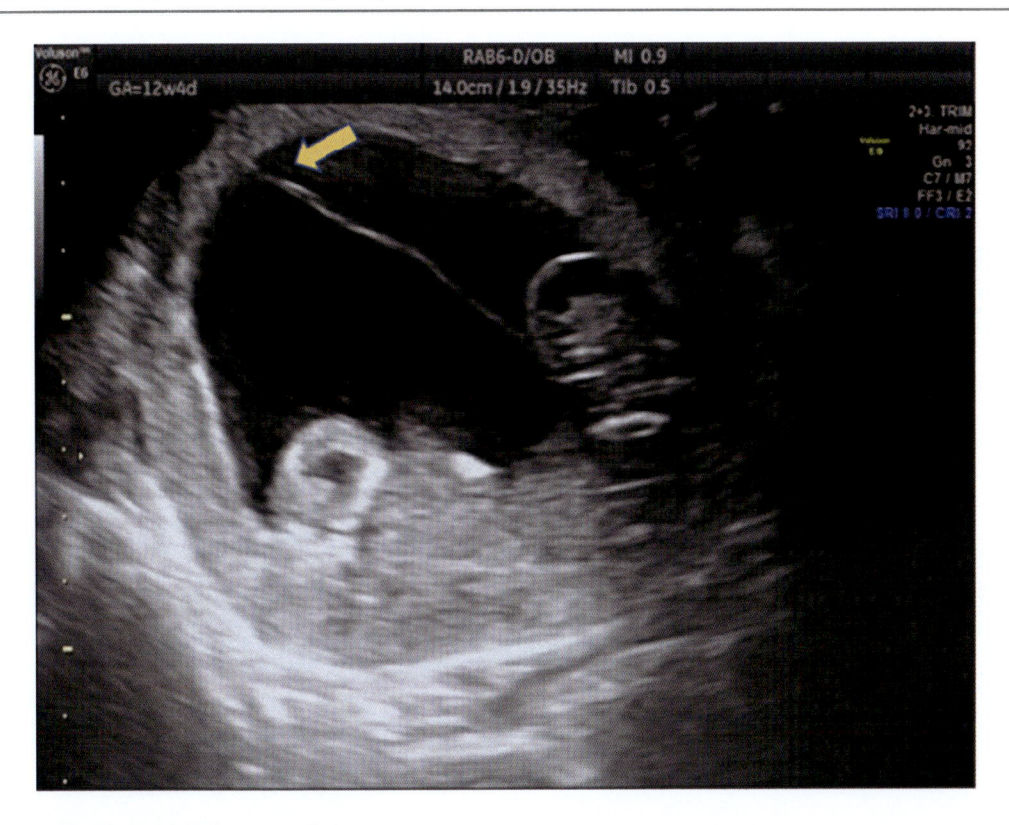

Fig. 10.31 Monochorionic twins—T sign

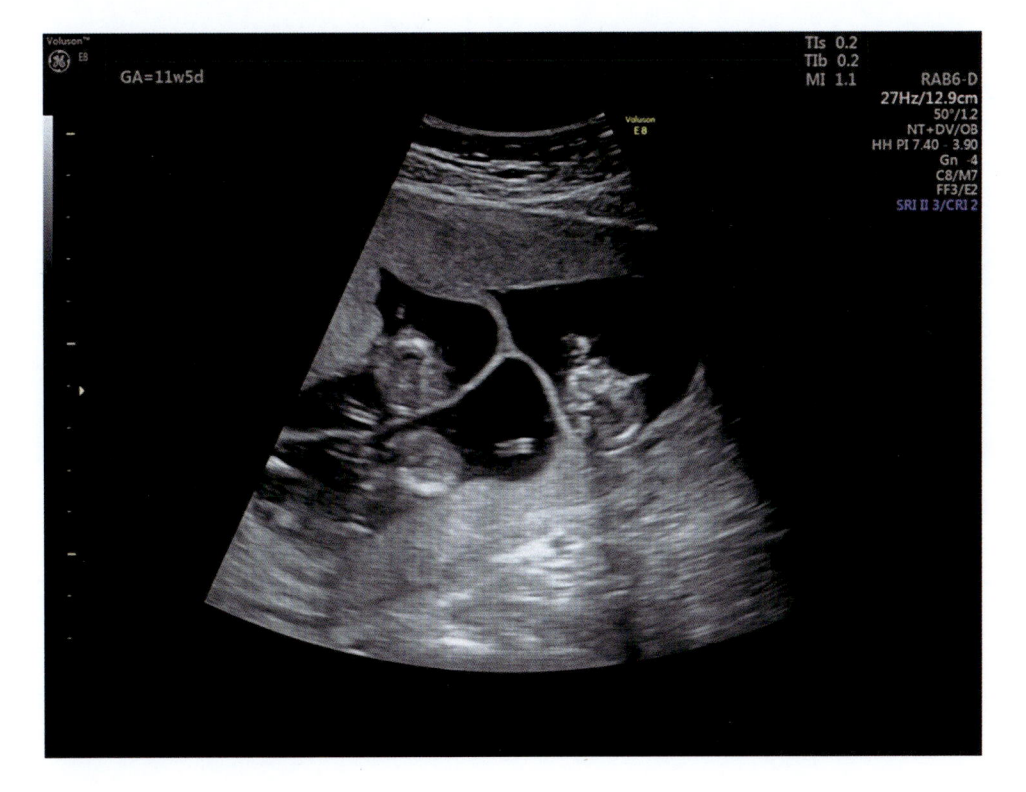

Fig. 10.32 Triamniotic triplets in the first trimester

10.6 Evaluation of Uterine Artery Doppler in First Trimester Scan

The uterine artery Doppler flow is an important parameter representing uteroplacental resistance and thus has become an effective marker for screening for risk of conditions related to uteroplacental insufficiency like maternal preeclampsia and fetal growth restriction. The evaluation of uterine artery Doppler flows in the first trimester is done by obtaining a sagittal section of the uterine cavity and then moving the probe slightly lateral at the level of the internal cervical os. The uterine artery is identified by color Doppler at this level and is interrogated with pulse wave Doppler using a sample gate of 2 mm and an angle of insonation less than 30°. The systolic peak velocity more than 60 cm/s confirms that the vessel is the uterine artery as shown in Fig. 10.33. This process is repeated on both (left and right) sides and the pulsatility indices of both uterine arteries are measured. The mean PI is used to calculate the risk of preeclampsia in the first trimester along with other biochemical and biophysical parameters.

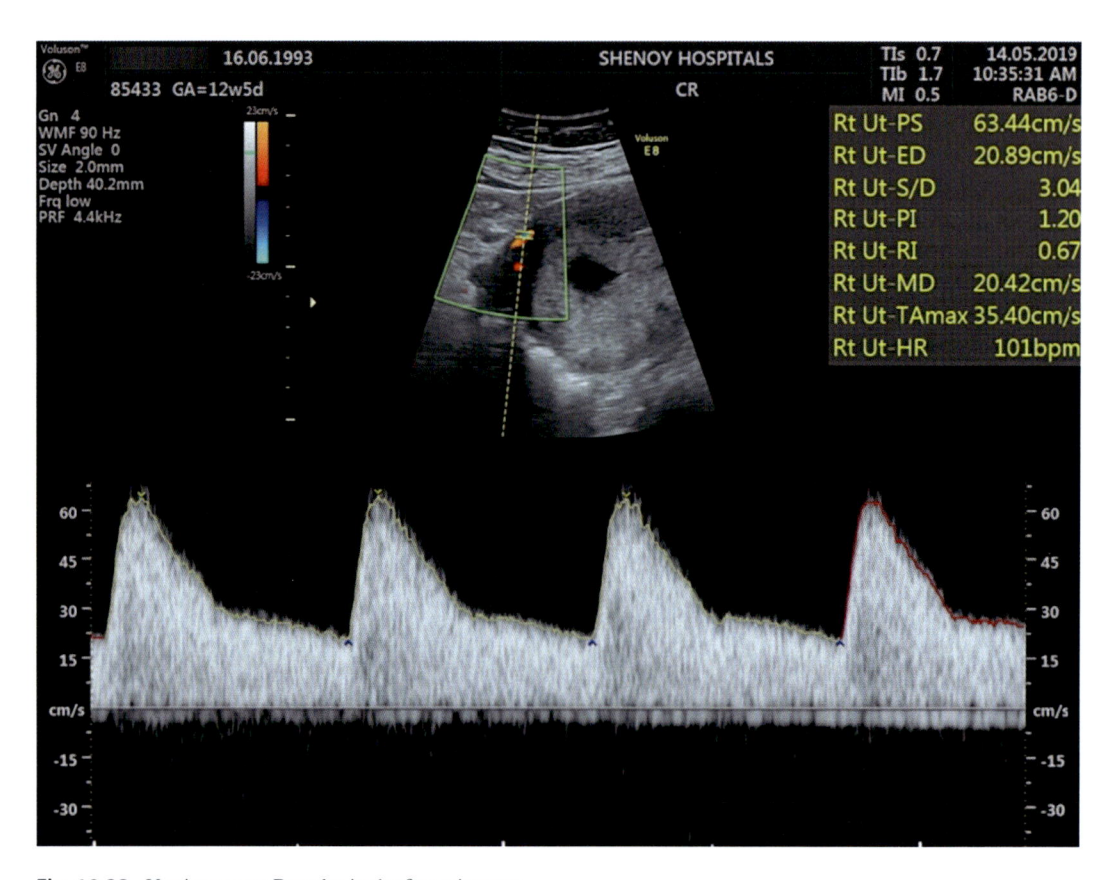

Fig. 10.33 Uterine artery Doppler in the first trimester

10.7 Evaluation of Maternal Cervix in First Trimester Scan

The evaluation of maternal cervix in the first trimester is ideally done transvaginally with an empty bladder. It is important to identify the internal and external os, cervical canal, and endocervical mucosa. The details of cervical length assessment are given in the chapter on cervical assessment in pregnancy (Chap. 12) (Fig. 10.34).

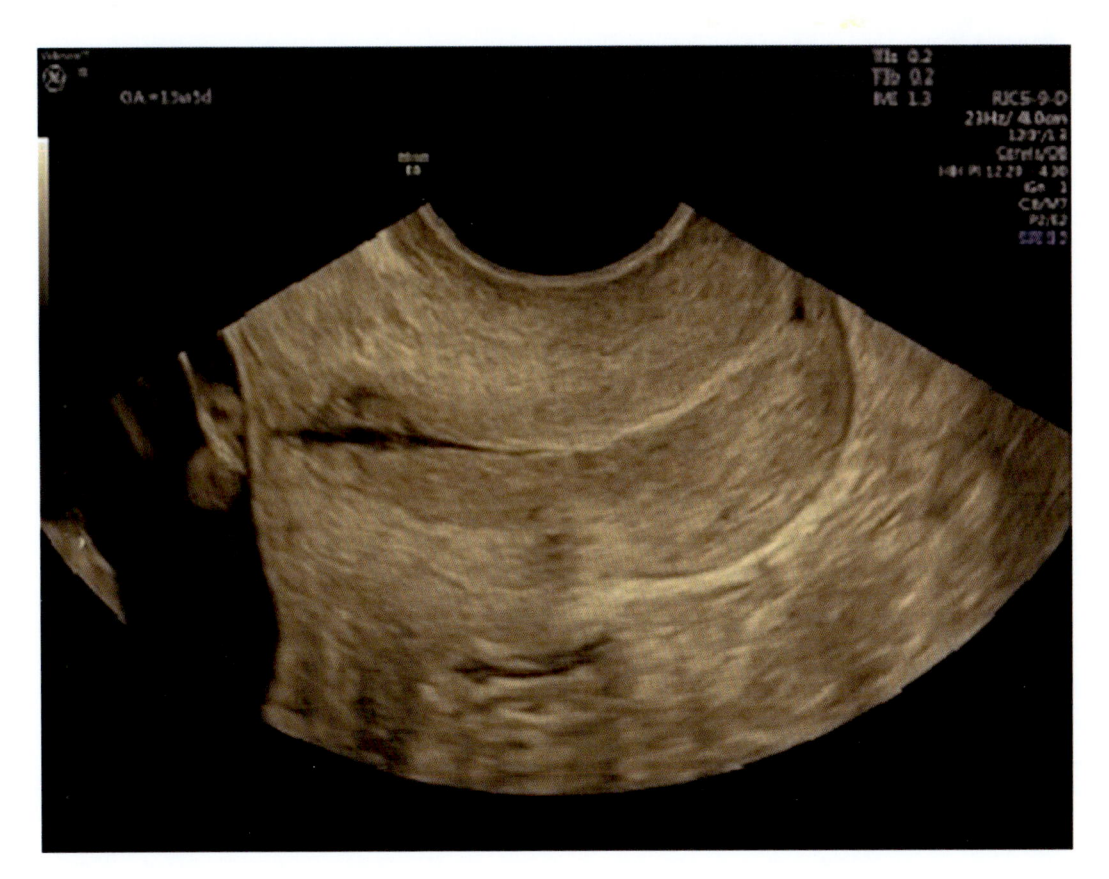

Fig. 10.34 Maternal cervix in the first trimester

Suggested Reading

First trimester scan guidelines on www.fetalmedicine.org.

Nicolaides KH. First-trimester screening for chromosomal abnormalities. Semin Perinatol. 2005;29:190–4.

Nicolaides KH. Turning the pyramid of prenatal care. Fetal Diagn Ther. 2011;29:183–9.

Nicolaides KH, et al. The 11-14 week scan. Baillieres Best Pract Res Clin Obstet Gynaecol. 2000;14:581–94.

Ratha C, Khurana A. "First things first": images for a proper nuchal translucency in the first trimester 11–13+6 weeks scan. J Fetal Med. 2014;1(2):1–3. https://doi.org/10.1007/s40556-014-0015-x.

Ratha C, Khurana A. "First things first": fetal nasal bone imaging in the first trimester 11–13+6 weeks scan. J Fetal Med. 2015;2(1). https://doi.org/10.1007/s40556-015-0034-2.

Multiple Pregnancy Evaluation in Fetal Medicine Clinic

11

Multiple pregnancy or multifetal pregnancy is a condition where there are more than one fetuses in the mother's womb at the same time. The most common type of multiple pregnancies is twin pregnancy and triplets, quadruplets, pentuplets, and so on are serially rarer to be seen. According to the classical "Hellin's rule," the incidence of twins was considered to be 1 in 89, and the incidence of other multifetal pregnancies appeared to be 1 in 89 raised to the power (n-1), where n is the number of fetuses in utero simultaneously. This was accepted for many years as long as nature was responsible for multifetal gestation due to wither multiple ovulation simultaneously or postzygotic splitting. In today's world, this law does not hold so good. The incidence of multifetal pregnancy has increased significantly in the last century primarily due to the advent of assisted reproductive techniques (ART) which rely heavily on multifollicular ovulation although other factors contributing to lifestyle changes and even better diagnostic techniques have contributed to the same. As early pregnancy ultrasound is gaining favor with obstetricians, most multifetal pregnancies are diagnosed in early pregnancy. Ultrasound has emerged as one of the most important diagnostic, prognostic, and even a therapy-guiding tool for multifetal pregnancy in present-day prenatal care protocols.

11.1 Establishing the Diagnosis and Chorionicity of Multifetal Pregnancy

Finding more than one fetal poles in the gravid uterus is the most unequivocal method of diagnosing multifetal pregnancy in today's medical practice. It can be done any time since early pregnancy (6–8 weeks), and the best time to unequivocally diagnose and allocate chorionicity to a multifetal pregnancy is before 14 weeks of gestation. The number of fetal poles can be counted and the pregnancy may be labeled as twins, triplets, quadruplets, and so on. However, clinically, this labeling remains incomplete unless the chorionicity or amnionicity is defined because these are important prognostic markers. In fetal medicine, multiple pregnancy nomenclature can only be complete if it includes three points:

1. Number of fetuses
2. Number of placentae (chorionicity)
3. Number of amniotic sacs (amnionicity)

Figure 11.1 shows some examples of the different types of multiple gestations based on amnionicity and chorionicity (DCDA, MCDA, MCMA, QCQA, TCTA)

© Springer Nature Singapore Pte Ltd. 2022
C. Ratha, A. Khurana, *Fetal Medicine*, https://doi.org/10.1007/978-981-19-6099-4_11

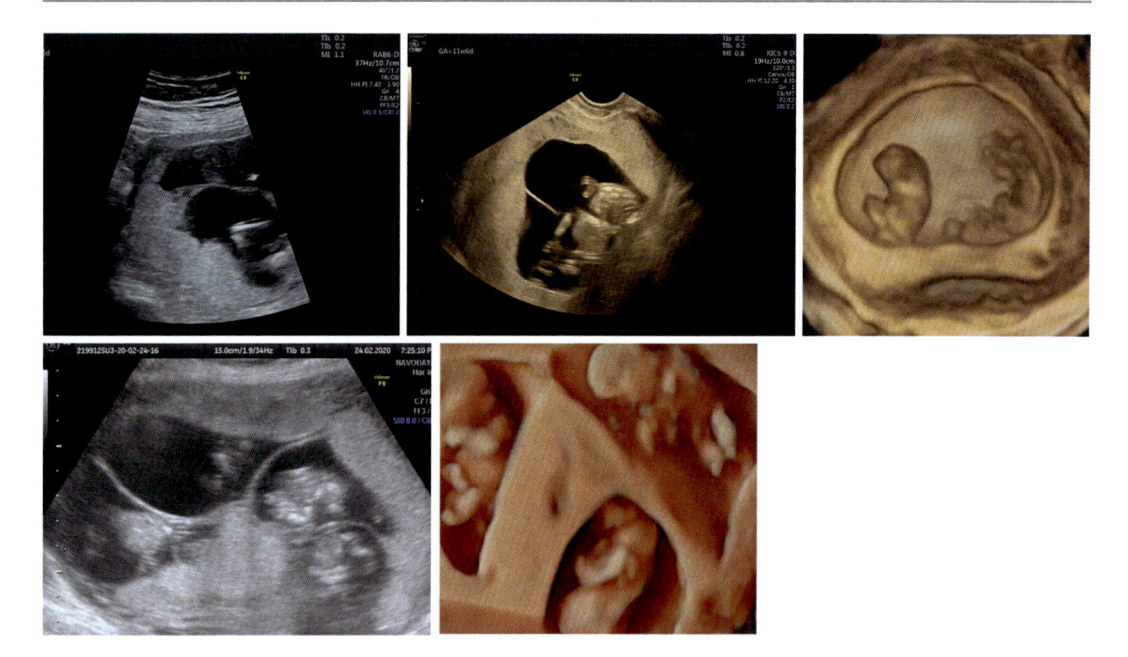

Fig. 11.1 Ultrasound appearance of multifetal gestation in first trimester

It is important to understand the rational basis of such classification rather than just learning the names. Although this fact has been stated time and again, over and over by experts, it is still not uncommon to find ultrasound reports and case notes on multifetal pregnancy where chorionicity and amnionicity are either not mentioned or erroneous due to nonadherence of some basic rules. One must realize that each fetus derives its nutritional and metabolic support from the placenta (chorion) so whenever there are more than one fetuses attached to one common placenta, this support has to be shared by two or more fetuses, and nature may not always be fair to each such that the "share" of individual fetuses may be unequal. This is a simple way of understanding why multifetal gestation is more than a mere mechanical overload on the womb. Also, each fetus is an individual entity and can have its own share of complications related to structure, development, chromosomal or genetic composition, or growth trajectory. This can lead to "discordance" in coexisting multiple fetuses and thus severe management dilemmas arise. The clinician will agree that CHORIONICITY remains the most important clinical criterion which will dictate management decisions in multifetal pregnancy.

Hence, BEFORE we proceed any further on the discussion of multiple pregnancy, we have to learn to establish CHORIONICITY.

The best time to determine chorionicity by USG is the first trimester of pregnancy when one can assign chorionicity with a sensitivity and specificity of 100% and 99.8%, respectively, as per current literature. In situations that each fetus has its own placenta, ultrasound will be able to demonstrate separate placentae or the "lambda sign" or "twin peak" sign (Fig. 11.2a, b) which is the hallmark of polychorionicity. When two fetuses are sharing one placenta, then the inter-twin membrane is seen arising from the fetal surface of the placenta without any intervening chorionic tissue—the "T sign" which indicates monochorionicity (Fig. 11.2c, d). These signs may disappear after 14–16 weeks of gestation and hence the need for checking them earlier on in pregnancy.

Once chorionicity is established, it is strongly recommended that this is well documented and preserved in the antenatal notes for future reference in case of any confusion because this is extremely a vital information in making critical decisions about multiple pregnancy management later. It is considered a good practice to take at

11.2 Dating of a Multifetal Pregnancy

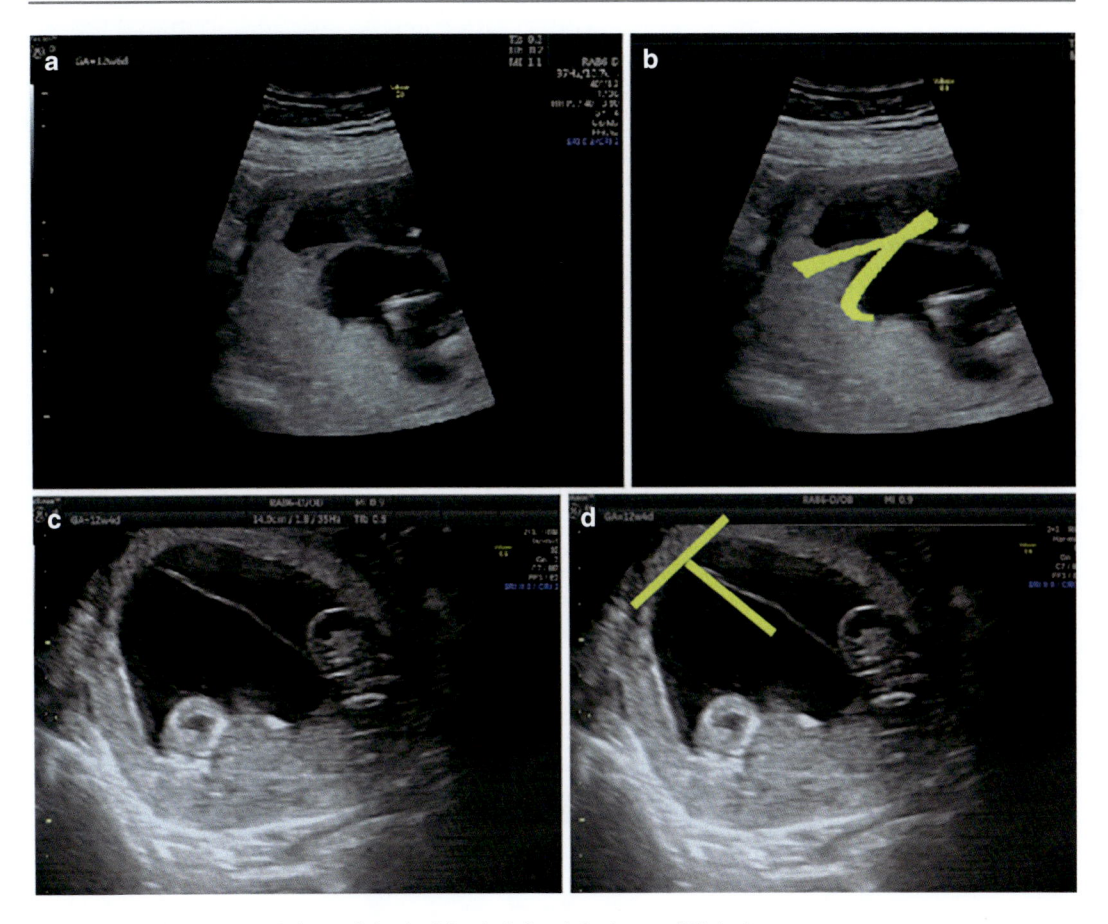

Fig. 11.2 (a–d) Ultrasound signs of chorionicity (a, b Lambda sign; c, d T sign)

least one picture of these important signs of chorionicity and keep the picture also for reference later. In any case that chorionicity is not established in early pregnancy and if the typical signs are lost by the time a clinician encounters the case, it is better to allocate "monochorionicity" and manage accordingly so as to not miss any potential complication.

11.2 Dating of a Multifetal Pregnancy

Accurate dating of a pregnancy is important in planning maternal and fetal care optimally. It is an accepted fact that dating of a pregnancy should be done by early pregnancy CRL as sometimes the mother's recollection of dates may not be accurate. In twin pregnancies, there may however be discrepancy in the CRL of two fetuses, and in such situations, the larger of the CRLs should be used to estimate gestational age. Similarly, in higher-order multiples, the CRL of the largest fetus is considered for dating as per the current guidelines. This is an area of active research and there may be some revision of protocol if alternate convincing evidence arises.

If the woman presents after 14 weeks' gestation, the larger head circumference should be used. Twin pregnancies conceived via in vitro fertilization should be dated using the embryonic age from fertilization. It is therefore important to take a detailed history of the periconception period to ascertain that the events that determine the dating of pregnancy are well documented and match the assigned gestational age calculation.

11.3 Systematic Labeling of Fetuses in Multifetal Gestation

Each fetus is identified and labeled in an unambiguous manner such that on serial evaluations at different points in time, the individual fetal parameters are correlated correctly without any confusion. This is of particular significance in follow-up of biometry as well as aneuploidy screening results allocation. Anatomical discrepancies may be easier to detect and distinguish between fetuses, but in structurally normal fetuses, there is scope for confusion unless labeling is unequivocal. Studies have shown that assigning laterality, placental position, and intertwin membrane orientation can help in systematically labeling twins as A and B (Fig. 11.3).

In higher-order multiples, it is useful to label the first fetus as the one closest to the cervix and then work clockwise and define the orientation, placental positions, and cord attachments of each fetus sequentially. This labeling is followed in all future examinations to ensure consistency of fetal evaluation.

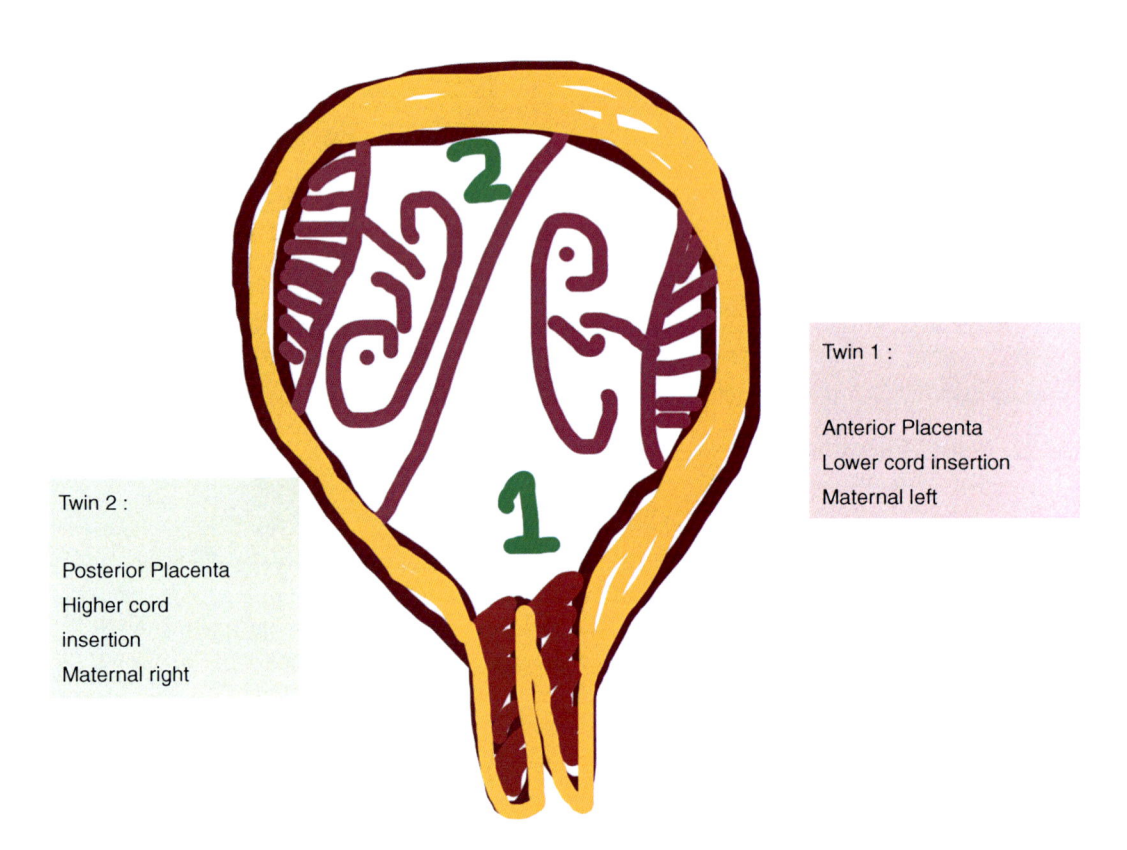

Twin 1:

Anterior Placenta
Lower cord insertion
Maternal left

Twin 2:

Posterior Placenta
Higher cord insertion
Maternal right

Fig. 11.3 Systematic labeling of twins

11.4 Aneuploidy Screening in Multifetal Pregnancy

In twin pregnancies, the first trimester combined screening test (NT scan along with serum biochemistry) can be used for risk assessment of aneuploidy after defining chorionicity.

It may be noted here that for all practical purpose, chorionicity is assumed to be a surrogate marker for zygosity while assigning risk of aneuploidy to multiple fetuses in a multifetal pregnancy. There is however a fundamental flaw in this approach because we must understand that even dichorionic twins may be monozygotic. If a zygote splits within the first 72 h, it may develop into two fetuses with two placentae and therefore continue as a dichorionic twin pair while both fetuses have originated from one zygote and are hence monozygotic. It is reasonable to accept monochorionic twins as monozygotic but all dichorionic twins are not definitely dizygotic. The problem is that we cannot assign zygosity by ultrasound and therefore we accept chorionicity as a surrogate marker for zygosity during risk allocation.

In DICHORIONIC twins, each fetus is allocated a separate risk based on its NT along with the maternal serum biochemistry. In MONOCHORIONIC twins, the average NT of both fetuses is considered as one entity which is combined with serum biochemistry to assign one risk to both fetuses with the assumption that this is a monozygotic pregnancy. The maternal serum biochemistry is only used in twins in the first trimester, but it cannot be used when dealing with higher-order multiple pregnancies as it is not reliable in those cases.

In higher-order multiples, the combination of maternal age and the aneuploidy markers at the NT scan should be used as biochemical screening becomes unreliable. Serum biochemical screening tests are not validated for triplets and higher-order multiples.

Figure 11.4 illustrates the use of NT in calculation of risk in multifetal pregnancies.

Twin pregnancies in the second trimester and higher-order multiple pregnancies should be offered aneuploidy screening based on ultrasound parameters as the primary method. In polychorionic pregnancies, each fetus gets an individual risk for aneuploidies, and there may be discordance in the NT values leading to discordant risks for both fetuses. It is important to inform women and their partners in advance of

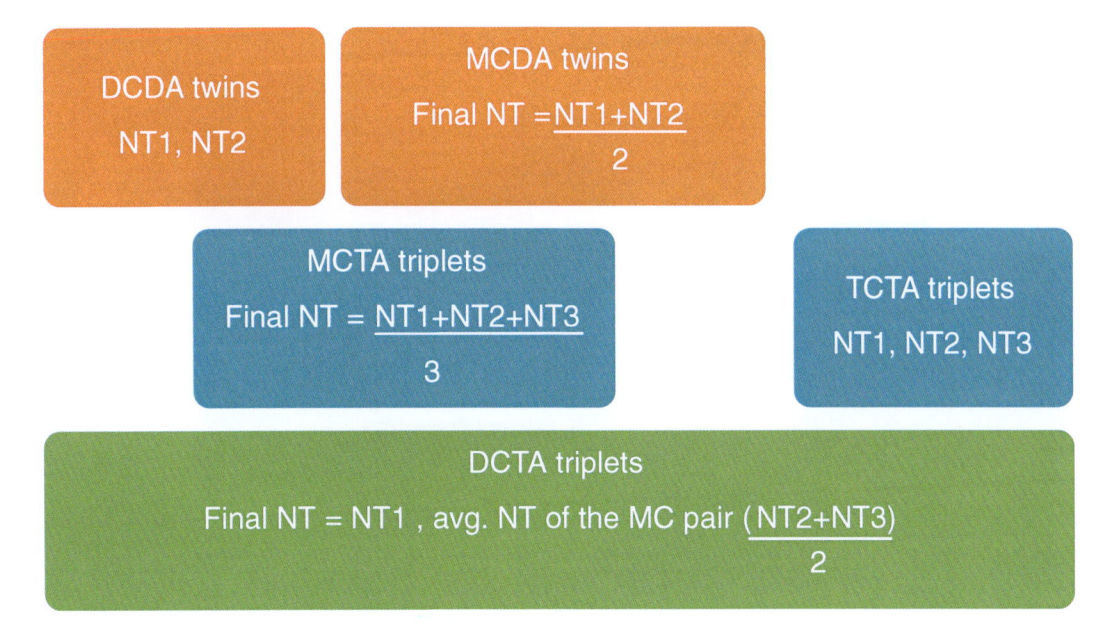

DCDA twins
NT1, NT2

MCDA twins
Final NT = $\dfrac{NT1+NT2}{2}$

MCTA triplets
Final NT = $\dfrac{NT1+NT2+NT3}{3}$

TCTA triplets
NT1, NT2, NT3

DCTA triplets
Final NT = NT1, avg. NT of the MC pair $\dfrac{(NT2+NT3)}{2}$

Fig. 11.4 Method of NT calculation for risk assessment in multiple pregnancy

the potentially complex decisions that they will need to make on the basis of the results of combined screening, bearing in mind the increased risk of invasive testing in twins, the possible discordance between dichorionic twins for fetal aneuploidy, and the risks of selective fetal reduction.

In monochorionic twins, as they are both theoretically assumed to have similar karyotypes, the risks are allocated after taking an average of the NT of both fetuses such that both have a similar risk for aneuploidy.

Cell-free fetal DNA can be offered in twin pregnancy after checking with the specific labs regarding this facility. This can act as a secondary screening method as it may reduce the need for unnecessary invasive testing. However, if the results of cell-free DNA suggest high risk of aneuploidy, invasive testing is warranted. As such this method is not validated for triplets or above. These are methods of screening for aneuploidies and help in allocating risk for aneuploidies for each fetus. In high-risk fetuses, ultrasound-guided CVS and amniocentesis help in confirming the fetal chromosomal status. A summary of a screening protocol is displayed in Fig. 11.5 about aneuploidy screening for twin pregnancies.

If such invasive procedures are contemplated, then it is better to check all the fetal sacs or placentae. This recommendation is based on the theoretical fact that even monozygotic pregnancies which split very early may develop into dichorionic gestation so chorionicity does not confirm zygosity. Details of invasive procedures are given in a subsequent chapter. In multiple pregnancy, special care must be taken to label the fetuses correctly and label their samples accordingly so that there is no confusion in interpreting the results and appropriate solutions may be provided in case of discordant results for fetal aneuploidy. In cases of confirmed aneuploidy in one fetus along with a normal co-twin, the parents may opt for selective fetal reduction. Only if the labeling of fetuses is accurate such a procedure can be carried out correctly.

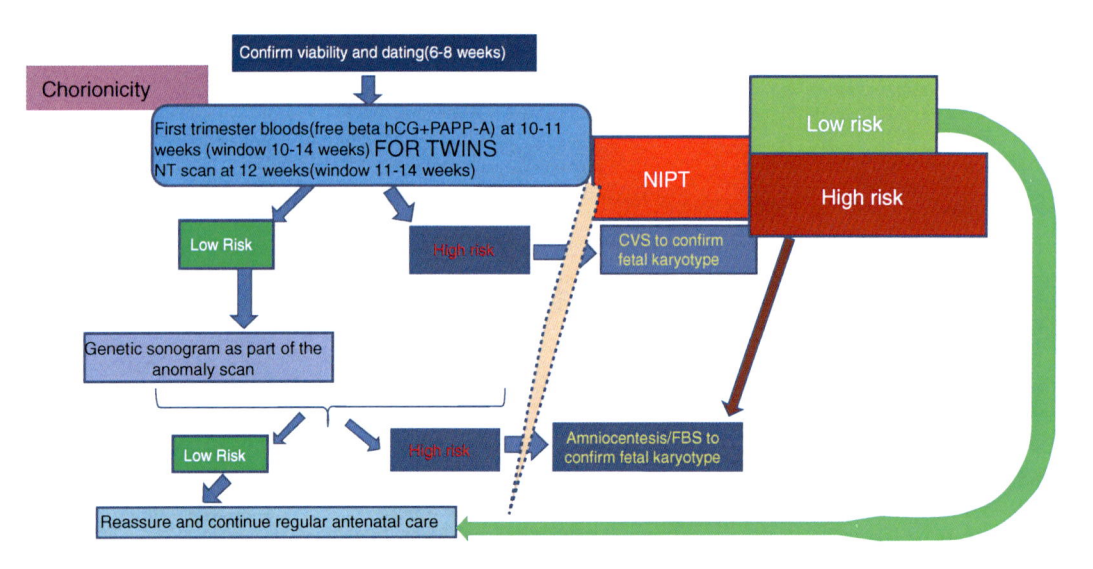

Fig. 11.5 Aneuploidy screening protocol for multiple pregnancies

11.5 Screening for Fetal Anomalies in Multifetal Pregnancy

The principles of ultrasound screening for fetal anomalies in the first and second trimester have been described in previous chapters. The same parameters have to be used for twins, triplets, and higher-order multiple fetuses too. The only important precaution to be exercised by the ultrasound operators is to carefully follow the structure of each twin separately as sometimes there can be an error of judgment due to fetal movements and the same fetus may get evaluated twice. To avoid such errors, a practical approach is to start with the first fetus and complete its evaluation before shifting focus to the next one. Utmost care and caution is needed during multifetal assessment to avoid any confusion. If during anytime of the scan the operator feels lost or is unsure of the fetus being evaluated, it is better to recheck the orientation and labeling and restart the examination if needed—much like the "recenter" application on Google Maps!!

These issues may seem mundane and one might wonder why a simple fact like this even merits a mention in a textbook for specialists! It is therefore vital to understand that while textbook pictures and theoretical learning deal with individual fetuses distinctly, during real-time scans, the fetuses are moving independent of each other and may even change position significantly while the scan is in progress. This poses a practical challenge to the operator. With experience and practice, such problems get minimized but it is always better to be prudent in this regard.

The incidence of structural abnormalities in multiple pregnancies is more than that found in singleton gestations. One or both of the co-twins may be affected in a twin pregnancy. If both twins are anomalous and the anomalies are not compatible with a good quality of life, it may be reasonable to consider termination of the pregnancy. Thus, timely screening for fetal anomalies in multiple pregnancies is important so that such issues can be detected at the earliest possible gestational age. The decision to continue or discontinue the pregnancy will depend on the type of anomaly and the decision of the parents so effective diagnosis and timely counseling must be arranged to plan further care. Figure 11.6 presents the possible plan of care when fetal anomalies are detected in twin pregnancy.

In case of any anomaly detected, the challenges of management in twin pregnancy are different and more complex than those faced in singleton gestations. In multifetal pregnancy, the potential effect of any intervention in the interest of an anomalous fetus puts the normal co-twin at some degree of risk. Some anomalies are lethal and may lead to fetal compromise in utero—while this may be acceptable in dichorionic gestation, a single fetal demise can be catastrophic in a monochorionic pair due to the complications of a shared placenta. Hence, the decisions to manage such problems are also based primarily on chorionicity and thereafter on the type of anomaly based on the system involved, its potential to affect the course of present pregnancy, and its subsequent viability and functional effects.

If a particular anomaly can lead to problems like polyhydramnios thus increasing the risk to the normal co-twin or if there is a high risk of intrauterine fetal demise in a monochorionic pair, selective fetal reduction may be done to ameliorate the effects of the anomalous fetus and improve the prognosis of the normal co-twin. Procedures like selective fetal reduction entail many considerations and risks, and these have been explained in detail in the chapter on invasive procedures.

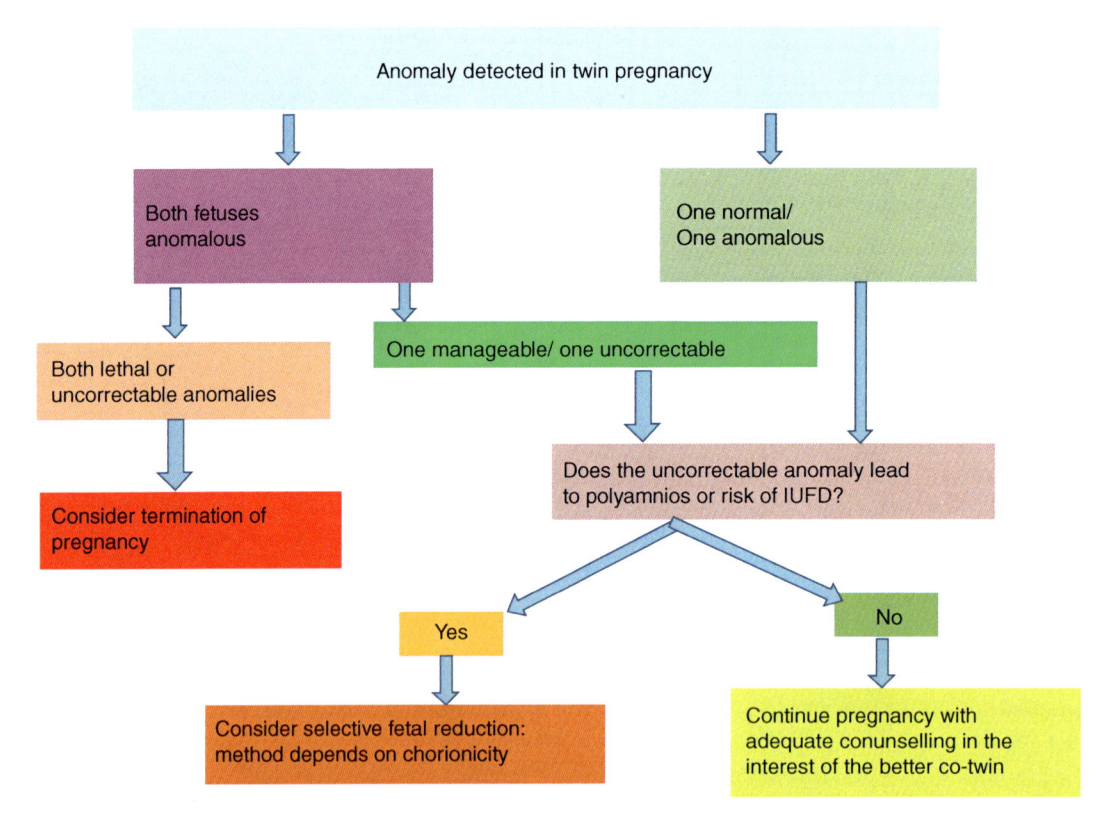

Fig. 11.6 Management plan for anomaly detected in twin pregnancy

11.6 Planning a Rational Follow-up for Serial Monitoring of Multiple Pregnancy

11.6.1 DICHORIONIC DIAMNIOTIC Twins

This is by far the commonest type of multifetal pregnancy encountered in clinical practice and accounts for 97–98% of such cases. The need and importance of determining chorionicity in early pregnancy have been explained earlier and are being reiterated only to reaffirm its importance.

An early pregnancy scan should be ideally done between 9 and 14 weeks of gestation, and the unequivocal evidence of dichorionicity like the "lambda" sign must be detected and documented in the patient's note for future reference in case she changes her center of care and books in another unit later in pregnancy.

A standard fetal care plan for DCDA twins can be formulated as shown in the following flowchart in Fig. 11.7. Individual issues like dating, labeling, and screening for aneuploidies and anomalies have been explained earlier. It has been established that although in the first and second trimesters, the growth rate of twins is not significantly different from that of singletons, there is usually slower fetal growth, even in uncomplicated twin gestations, in the third trimester, as compared to uncomplicated singleton fetuses. Twin pregnancies are more likely to be affected by fetal growth restriction, and therefore such pregnancies should be monitored with serial ultrasound examinations for growth and Dopplers in the third trimester.

In uncomplicated DCDA twin pregnancies, with adequate feto-maternal surveillance, pregnancy can be continued till term, and at term the obstetrician can plan the time and mode of delivery based on obstetric indications.

DICHORIONIC TWINS: Follow up protocol

- 6-8 weeks → Viability, dating and number of fetuses
- 11-14 weeks → Systematic Labelling of fetuses, Chorionicity, Aneuploidy screening
- 18-20 weeks → TIFFA, Biometry, AF volume, Cervical length
- 24-26 weeks
- 28-30 weeks
- 32-34 weeks
- 36-37 weeks

→ Growth and Doppler, AF volume

Uncomplicated: Plan for delivery at term
Mode of delivery: Obstetric indications

Complicated DCDA: selective IUGR -
Mild discrepancy/advanced gestation (>32 weeks) — try to continue pregnancy as long as possible to achieve better fetal maturity

Severe discrepancy/early gestation (<26 weeks) — consider continuing in the interest of better maturity for the better growing co twin even at risk of IUFD of the IUGR fetus

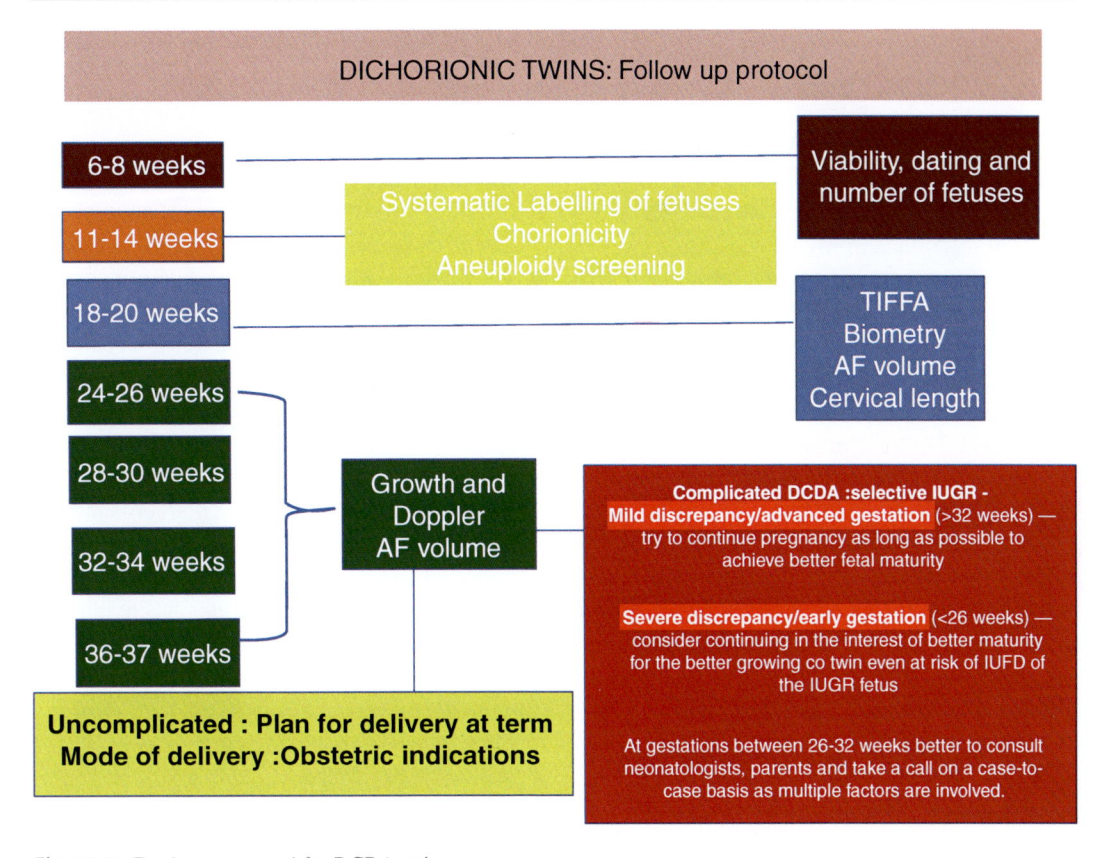

At gestations between 26-32 weeks better to consult neonatologists, parents and take a call on a case-to-case basis as multiple factors are involved.

Fig. 11.7 Fetal care protocol for DCDA twins

If one or both fetuses are not growing optimally, on serial follow-up, FGR or discordant growth may be detected in DCDA twins. "Discordance" in fetal growth in twins is defined as any of the following parameters:

1. In the first trimester, discrepancy of ≥20% in the CRL (crown-rump length) may be observed and is predictive of later weight discordance.
2. An intertwin AC (abdominal circumference) difference ≥20 mm, irrespective of gestational age, has been reported to have 83% positive predictive value to detect a difference in birth weight ≥20%.
3. The percentage of the intertwin weight difference in comparison to the weight of the larger twin: (difference of EFW of twins/EFW of larger fetus X 100)%. Discordance of 20% or more is considered clinically significant and suggests selective FGR.

Discordant growth in twins presents a major clinical dilemma for the managing team. A fine balance has to be achieved between allowing the pregnancy to continue so that better maturity is achieved especially for the normal or better growing co-twin and the risks of fetal compromise that may become palpable for the smaller fetus implying added dangers of adverse effects on neurodevelopmental outcome due to in utero hemodynamic and possibly, metabolic compromise.

The decision to deliver discordant DCDA twins is dependent on the extent of discrepancy such that if a fair prognosis for intact survival exists for both fetuses, an elective preterm delivery may be justified for the normal growing co-twin to prevent further in utero compromise of its growth-restricted partner. However, if there is severe discordancy in early gestation, it may be reasonable to continue pregnancy in the interest of the normal co-twin even at the risk of an intrauterine fetal demise (IUFD) of the growth-restricted fetus.

11.6.2 MONOCHORIONIC DIAMNIOTIC Twins

Monochorionic diamniotic (MCDA) twins are the second most common variety of multifetal pregnancies encountered in clinical practice. The most important difference in MC and DC twins is the common placenta between two fetuses in the MC pair unlike DC twins where each fetus has its own independent placenta. Therefore, the chances of complications are higher and the type of problems faced by monochorionic twins is rather unique.

The need for closer monitoring of monochorionic pregnancies has been realized, and the follow-up protocol for any monochorionic pregnancy recommends at least two-weekly reviews from 16 weeks of gestation onward. The situation would change if any complication was associated, but as a general consensus, uncomplicated MC twins can be followed up based on the plan displayed in Fig. 11.8.

The sharing of placenta by two fetuses leads to some unique complications in MC twins, and understanding the basic pathophysiology of these complications is vital to planning reasonable care for these conditions. The placental size, position, and architecture are definitely important in prognosticating any pregnancy, but its typical vasculature is the most important determinant of prognosis of a MC pregnancy. As explained earlier in this chapter, sharing the placenta in terms of its area and vascularity can inherently lead to "discordance" in natural allocation of resources to the twins and therefore increase the possibility of fetal problems.

The placenta is a very vascular organ with multiple interconnecting or "anastomotic" vessels formed during its development. When two fetuses are connected through the placenta, these interconnections or anastomoses form pathways or "shunts" capable of bidirectional blood flow, but the direction depends on the pressure gradient

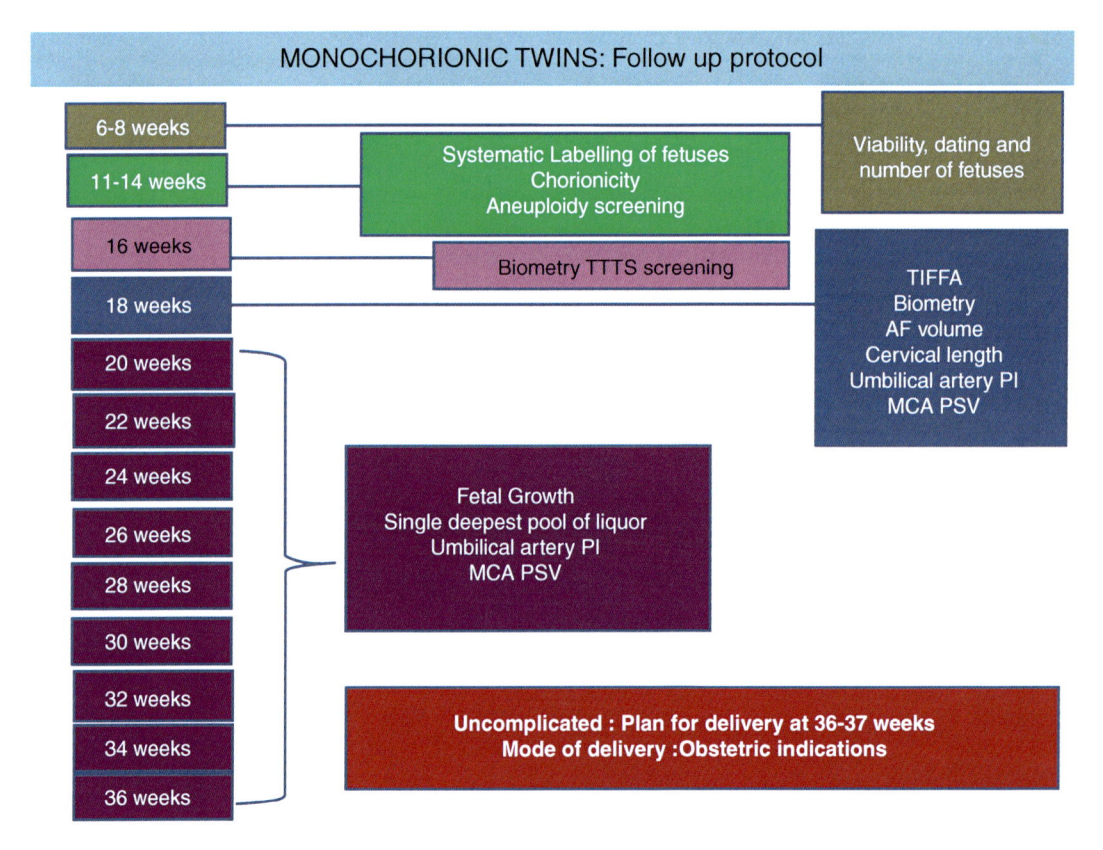

Fig. 11.8 Fetal care protocol in uncomplicated MC twins

across these vessels. There are three types of "shunts" that are possible:

1. Arterioarterial (A-A) shunts
2. Venovenous shunts (V-V) shunts
3. Arteriovenous (A-V) shunts

Figure 11.9 shows the monochorionic placenta with different types of anastomoses. The pressure gradient across A-A or V-V shunts is minimal such that they do not cause much hemodynamic changes, but the A-V shunts have a definite pressure gradient such that the blood flows preferentially from the arterial to the venous side.

If such shunting is "balanced" across two fetuses who share a placenta (monochorionic), then the pressure compensation maintains circulatory balance, but if these shunts are "unbalanced," then blood tends to flow toward the fetus which has more venous connections. Thus, blood is "pumped" toward one fetus preferentially—the fetus which is toward the "venous" predominance becomes the "recipient," while the fetus toward the "arterial" predominance becomes the "donor." Blood thus flows from the donor to the recipient leading to the condition known as "twin-to-twin transfusion syndrome" or TTTS. TTTS affects about 15% of all monochorionic twin pregnancies and is a result of unbalanced AV anastomoses in the placenta. Figure 11.10 illustrates the pathophysiology of TTTS.

The donor becomes progressively hypovolemic, oliguric, and growth restricted. The recipient becomes overperfused and at risk of cardiac failure. Both fetuses are at risk of mortality in this condition, if left untreated. TTTS is classified into five stages based on a system of staging proposed by Prof. Ruben Quintero in 1999. These stages are the following:

- Stage I: Significant difference in amniotic fluid volumes (polyamnios-oligoamnios)

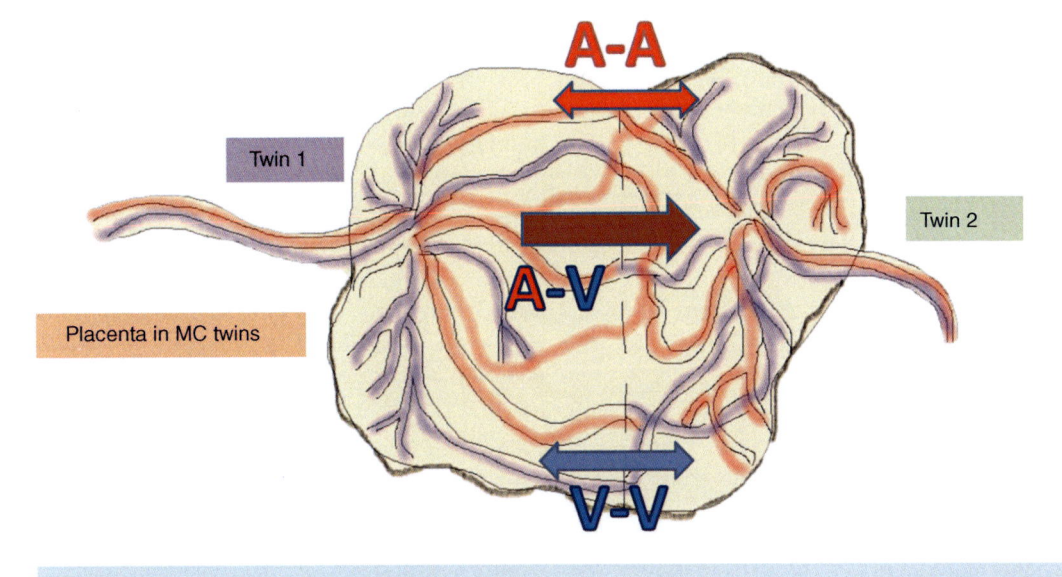

A-A anastomosis : equal pressures – bidirectional flow

V-V anastomosis : equal pressure – bidirectional flow

A-V anastomosis : Pressure gradient - unidirectional flow from A to V

Fig. 11.9 Monochorionic placenta with vascular anastomoses

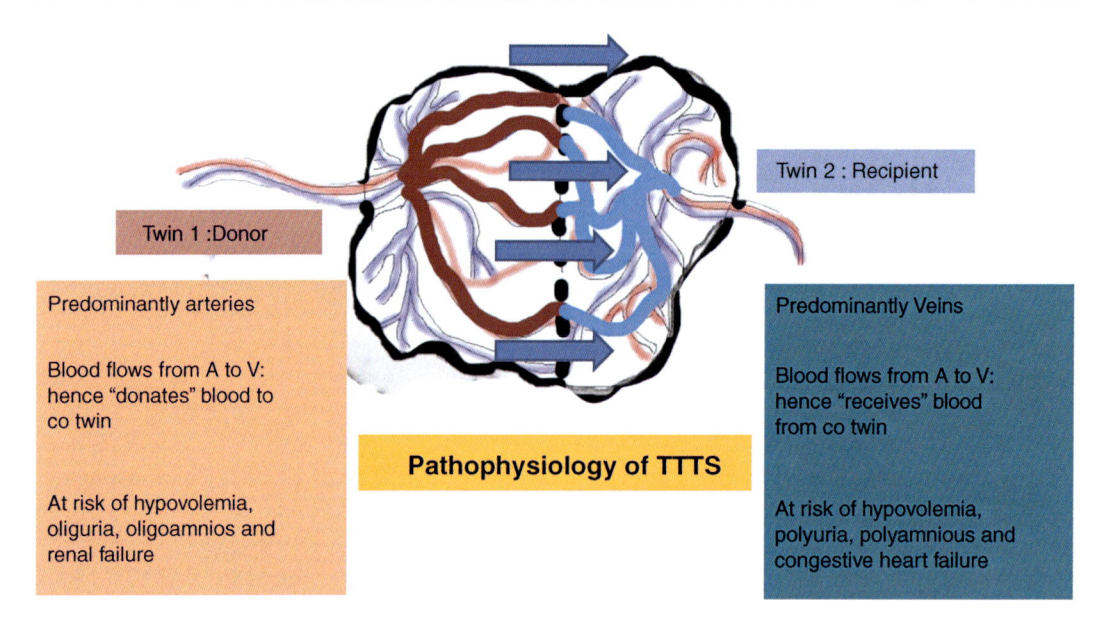

Fig. 11.10 Pathophysiology of twin-to-twin transfusion syndrome

between the two sacs but urine still visible within the donor twin's bladder during ultrasound. There is a 40% risk of fetal mortality.
- Stage II: In addition to the features of stage I, the donor's bladder is "empty" as no urine is detected in the bladder during scans. Fetal Dopplers are normal so far.
- Stage III: In stage III, abnormal Doppler studies of the umbilical artery, ductus venosus, or umbilical vein are seen in addition to stage II features.
- Stage IV: Ascites or frank hydrops in either twin. The risk of fetal mortality increases to 60% by now.
- Stage V: Demise of either fetus. In case there is one surviving twin, there is a 19–26% risk of neurological morbidity in this fetus.

The progression of TTTS through these stages is a logical sequence of events that happen due to the drastic hemodynamic imbalance in the donor and recipient as shown in the table below (Table 11.1).

It is imperative that all ultrasound scan reports pertaining to monochorionic twins must mention the presence or absence of TTTS signs in addition to the general issues of viability and biometry. In particular, all scan reports of MC twins should mention the comparative fluid levels in both sacs (whether normal/oligo/poly) and the presence or absence of fetal bladder and the fetal Doppler features as the preliminary features which help in diagnosing TTTS. Once TTTS is diagnosed and staged, management of the condition is another challenge. Stage I TTTS may be managed conservatively with serial review, but stage II or III warrants definitive treatment like LASER photocoagulation of anastomotic vessels in the placenta. This procedure helps in effectively "dichorionizing" a monochorionic placenta and hence is an effective treatment of TTTS which allows salvaging both the fetuses. It is however a very skill-intensive procedure and should be undertaken only by operators specifically trained for the same. Details of such fetal therapeutic procedures are discussed in a separate chapter later in the book.

In some cases single fetal salvage may be done by Radiofrequency ablation or Bipolar cord coagulation of the worse affected twin. Decisions regarding which procedure to be performed and when have to be considered with the merits of each individual case and cannot be randomly generalized.

The important point to remember here is that TTTS potentially affects both donor and recipi-

Table 11.1 Stage-wise progression and ultrasound findings in TTTS

TTTS Stage	Donor physiology	Recipient physiology	USG findings
Stage I	Receives less blood flow, decreased GFR, decreased urine output although renal functions are maintained	Receives more blood volume, hyperdynamic circulation, polyuria	Donor: Oligoamnios, small bladder Recipient: Polyamnios, large bladder
Stage II	Receives further less blood flow, decreased GFR, critically decreased urine output such that renal functions are affected and almost no urine is formed, fetal growth restriction starts to set in	Receives more blood volume, hyperdynamic circulation, polyuria, and increased stress on the fetal heart	Donor: Severe oligoamnios, absent bladder echo Recipient: Polyamnios, large bladder
Stage III	Fetal growth restriction sets in with anuria and abnormal umbilical artery dopplers	Early signs of cardiac compensation to the hyperdynamic state and hypervolemia are seen	Donor: FGR, umbilical artery dopplers PI is raised or AREDF seen Recipient: Cardiomegaly, tricuspid regurgitation, abnormal ductus venosus flows
Stage IV	Severe FGR with renal compromise	Cardiac decompensation, congestive heart failure	Donor: Severe FGR with anuria Recipient: Hydrops fetalis
Stage V	Death or risk of residual neurological morbidity if alive		USG signs of neurological damage may not present immediately but take several weeks to manifest

ent adversely, and if left untreated, both fetuses are at risk of morbidity and mortality. Death of any one fetus in a MC pair causes a risk of neurological deficit to the surviving co-twin because there is some exsanguination from the live fetus to the dead co-twin at the time of the latter's demise. This leads to a transient ischemia in the tissues of the surviving fetus, and since brain is very sensitive to hypoxia, it may get irreversibly affected in some cases accounting for 19–26% risk of neurological morbidity in these cases. Therefore, any intervention toward fetal therapy must be attempted only before a fetal demise because these adverse events occur at the time of the fetal demise and even if subsequent procedures are done, the risk for residual neurological damage exists. The basic premise of therapeutic procedures is to disconnect the circulations of the fetuses, and this is only meaningful if done when both have their inherent circulations active. Although the result of some procedures like radiofrequency ablation and bipolar cord cauterization is the demise of one fetus, this iatrogenic reduction is beneficial to the live co-twin because as the connecting vascular channels are sealed, there is no exsanguination into the other's circulatory pathways and therefore the risk of neurological damage is minimized.

11.7 Twin Reversed Arterial Perfusion (TRAP) Sequence

This is another unique complication associated with MC twins where one fetus is normally formed but the other one is an acardiac, amorphous mass which does not have a heart of its own (hence "acardiac") and its circulation is based on abnormal arterioarterial and venovenous anastomoses that is supported by the cardiac activity of the "pump twin." As shown in Fig. 11.11, the pathophysiology of the TRAP sequence is based on the "reversed arterial perfusion" of the acardiac mass. This mass receives blood through the umbilical artery that in turn is filled by blood from the heart of the normal twin. The blood is returned by the umbilical vein, and through the placenta, this again circulates to the other fetus, thus putting the "pump twin" at risk of congestive heart failure due to hyperdynamic circulation, while this acardiac mass may grow into bigger proportions. The

Pathophysiology of TRAP sequence

Normal twin
Inflow: Umbilical vein
Outflow: Umbilical artery
Pumb: fetal heart

Acardiac twin
Inflow: Umbilical artery
Outflow: Umbilical vein
Pumb: No internal pump, supported by noraml twin's heart

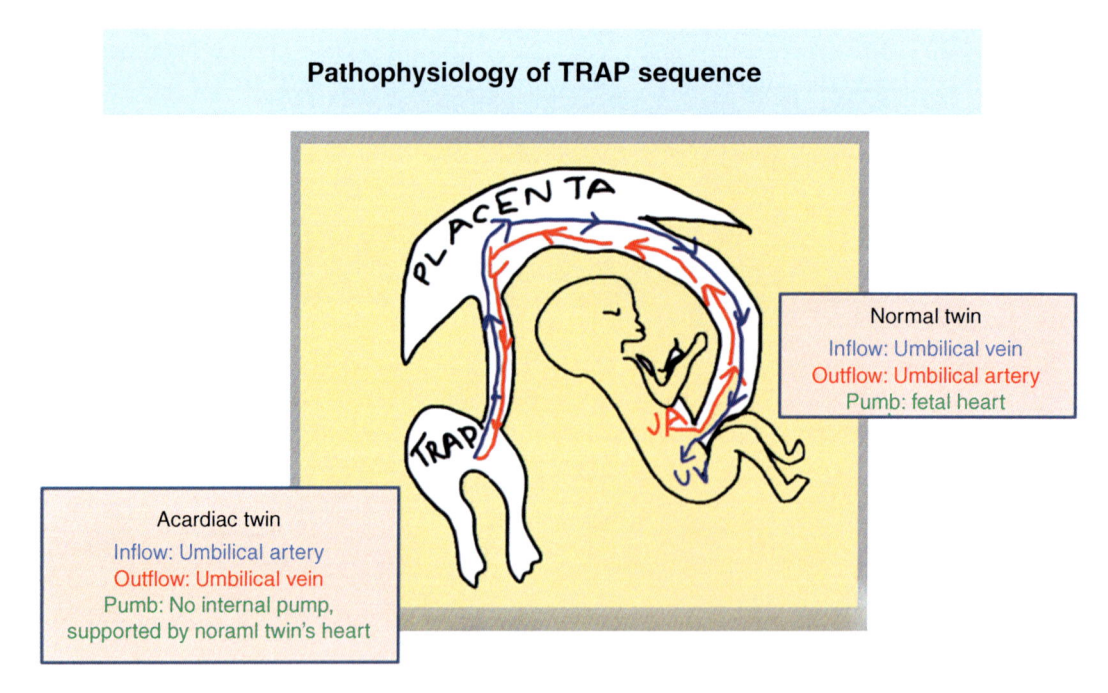

Fig. 11.11 Pathophysiology of the TRAP sequence

TRAP itself may have different names based on the parts formed or absent, e.g., acephalus, anceps, acormus, or truly amorphous. Like all monochorionic complications, this is also a double whammy—the pump twin may develop hydrops due to volume overload, and the acardiac mass may grow so much that delivering it will become challenging as it may not have the "limb handles" or any structure that can be grasped easily to deliver. In some cases, the TRAP may spontaneously cease growing if the arterial supply is hampered naturally. Many of these pregnancies continue successfully, but if the acardiac mass continues to grow in size and vascularity, co-twin demise is the result of the sequence of changes. In such cases, fetal salvage may be done by ablating the vessels of the acardiac twin by either LASER or RFA or BPCC. The details of these procedures are given in the chapter on fetal therapy.

It is important to be aware of this condition as many times the presence of a second mass without cardiac activity is erroneously diagnosed as a missed miscarriage of one twin, and subsequently when this presumably nonviable fetus starts growing in dimensions and even developing skeletal elements, then it leads to clinical dilemma due to ignorance of the cause (Figs. 11.12, 11.13, and 11.14).

When diagnosed early and correctly, a reasonable plan of care can be formulated to lead to a good perinatal outcome.

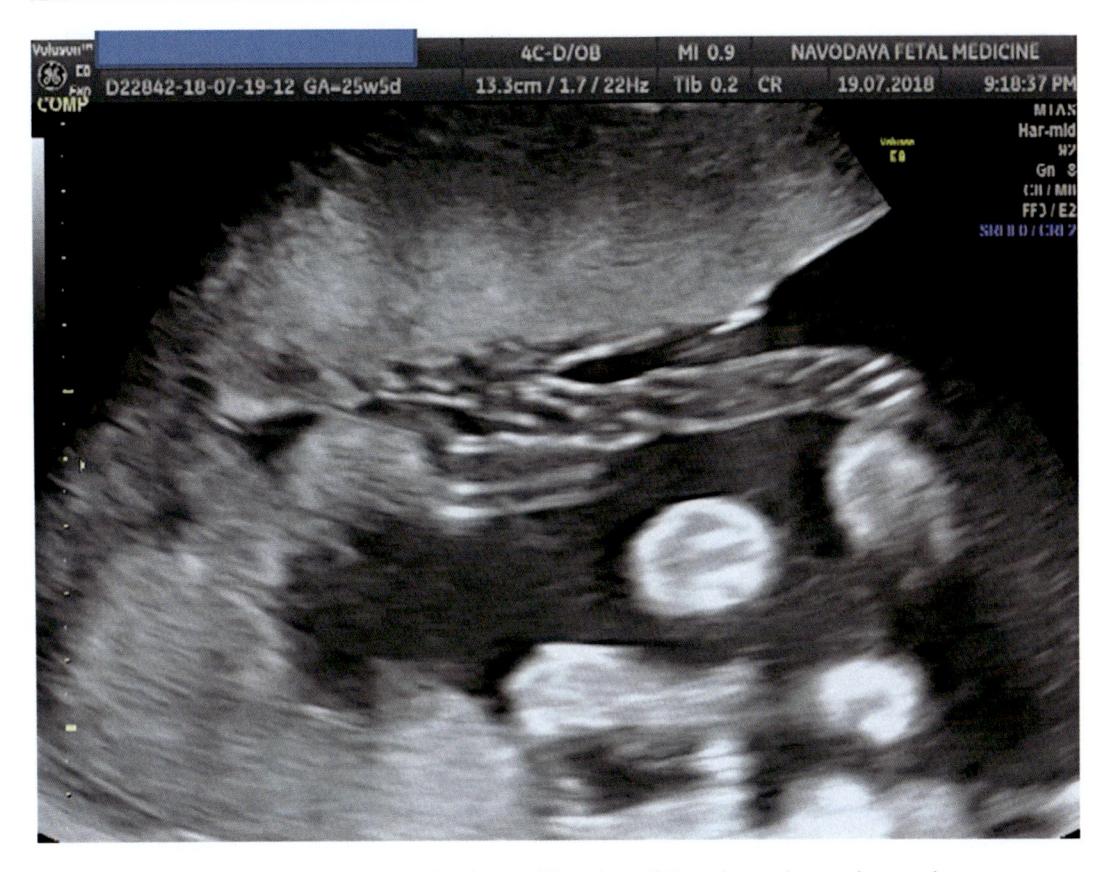

11.7 Twin Reversed Arterial Perfusion (TRAP) Sequence 119

Fig. 11.12 Monoamniotic twin pregnancy showing cord insertions of the twins, no intervening membrane

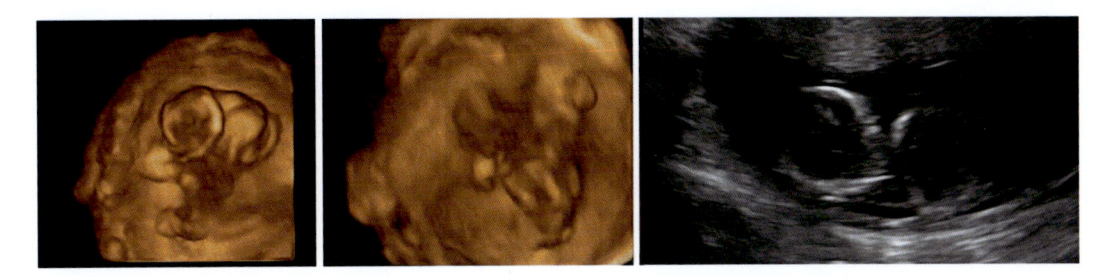

Fig. 11.13 Conjoined twins

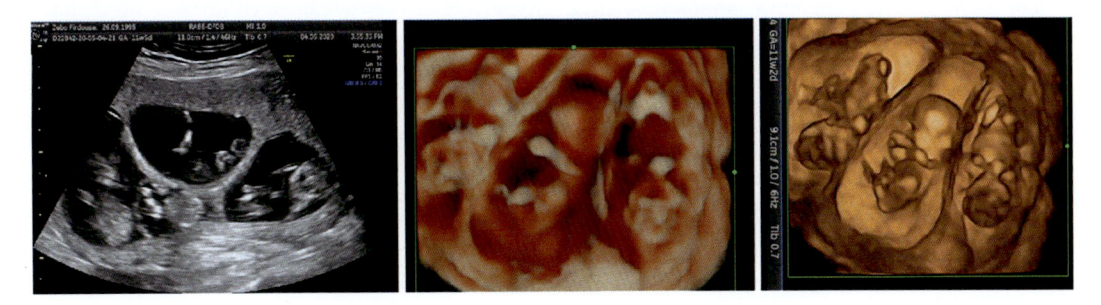

Fig. 11.14 Higher-order multiple gestation

11.8 Monochorionic Monoamniotic (MCMA) Twins

Monochorionic twins are monozygotic twins that split after 72 h of fertilization such that they retain a common placenta. MCDA twins (common placenta-different sacs) result from splitting between 3 and 8 days. If the zygote splits between 8 and 12 days, then it results in MCMA (common placenta and common sac).

As a simple analogy, DCDA twins have their own rooms and own kitchens, while MCDA twins have separate rooms but a common kitchen—hence the problems of unequal sharing and distribution!! MCMA twins share not only the kitchen but also their room!! The MCMA twins may have further unique problems like "cord entanglement" which can be benign if it remains loose and does not disrupt circulation or may cause intermittent hypoxic episodes and is potentially lethal causing intrauterine fetal demise of one or both co-twins.

Diagnosis of a monoamniotic twin pregnancy is based on exclusion of the possibility of an intervening membrane between the fetuses, and sometimes it may take more than one occasion to firmly establish this diagnosis. Presence of cord entanglement is a confirmatory sign, but nonvisualization of the membrane despite a thorough search in a monochorionic twin pregnancy latest by 11–14 weeks' scan should enable one to confirm the diagnosis of MCMA pregnancy. Approximately 1% of monozygotic twins are monoamniotic and the overall incidence is about 1 in 12,500 births. Perinatal mortality is high in MCMA twins due to cord entanglement (in almost 50% cases), congenital anomalies, preterm birth, or even twin-twin transfusion syndrome, which is difficult to diagnose and managed in these cases.

There is no effective method of monitoring MCMA twins to prevent cord entanglement or consequent fetal demise, and hence many professional bodies recommend elective delivery by caesarean section at 32 weeks after steroid over for fetal lung maturity. This approach is definitely not ideal and controversial, but considering the unique and unpredictable nature of clinical problems in the context of MCMA twins, such management may be justifiable.

11.8.1 Conjoined Twins

If a single zygote splits into two fetuses after 13 days of fertilization, complete separation is not achieved, and the two fetuses are joined to each other and often found to be sharing organs too. Depending on the common, shared organs, conjoined twins may be called craniopagus, thoracopagus, ischiopagus, etc.

If multiple fetal parts are seen on ultrasound scan and found to be moving simultaneously with no relative motion, conjoined twins are suspected. A thorough ultrasound imaging eventually confirms the diagnosis which is corroborated by the presence of a four-vessel umbilical cord.

The prognosis of conjoined twins is uniformly bad and postnatal complex surgery is warranted to separate them—the results of which have not been very encouraging. Most parents opt to discontinue pregnancies with conjoined fetuses and hence an early diagnosis becomes clinically an important issue. Delivering a conjoined pair of twins is a technical challenge as the size of the fetuses grows and can cause serious damage to maternal structures in the process of vaginal expulsion or caesarean section. A "bifid" fetal pole in early pregnancy is an early indicator of the possibility of "conjoined" twins. By 11–14 weeks, again this diagnosis can be unequivocally established although it may be possible earlier too.

11.9 Higher-Order Multiples (Triplets, Quadruplets, and So on)

The incidence of higher-order multiple is rising steadily especially due to assisted reproductive techniques that cause "superovulation" or multiple embryo transfers during IVF. Higher-order multiples pose severe challenges to the clinical management not only due to exaggerated mechanical effects of a pregnancy with more than two fetuses but also due to some specific issues like lack of robust aneuploidy screening methods, technical difficulties in scanning each individual fetus for anomalies, increased risk of preterm birth, and add-on problems of "monochorionicity" if some fetuses are sharing their placentae.

Higher-order multiple pregnancy must be diagnosed early, and assessment of number of fetuses and chorionicity should be clearly completed by 11 weeks. Labeling of these fetuses is done by identifying the first sac closest to the cervix and then moving anticlockwise or clockwise from thereon and defining each placental position, cord insertion, and fetal orientation. Potential problems with higher-order multiples must be discussed in detail with the parents in early pregnancy.

Care for higher-order multiple should be arranged in close coordination of a fetal medicine center and an obstetric care center with a tertiary level neonatalogy backup. Aneuploidy screening is scan-based and biochemical tests do not perform well in higher-order multiples. Offering serial two-weekly scans is justified as clinical assessment of growth is fallacious in these cases. Maternal discomfort can be considerable and despite recommended precautions, the risk of preterm birth is above 30%.

In order to improve perinatal outcomes in higher-order multiples, iatrogenic fetal reduction to twins is a justifiable option, and the technique is discussed in the chapter on prenatal interventions (Chap. 15).

> **Key Learning Points in Multiple Pregnancy**
> 1. Multiple pregnancy incidence has increased significantly due to multiple reasons and is a regular entity in fetal medicine clinics.
> 2. Identification, prognostication, and management of multiple pregnancy cases pose a daunting challenge to clinicians.
> 3. CHORIONICITY is the most important prognostic factor in multifetal pregnancy and MUST be established by the first trimester of pregnancy.
> 4. Dating, risk assessment, and serial fetal surveillance in multifetal pregnancy are based on protocols defined by chorionicity.
> 5. Systematic labeling of multiple fetuses helps in proper monitoring of the fetuses in serial assessments.
> 6. Monochorionic pregnancies carry risk of specific complications and need specialized management.
> 7. Higher-order multiple pregnancies need careful identification and management.

Suggested Reading

Algeri P, et al. Selective IUGR in dichorionic twins: what can Doppler assessment and growth discordancy say about neonatal outcomes? Med: J. Perinat; 2017.

Dias T, et al. First-trimester ultrasound determination of chorionicity in twin pregnancy. Ultrasound Obstet Gynecol. 2011;10(1):89.

Khalil A, et al. ISUOG Practice Guidelines: role of ultrasound in twin pregnancy. Ultrasound Obstet Gynecol. 2016;47:247–63.

Lewi L, et al. Clinical outcome and placental characteristics of monochorionic diamniotic twin pairs with early- and late-onset discordant growth. Am J Obstet Gynecol. 2008;199:511.

Placenta, Cord, Amniotic Fluid, and Cervix

12

The human placenta is a pregnancy-specific organ that is the connecting bridge between the mother and the fetus. The placenta provides a platform for exchange of oxygen and nutrients for the fetus and is a vascular structure that also regulates fetal hemodynamics as a pressure and volume interface. The placenta is the first organ to form in the feto-maternal unit as it is required for supplying the bioenergetic needs of the developing fetus. The placenta itself is a temporary organ, but its effects on the life of the fetus as well as the mother are coming to be recognized as extremely important and long-standing after more and more studies are being conducted on the molecular basis of maternal-fetal health. There is a wealth of information available about the evolution, metabolomics, and genomics of the placenta which is now considered central in the mechanism of fetal development and maternal adaptations to pregnancy.

It is always interesting to delve a bit into the basics of biology which establish a link of our understanding of human life as part of the evolutionary story of living beings. We remember that we are part of the group of "mammals" in the animal kingdom. Some interesting trivia about the placenta are given in Box 12.1. which are worth a quick recapitulation at this stage.

Box 12.1: Interesting Trivia About the Human Placenta
- Human beings are "viviparous" mammals—they give birth to their little ones as opposed to "oviparous" animals which lay eggs and hatch them externally. The placenta is the organ which allows in vivo growth of the human fetus.
- Human "placental" tissues include *amnion, chorion, and allantois* which represent the amniotic sac, placenta, and umbilical cord, respectively.
- The placenta is *discoidal* and *hemochorial*.
- The presence of live ectopic pregnancies indicates that *placenta, not uterus, is the critically important factor in maternofetal physiology*.
- The *placenta, though transient, is considered a highly "mutable" organ*. The higher evolution of the placenta in the "eutherian" mammals has enabled an evolutionary advantage leading to differentiation of several taxonomic orders.

© Springer Nature Singapore Pte Ltd. 2022
C. Ratha, A. Khurana, *Fetal Medicine*, https://doi.org/10.1007/978-981-19-6099-4_12

12.1 Evaluation of the Placenta in Pregnancy

The placenta can be evaluated by ultrasound, and the appearance of this organ changes progressively during different stages of pregnancy. Figure 12.1 shows how the placenta appears as a small hyperechoic area near the fetal pole in early pregnancy and gradually develops as a well-defined entity by the end of the first trimester.

In the late first trimester, the size of the placenta in comparison to the uterine cavity is such that it is spread over more than half of the longitudinal axis and hence may appear invariably "low lying" although it may not be a truly placenta previa. It is therefore better not to label the position of the placenta in the first trimester. It suffices to mention "normal appearances" of the placenta in the first trimester unless there are some distinctly disturbing features as shown in Fig. 12.2a, b.

This appearance of small cystic spaces in a bulky placental mass is suggestive of molar changes and warrants a battery of investigations. A highly elevated hCG level in maternal serum corroborates the diagnosis although confirmation is only by histopathological examination of the placenta. Although a complete mole warrants evacuation of the uterus, a partial mole or a coexistent twin fetus with a complete molar pregnancy may present management dilemmas in the pregnancy.

Such pregnancies must be managed in centers with expertise to address all the complications which include fetal aneuploidy, severe fetal growth restriction, early preeclampsia, and invasive mole. Detailed counseling and thorough follow-up is necessary in these cases.

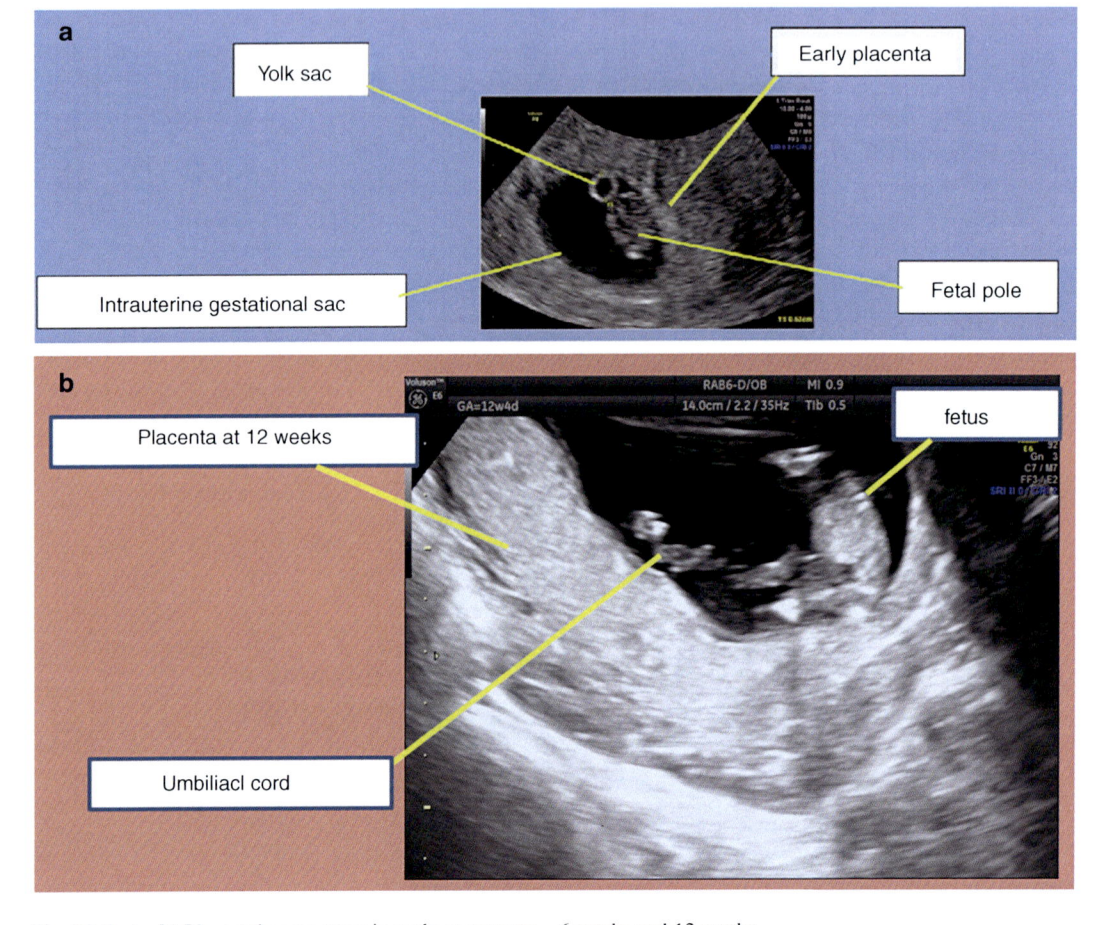

Fig. 12.1 (a, b) Placental appearance in early pregnancy—6 weeks and 12 weeks

12.3 Location and Edges

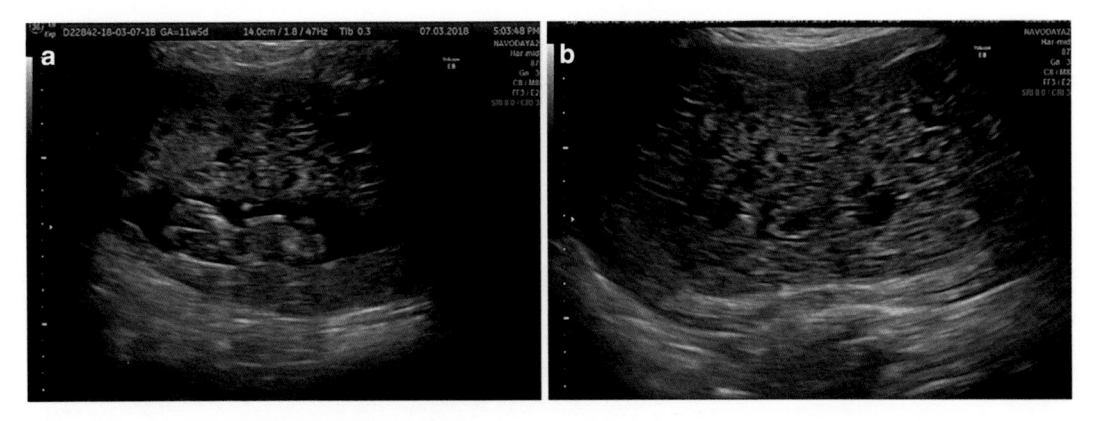

Fig. 12.2 (a) Partial molar placenta. (b) Complete molar placenta

12.2 Placenta in Second Trimester

By the second trimester, the placenta is a well-defined organ seen on ultrasound, and it is imperative that a proper placental evaluation accompanies fetal evaluation during the midtrimester fetal scan. The points to be noted with respect to the placenta and mentioned in the report of a second trimester pregnancy scan are placental location, size, any remarkable morphologic changes, cord insertion, and associated cord issues. "Grading" of the placenta which was done in earlier times is no longer part of placental evaluation.

12.3 Location and Edges

The placenta may be present on the anterior (Fig. 12.3a), posterior (Fig. 12.3b), or lateral walls of the uterus as observed during the scan, and its lower edges must be defined with respect to the internal os of the cervix.

A "low-lying" placenta (Fig. 12.4) is defined as one where the lower edge is seen within 3 cm from the internal os or may even be partially or completely covering it as in placenta previa. A complete placenta previa (Fig. 12.5) is an important diagnosis to make although partial previas and other types of "low-lying" placentae are expected to "move" away from the internal os as the pregnancy progresses due to development of the lower uterine segment. Therefore, these cases need to be reassessed in the third trimester, around 32 weeks, to check the placental location and modify care as needed.

It is important to alert the obstetrician about a low-lying placenta in any case so that a rational follow-up may be maintained. If the lower edge of the placenta is seen clearly on transabdominal scanning, then it is highly reassuring. However, in case of any doubts at all, especially in posterior placentae, a transvaginal assessment must be done in order to correctly assign placental location.

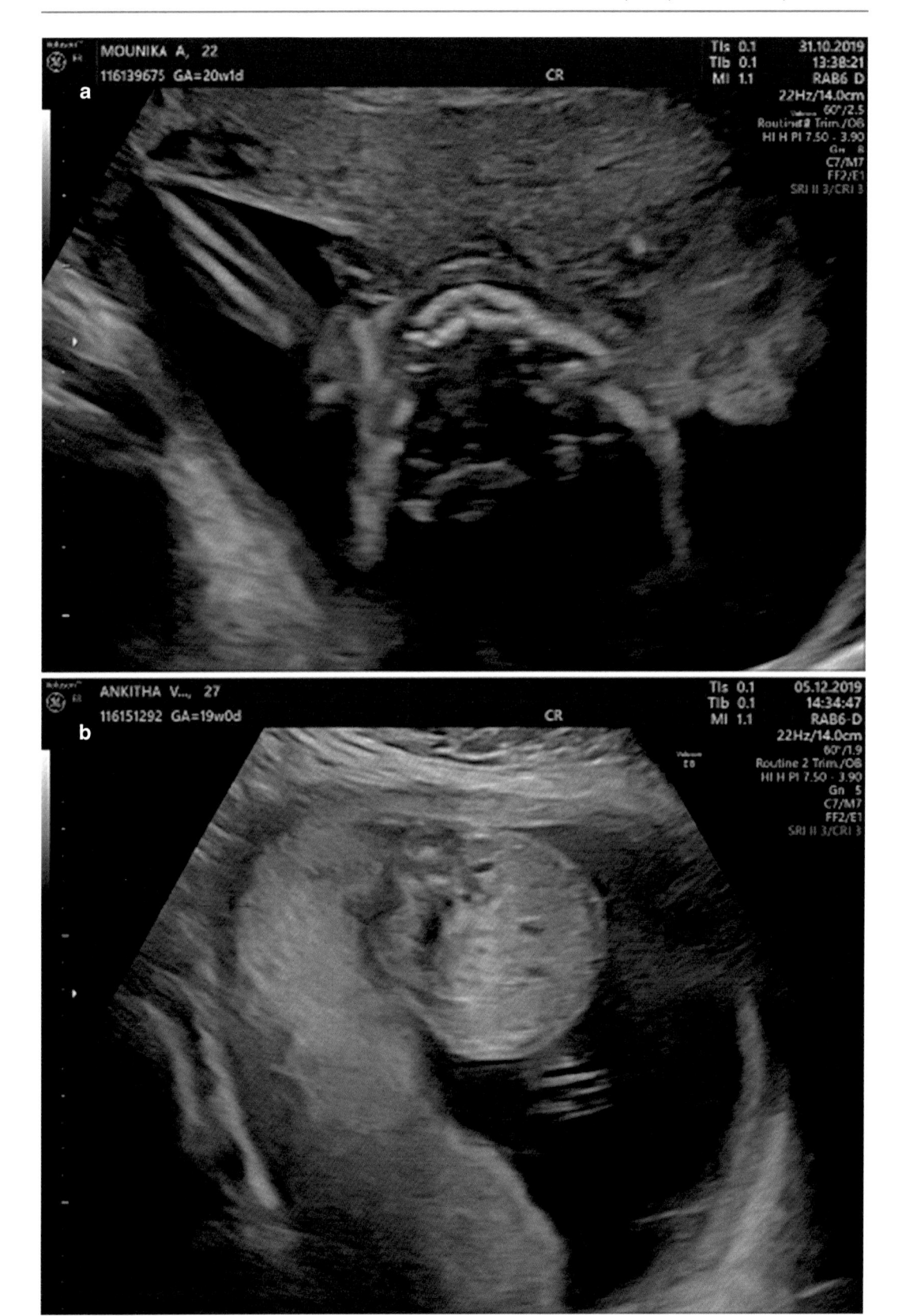

Fig. 12.3 (a) Anterior placenta. (b) Posterior placenta

12.3 Location and Edges

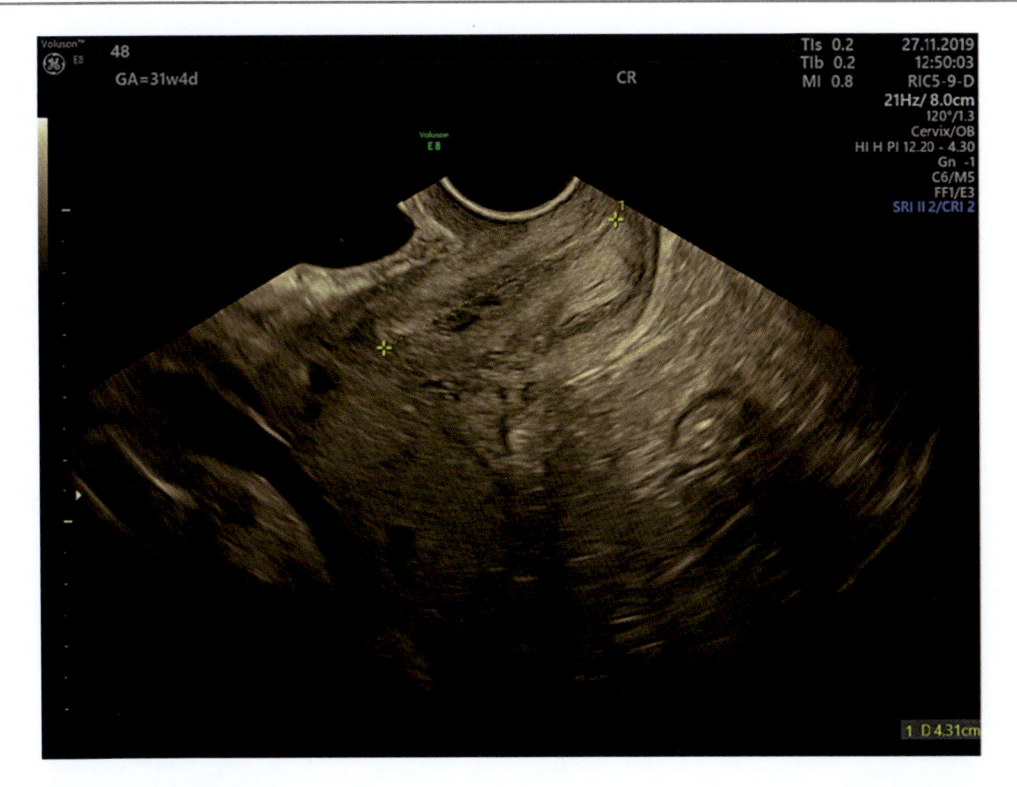

Fig. 12.4 Low-lying placenta

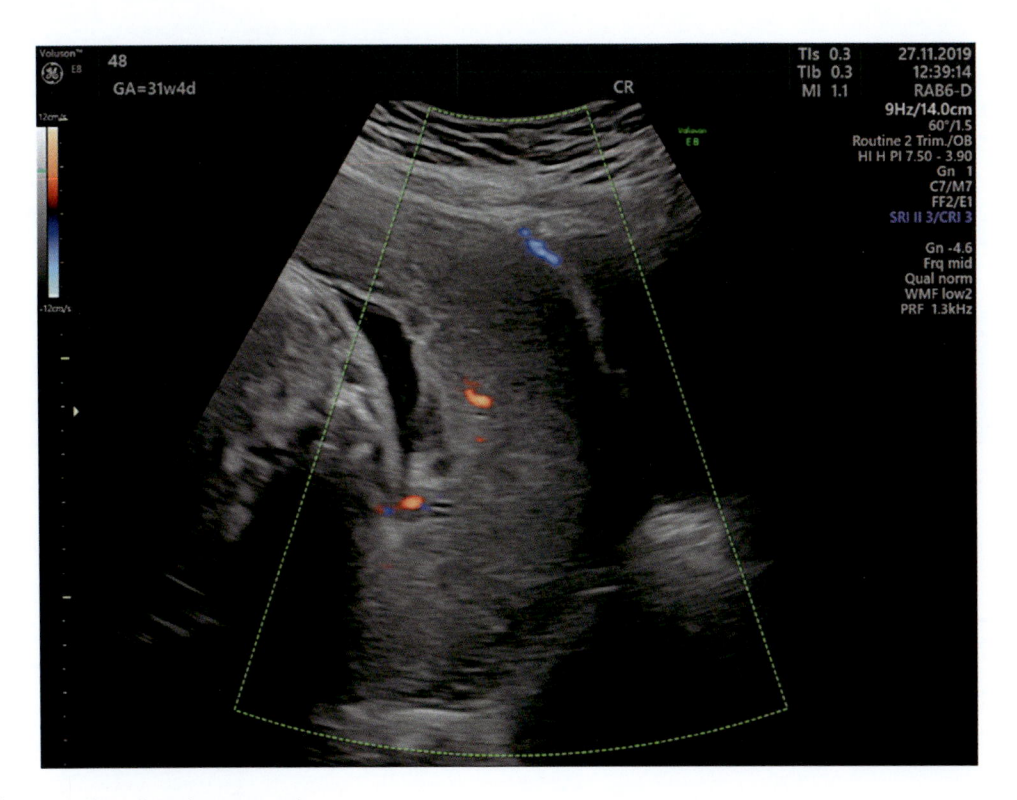

Fig. 12.5 Complete placenta previa

12.4 Size

Assessment of placental size is generally subjective during antenatal ultrasound. The size of the placenta typically correlates with fetal size but there is scope for a large degree of variation too. A relatively large placenta for birth weight may indicate that the placenta was compensating for inefficient transport mechanisms due to defects at the cellular level. However, a small placenta also indicates restriction in provision of nutrients to the fetus. A review of literature reveals that both low and high placental weight with respect to fetal weight are associated with fetal growth restriction and even have been correlated to later hypertension and cardiovascular disease.

When the thickness of the placenta is more than 5 cm, it is classified as a "large placenta" (Fig. 12.6). Such large placentae are commonly seen in cases of fetal hydrops, intrauterine infections, fetal anemia, or maternal diabetes. If all such associations are ruled out, it may be a physiological variant too.

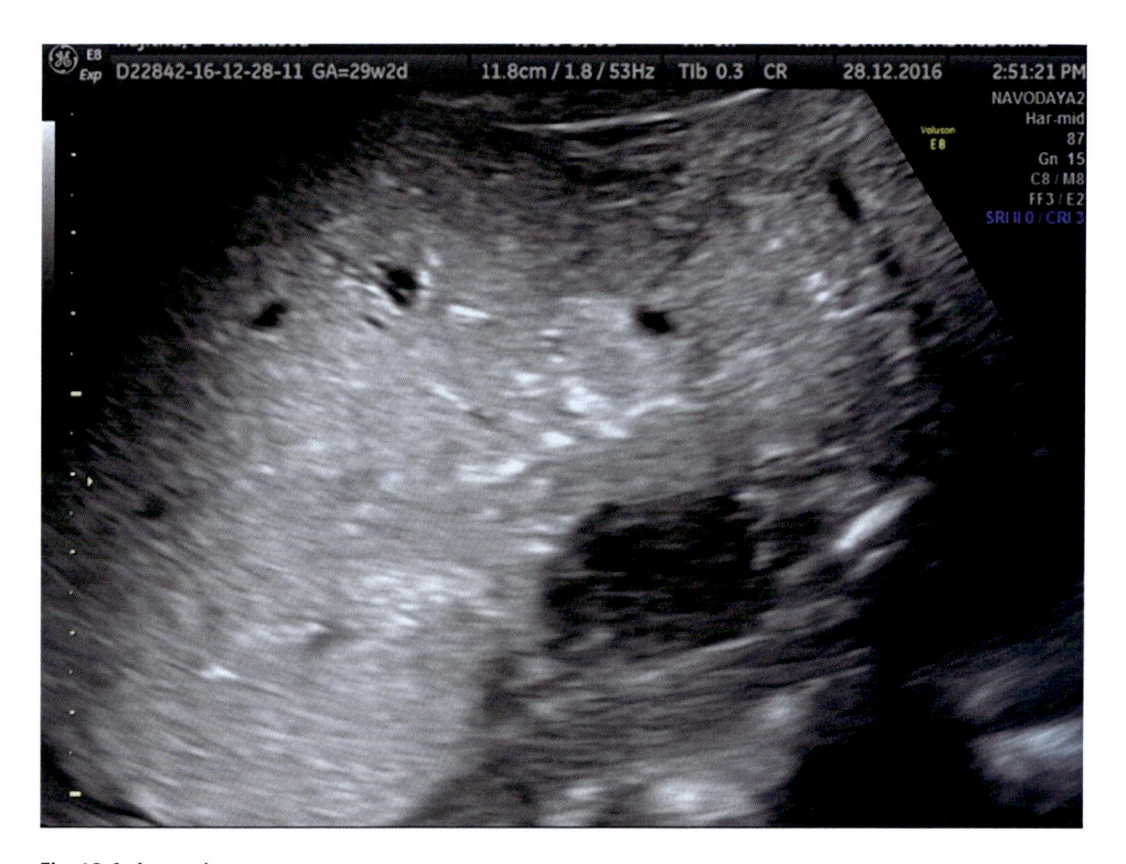

Fig. 12.6 Large placenta

12.5 Morphology of the Placenta

The "normal" appearance of the placenta has been discussed in an earlier section, and we will delve a bit into the details of the structural evaluation of a placenta during the midtrimester scan (Fig. 12.7).

The distinct, hypoechoic basal layer is indicative of a normal interface in the myometrium, whereas absence of this layer beneath the placenta raises the possibility of morbid adherence. Presence of placental lakes, obvious "dropout areas" in uterine myometrium, and vascular connections across the myometrio-chorial interface are factors corroborating the diagnosis of morbidly adherent placenta. The common risk factors for morbid adherence are cases with previous uterine surgery or scars (caesarean sections, transcavitary myomectomy or curettage, etc.) and low-lying placentae. In low-lying placentae, a thorough assessment of the vesicouterine interface should be done to look for these signs, and color Doppler (Fig. 12.8a–d) with multiplanar imaging can help in such assessment.

Based on the above factors, recently, an ultrasound-based classification of placenta accreta spectrum (PAS) has been suggested (Ref: Cali et al.) which appears to be feasible and also correlates with the severity of adverse clinical outcomes as the stage progresses. Table 12.1 lists the different features of the progressive stages of PAS (0–3).

Whenever morbid adherence is suspected, it is prudent to alert the obstetrician to be prepared during the process of delivery anticipating risks and the need for added interventions. MRI has been suggested by some authors to aid in the ultrasound diagnosis of morbid adherence, but the sensitivity of both is limited by multiple factors and hence it is better to be prepared for clinical emergencies in such cases.

Some other placental conditions encountered in clinical practice that can be diagnosed on antenatal ultrasound are chorangiomas (Fig. 12.9) and placental cysts (Fig. 12.10).

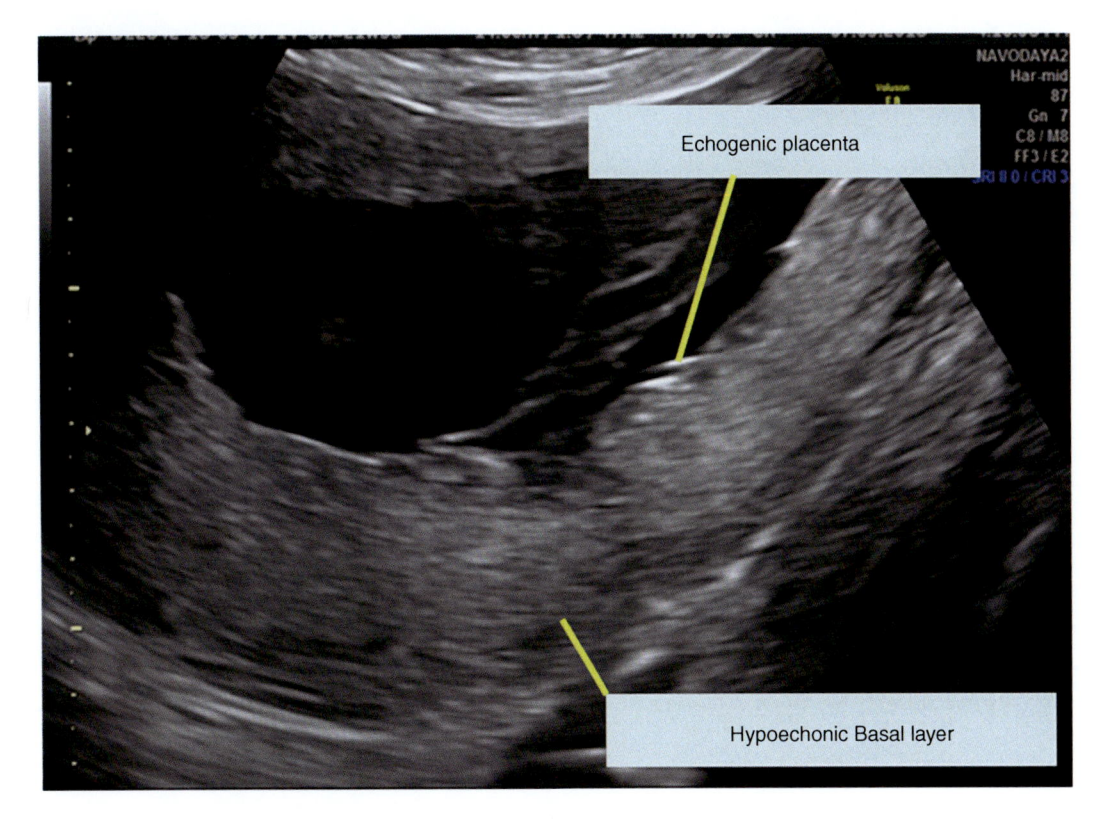

Fig. 12.7 Normal placental morphology

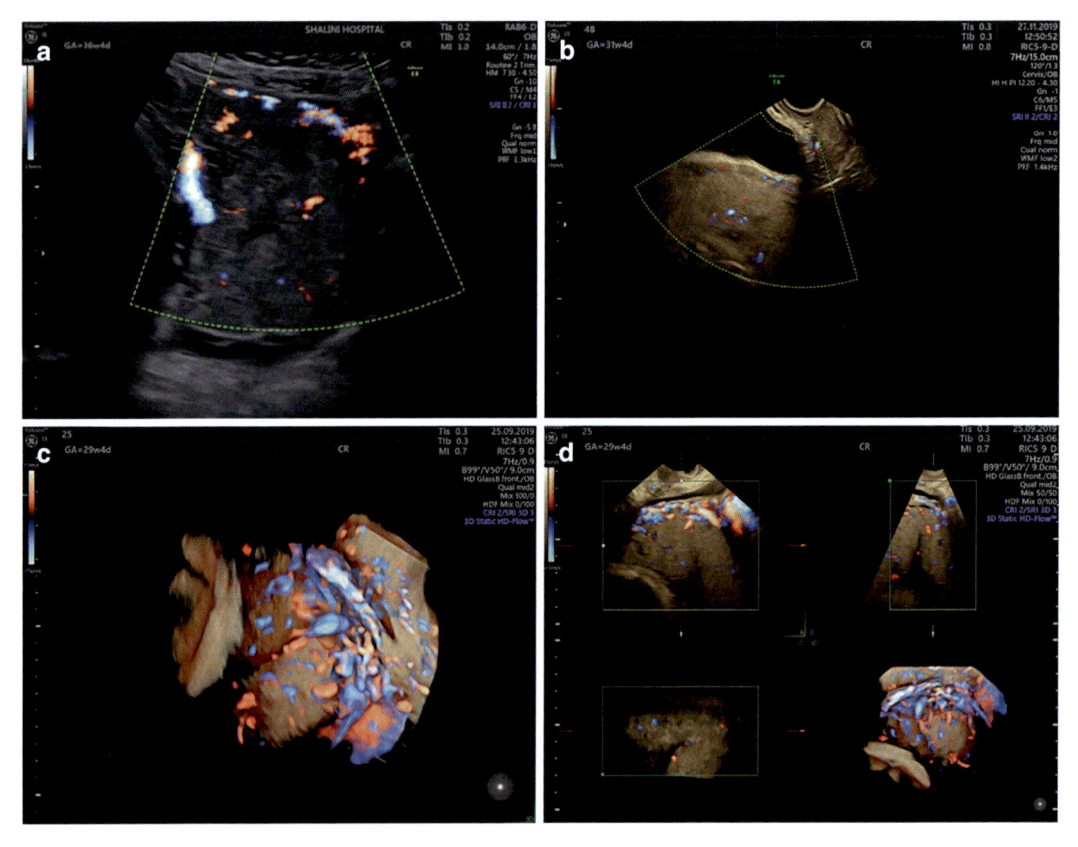

Fig. 12.8 (a–d) Assessment of placenta to rule out morbid adherence

Table 12.1 USG-based classification of PAS (Ref: Cali et al. Prenatal Ultrasound Staging System for Placenta Accreta Spectrum Disorders. Ultrasound Obstet Gynecol. 2019 Jun;53(6):752–760)

PAS0	Placenta previa with no US signs of invasion or placenta previa with placental lacunae but no evidence of abnormal uterine-bladder interface
PAS1	Presence of at least two ultrasound signs among placental lacunae, loss of the clear zone, or bladder wall interruption
PAS2	PAS1 + uterovesical hypervascularity
PAS3	PAS1/PAS2 + evidence of increased vascularity in the inferior part of the lower uterine segment potentially extending in the parametrial region

While placental cysts are relatively benign, chorangiomas either can be asymptomatic or may contribute to hyperdynamic circulation in the fetus leading to polyhydramnios and a risk of fetal hydrops necessitating interventions like occluding its feeding vessel to stop its growth and effects.

Sometimes, echogenic rims are seen lining the placental cotyledons (Fig. 12.10), and this is considered as a sign of placental ageing by some authors in the literature of yester years. Now it is known that such appearance of placenta does not directly correlate with clinical outcomes, and hence clinical decision-making based on these placental appearances is not recommended.

12.5 Morphology of the Placenta

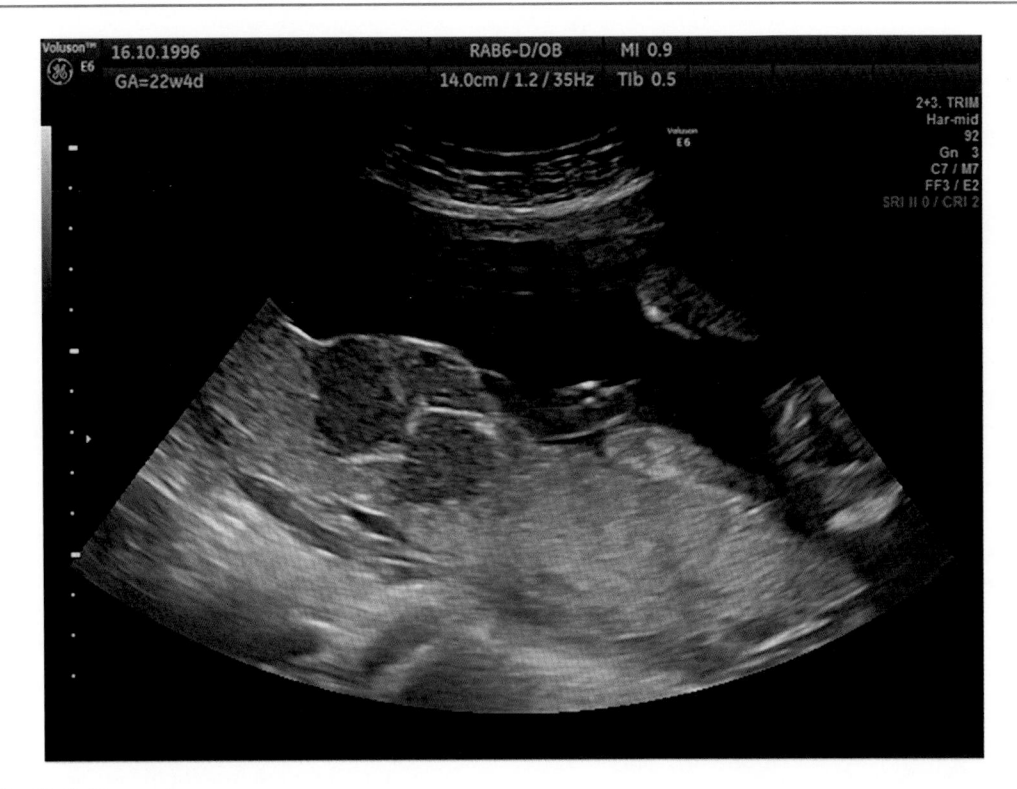

Fig. 12.9 Chorangioma

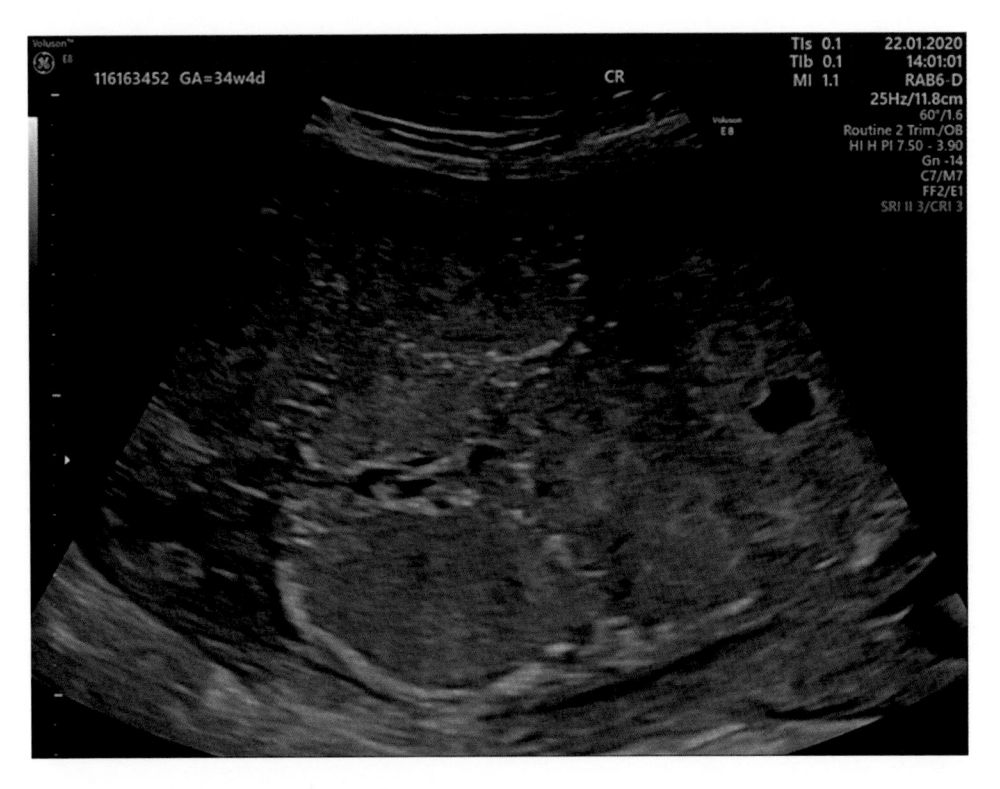

Fig. 12.10 Echogenic rims in placental cotyledons

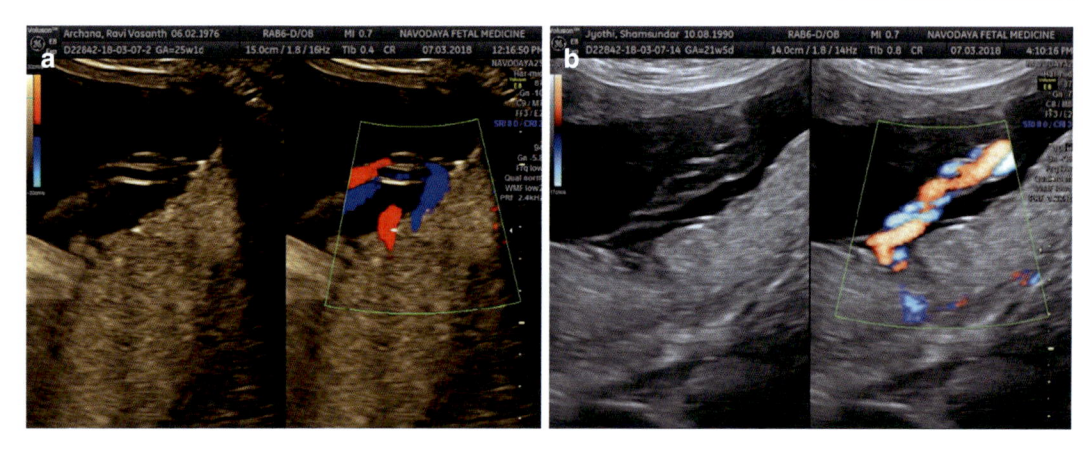

Fig. 12.11 Marginal cord insertion (**a**) as compared to central insertion (**b**)

12.6 Umbilical Cord Insertion

Umbilical cord insertion site on the placenta also must be checked as part of the placental evaluation because the insertion site has clinical significance. The site of cord insertion can be investigated by making a transverse sweep across the uterine cavity from the fetus toward the placenta. Majority of placentae (90–91%) have a "central" or eccentric cord insertion. There may be abnormalities like marginal (7%) or velamentous (1–2%) insertions which are associated with high risk for poor fetal outcomes (Fig. 12.11). Marginal insertion is defined as the cord inserted less than 2 cm away from an edge of the placenta, while velamentous insertion is defined as insertion of the cord in the membranes rather than the bulk of the placenta.

12.7 Assessment of Umbilical Cord Morphology

The assessment of the structure of the umbilical cord is also important along with its insertion site. This umbilical cord is the only connection between the mother and the fetus and allows for transport of oxygen, nutrients, and metabolites. The length and flexibility of the umbilical cord make it possible for the fetus to move freely in the amniotic cavity while maintaining its nutrition and other functions. This free movement is necessary for optimum psychomotor development of the fetus. The length of the normal umbilical cord is anything between 50 and 75 cm, but it is difficult to assess the exact length—especially in long cords. Very short umbilical cords may be suspected if the fetus is not freely moving at around the uterine cavity, and this is sometimes seen with body stalk anomalies.

The normal umbilical cord of the fetus has three vessels—two umbilical arteries and one umbilical vein. Usually, the left umbilical vein remains patent throughout fetal life, while the right umbilical vein naturally regresses by the seventh week of gestation.

The normal umbilical cord configuration is seen either by using color flow across the transverse section of lower abdomen demonstrating two perivesical umbilical arteries (Fig. 12.12) or as a transverse section of the free loop of the cord (Fig. 12.13) demonstrating the "Mickey mouse" sign.

12.7 Assessment of Umbilical Cord Morphology

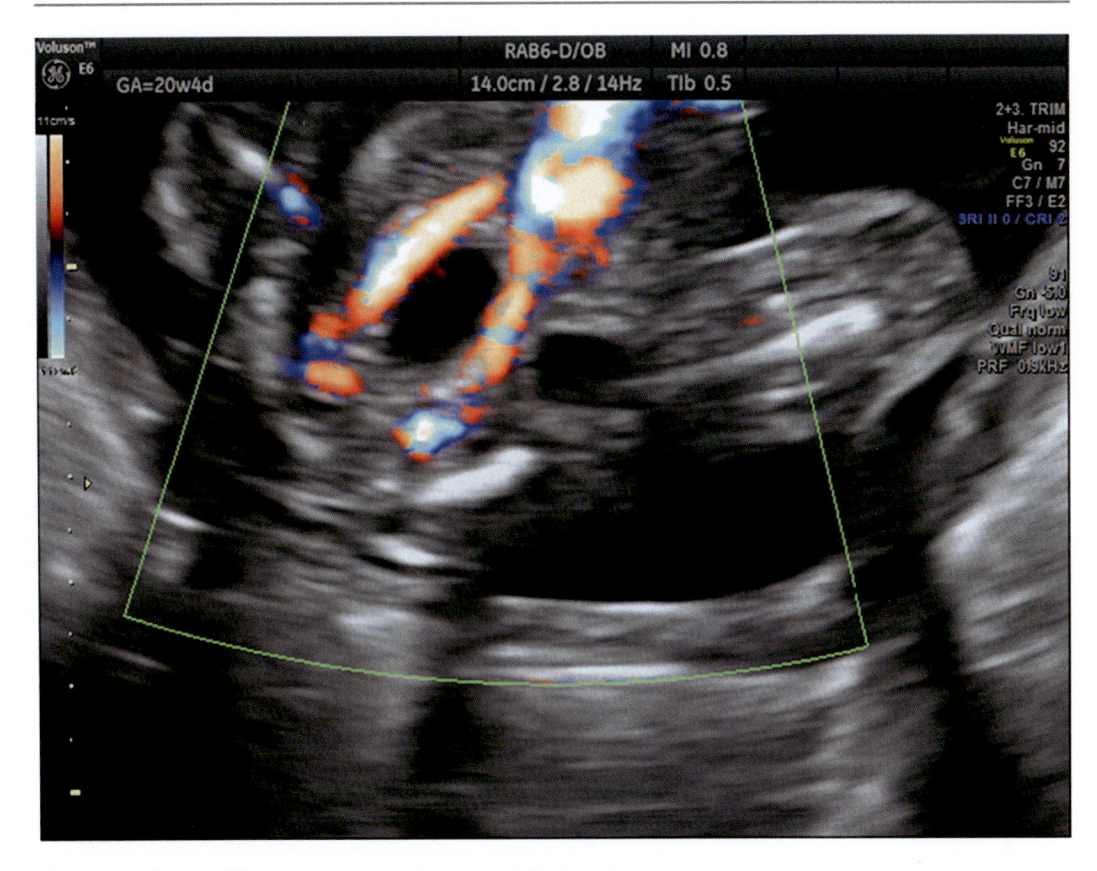

Fig. 12.12 Two umbilical arteries continuing into umbilical cord

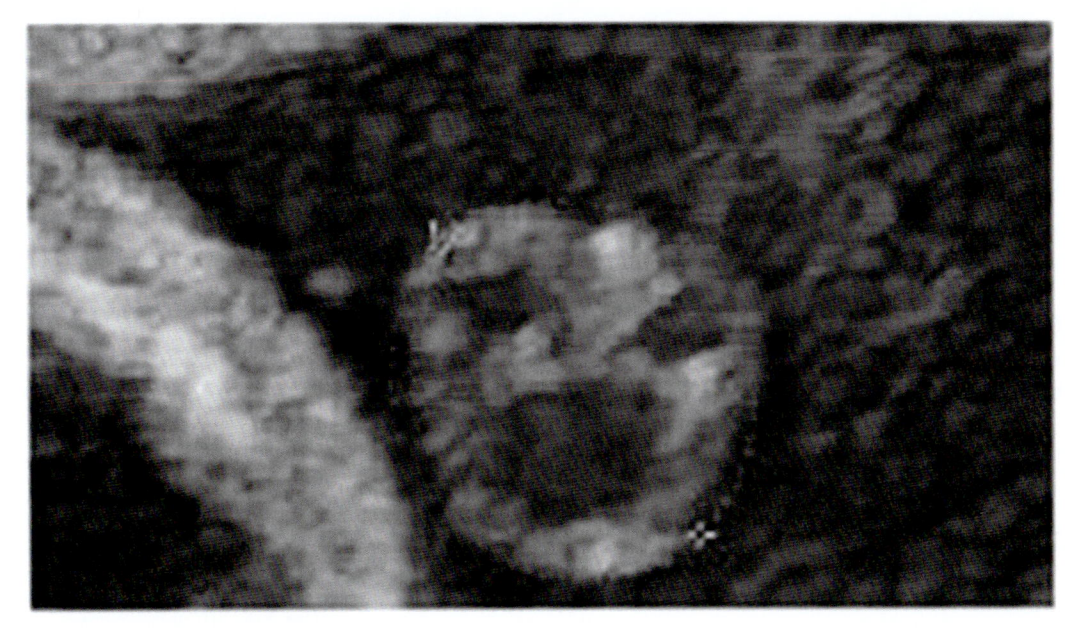

Fig. 12.13 Mickey mouse sign

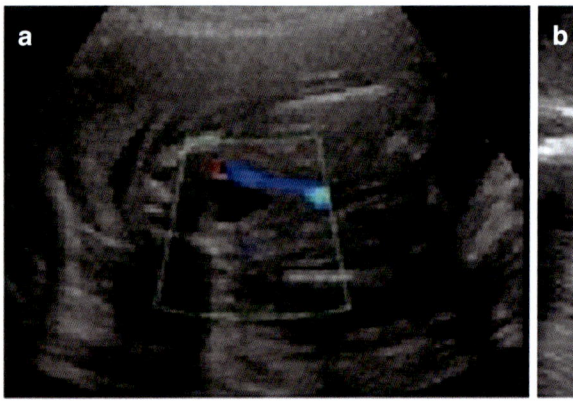

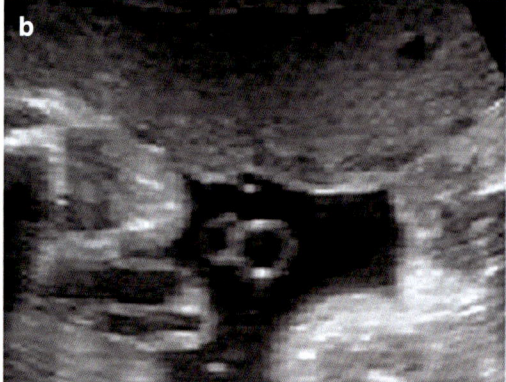

Fig. 12.14 (a, b) SUA

12.8 Single Umbilical Artery

Umbilical cord abnormalities can have important prognostic implications for perinatal outcome. One of the common abnormalities is the finding of a single umbilical artery (SUA) whereby the cord has only two vessels—one artery and one vein. The reported incidence of SUA varies from 0.5% at the time of second trimester prenatal ultrasound and in umbilical cord specimens from live-born infants to 2.1% in fetal deaths, autopsies, or aborted fetuses.

The cause of a SUA could be either a primary agenesis or a secondary thrombotic atrophy of one umbilical artery or the persistence of the original single allantoic artery of the body stalk. Depending on the cause, the prognosis would vary, but it is not realistically possible to definitively establish this cause during antenatal scans.

The diagnosis of SUA is based on the findings of the perivesical view revealing only one patent vessel or two lumens seen on transverse section of the cord (Fig. 12.14a–b).

Diagnosis of a single umbilical artery (SUA) leads to a lot of anxiety, but it is important to remember that is most commonly (70%) a normal variant unless proved otherwise. SUA is an indication to ensure that there are no other associated structural anomalies (30%) as it may be associated with multisystem abnormalities of the VACTERL group and those associated with trisomy 18. SUA is also associated with a risk of SGA fetus and hence warrants serial growth follow-up. Once all of the above are sorted, parents can be reassured that majority of the babies with SUA will have a normal antenatal course and a good postnatal outcome.

12.9 Persistent Right Umbilical Vein

This happens rarely and is seen in 0.08–0.5% cases. The diagnosis of persistent right umbilical vein (PRUV) is tricky as the umbilical cord on cross section has three vessels and the two arteries are demonstrated perivesically in the normal manner. However, the clincher for diagnosis is to notice the course of the umbilical vein intraabdominally—it curves toward the stomach in the transverse abdominal view instead of curving away from the stomach (Fig. 12.15).

The extrahepatic PRUV has a poorer prognosis as it is often associated with absent DV leading to high risk of fetal hydrops. The intrahepatic PRUV may have a fairly good prognosis (Fig. 12.16).

Other umbilical cord abnormalities like cord cysts (Fig. 12.17) and umbilical vein varices may be seen on antenatal ultrasound.

Problems like true knots (Fig. 12.18) are commonly evident only after delivery in most cases as detection of true knots in utero is more of a chance finding and practically one cannot interrogate the

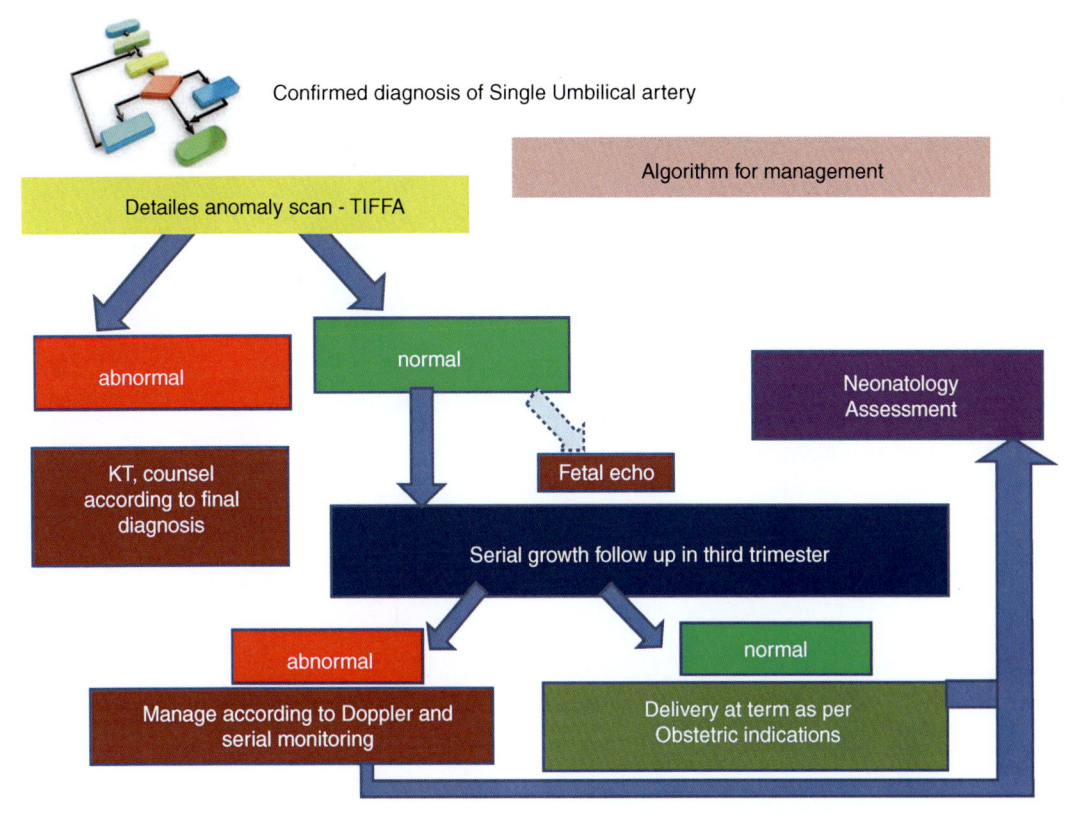

Fig. 12.15 Algorithm for follow up after diagnosis of single umbilical artery

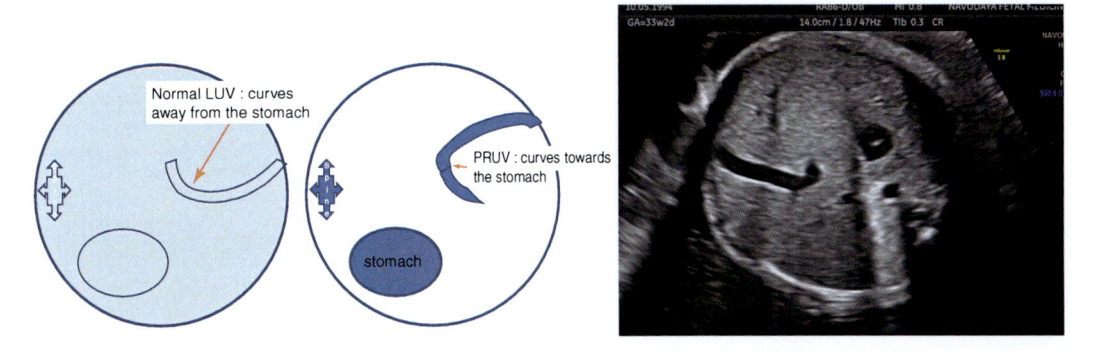

Fig. 12.16 PRUV

entire length of the umbilical cord in all cases, at all gestations. Most of the times, knots in the cord are incidental diagnoses and may be missed despite regular scans if the affected part of the cord is not in the visual field of the operator.

Another aspect commonly associated with umbilical cord anatomy is the degree of coiling—hyper- or hypocoiling. The cord "coiling index" remains a rather subjective and debatable entity, and literature is divided on whether umbilical cord coiling is a cause or effect of fetal problems.

In addition to all the above findings is the incidental finding of a "nuchal cord"—a loop of cord either around or across the fetal neck. This is just an observation and should not be the sole guide decisions regarding delivery. This is considered a

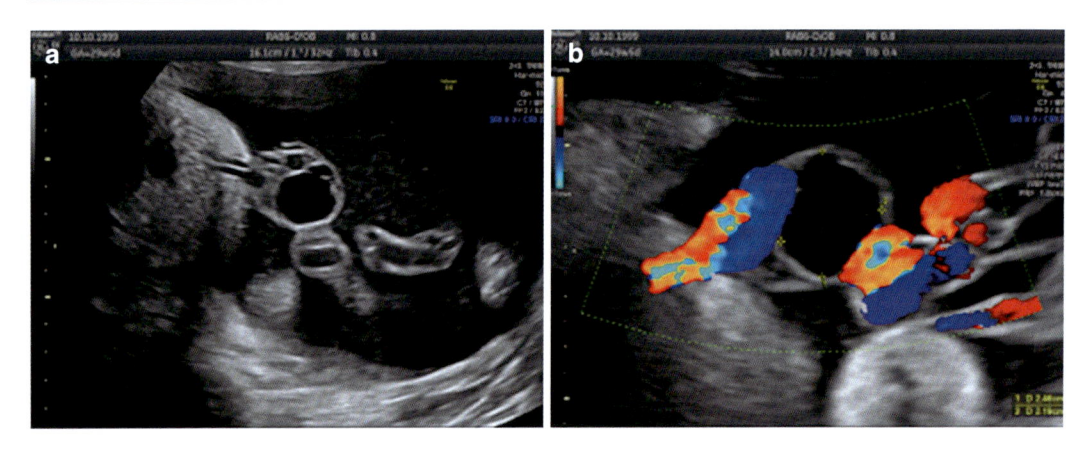

Fig. 12.17 Umbilical cord cyst: (**a**) gray scale, (**b**) color Doppler

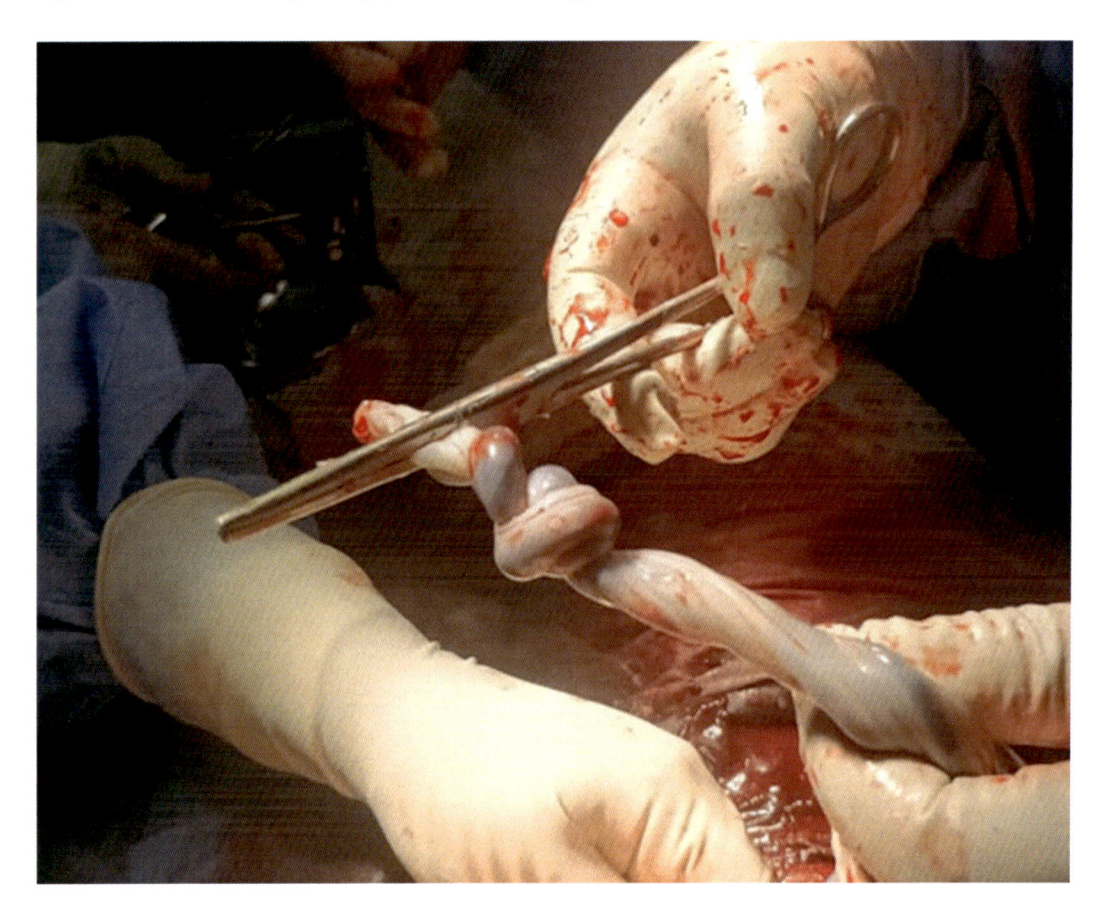

Fig. 12.18 True knot in umbilical cord discovered after delivery

normal variation in the cord position—it may slip off or may cause tightening in labor which will anyway be detected as fetal heart rate pattern abnormalities during intrapartum monitoring and then the decisions to deliver may be justified.

The examination of the umbilical cord is an important part of fetal ultrasound, and the detection of cord abnormalities should prompt a thorough fetal examination as these conditions could result in fetal growth restriction and even fetal death. Early diagnosis and surveillance can minimize fetal mortality and help make decisions. The isolated cord abnormalities generally have a good prognosis.

12.10 Amniotic Fluid

Amniotic fluid is the liquor in the amniotic cavity which provides spaces, buoyancy, mechanical cushioning, and temperature maintenance of the fetal environment. In early pregnancy, most of the amniotic fluid is formed by the placenta and its membranes, while after 16 weeks of gestation, the fetal urine becomes a major contributor. Assessment of amniotic fluid levels is part of every fetal assessment. In the first trimester, the assessment is rather subjective, but in the second half of pregnancy, a quantitative amniotic fluid assessment can be made based on either a "single deepest pool" (Fig. 12.19) or a four-quadrant amniotic fluid index (Fig. 12.20).

Both methods are acceptable methods of assessing amniotic fluid but it is important that the normal values be adjusted based on the method used.

The normal range of AFI based on SDP is 2–8 cm while that on 4Q AFI is 5–25 cm. Values less than normal are called "oligoamnios" (Fig. 12.21) and more than normal is known as "polyamnios".

The common causes of oligoamnios are hypoperfusion of fetal kidneys due to fetal growth restriction or fetal anomalies like bilateral renal agenesis or donor twin in TTTS. Polyamnios on the other hand may be due to fetal, maternal, or placental causes. Fetal anomalies like open neural tube defects, cleft lip and/or palate, anterior abdominal wall defects, and neuromuscular disorders leading to fetal akinesia, fetal GI obstructions, fetal anemia, or recipient twin in TTTS may have polyamnios. Maternal factors like hyperglycemia due to uncontrolled diabetes and placental chorangiomas can cause polyamnios.

With this background, it may be understood that reporting only "oligoamnios" or "polyamnios" in an antenatal scan leaves scope for a lot more information pertaining to the suggested cause of these problems. It is therefore imperative on the reporter to make a note of fetal anatomy, placental morphology, and possibility of

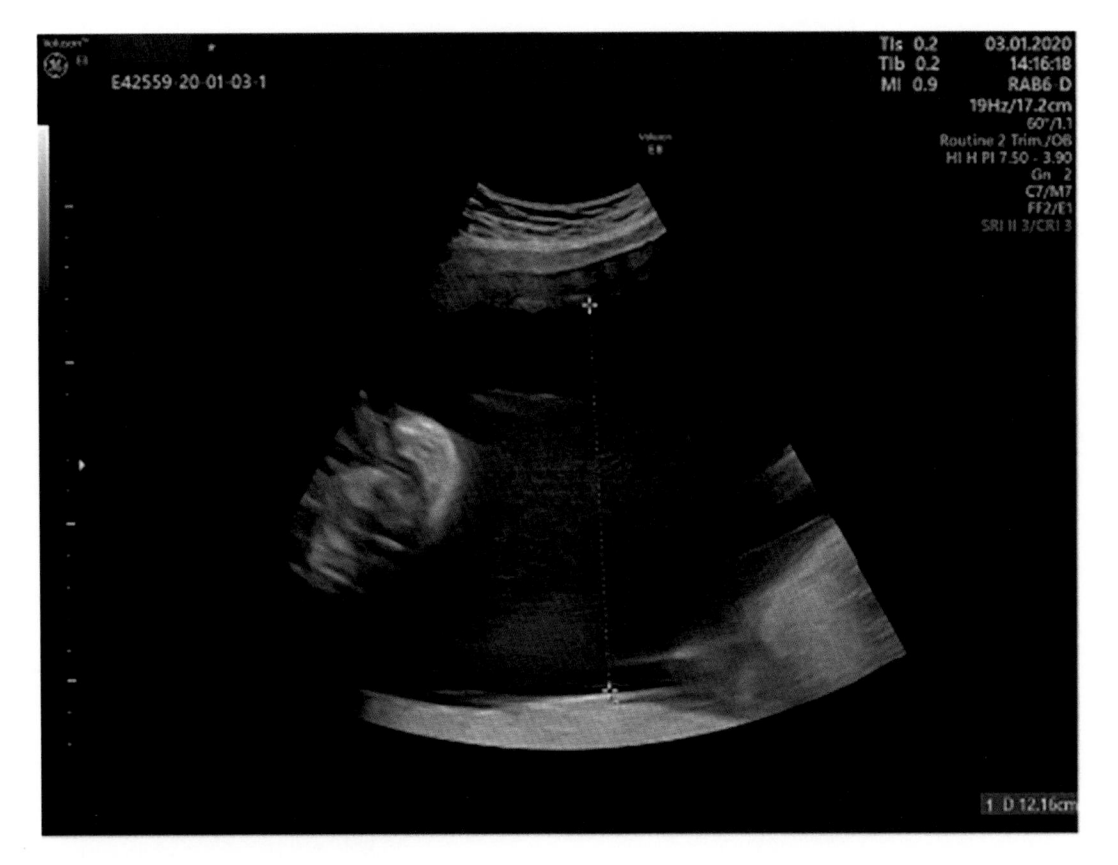

Fig. 12.19 SDP

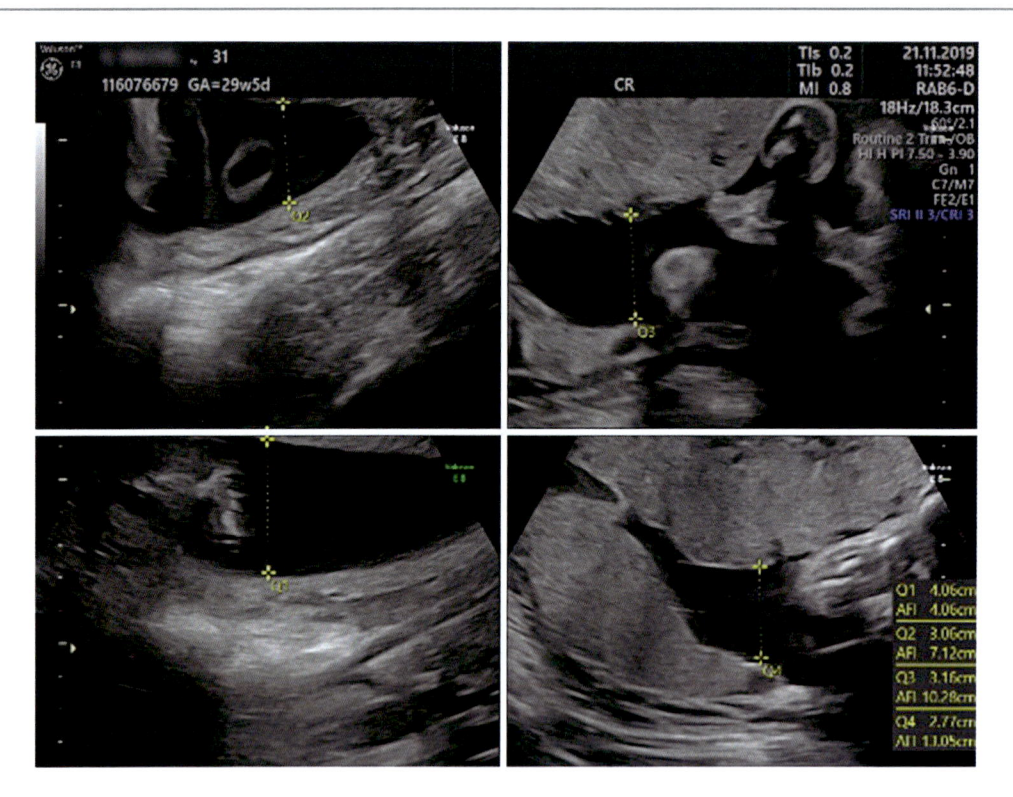

Fig. 12.20 4Q AFI

No measurable liquor pocket

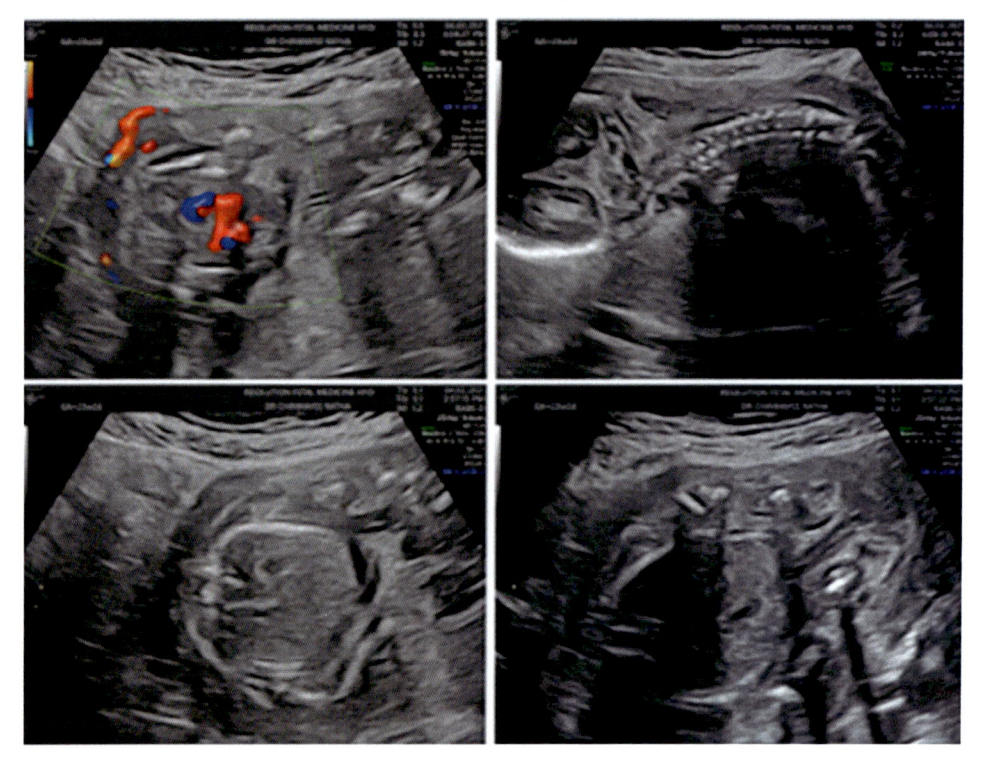

Fig. 12.21 Severe oligoamnios

fetal growth restriction or hypoperfusion or even macrosomia to indicate any plausible etiological conditions. In an average grown fetus with no other associated features as described above, mild liquor disturbances may be physiological.

However, even when unexplained, severe oligoamnios or polyamnios could be potentially lethal. Severe oligo leads to postural limb defects and pulmonary hypoplasia, while severe poly puts the fetus at risk of preterm birth along with maternal health risks due to overdistension of the uterus. Such cases have to be dealt with by a dedicated maternal-fetal medicine team of experts with adequate investigations, counseling, and follow-up.

12.11 Assessment of Cervix

The length and integrity of the maternal cervix are important determinants of in utero safety of the pregnancy. A short cervix places the woman at a high risk of preterm birth. Cervical assessment is done most accurately by the transvaginal method with a high frequency (5 MHz). By gently placing the probe in the anterior vaginal fornix, a sagittal view of the cervix is obtained (Fig. 12.22).

The internal os, external os, cervical canal, and endocervical mucosa are identified without exerting undue pressure on the cervix with the probe because this will falsely elongate the cervix.

Sometimes, one may find a short cervix (Fig. 12.23) with or without funneling of membranes. A cervical length of less than 25 mm at 24 weeks on TVS in singleton pregnancy increases the risk of preterm birth by sixfold and the risk escalates with the degree of shortness.

Cervical funneling may add to the risk and funneling is progressively seen, characterized by the appearance of membranes at the level of internal os resembling the alphabets—Y, V, and U (Fig. 12.24a–c), respectively.

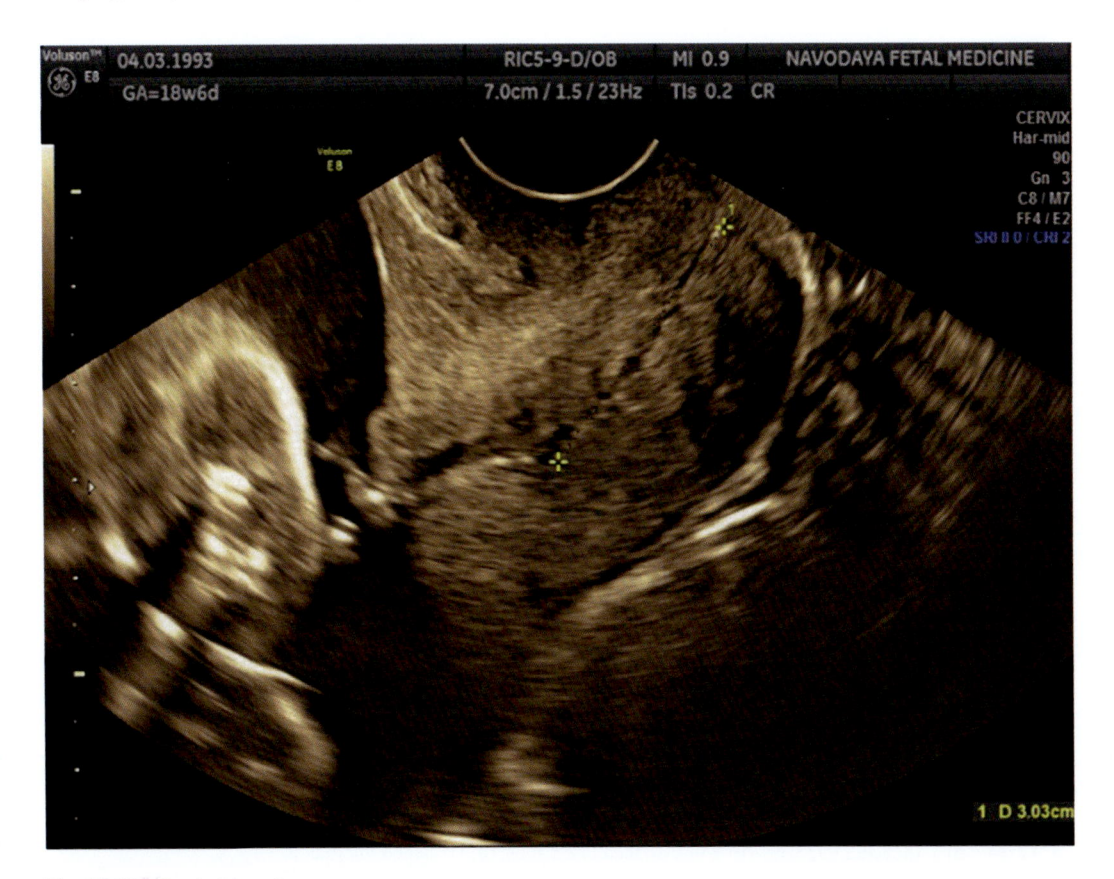

Fig. 12.22 Cervical length

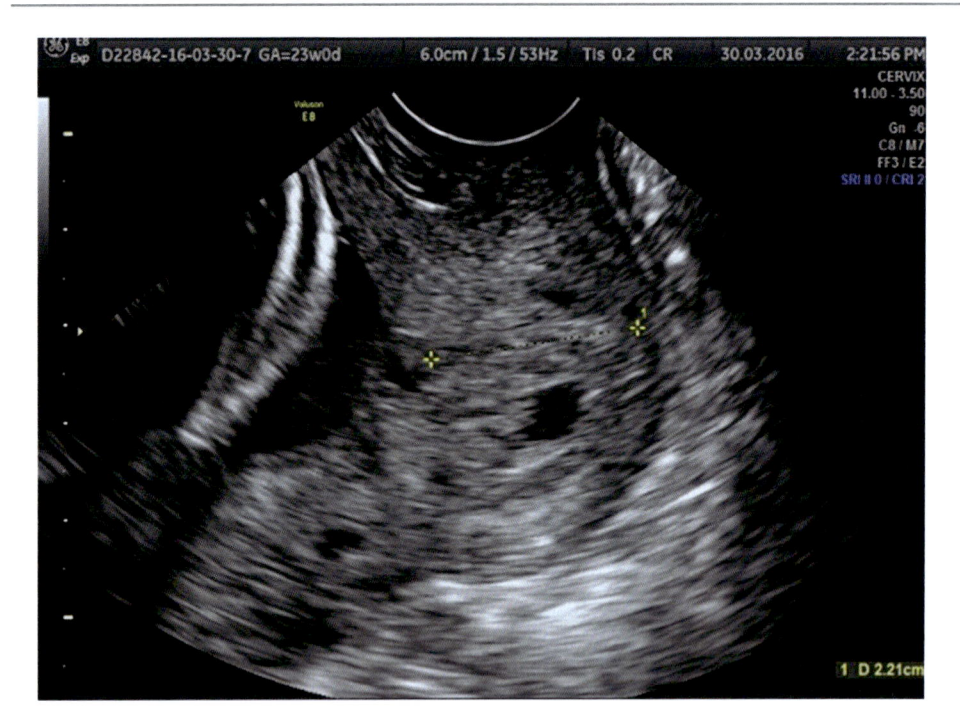

Fig. 12.23 Short cervix without funneling

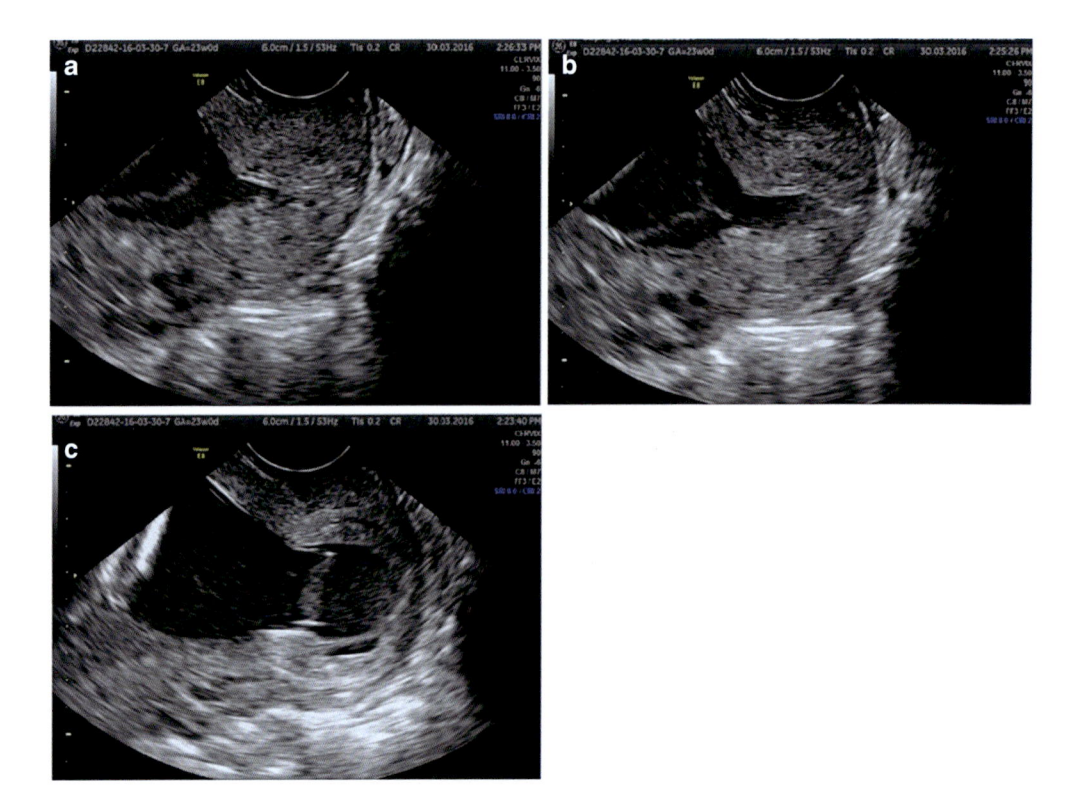

Fig. 12.24 (**a**) Y-shaped internal os. (**b**) 24b V-shaped internal os. (**c**) U-shaped internal os

Key Learning Points in Placenta, Cervix, and Cord Issues

1. Evaluation of the placenta is vital to prognosticating pregnancy outcome—at every stage of pregnancy, there are objective methods of evaluating the placenta, and these features should be included in the obstetric scan report.
2. Placental position and signs of morbid adherence must be noted during all obstetric scans.
3. Umbilical cord variations and anomalies add information that can alter the prognosis and follow-up protocol in pregnancy.
4. Amniotic fluid assessment can be done objectively in the second half of pregnancy, and liquor abnormalities are associated with adverse pregnancy outcomes.
5. Cervical length by TVS is an important predictor of preterm birth.

Suggested Reading

Baergen RN. Pathology of the umbilical cord, in manual of pathology of the human placenta. 2nd ed. New York: Springer; 2011.

Cali, et al. Prenatal ultrasound staging system for placenta Accreta Spectrum disorders. Ultrasound Obstet Gynecol. 2019 Jun;53(6):752–60.

Cervical assessment guidelines as given in the website of the Fetal Medicine Foundation, UK. www.fmf.org.

Desforges, et al. Placental nutrient supply and fetal growth. Int J Dev Biol. 2010;54(2–3):377–90.

Jansson, et al. Role of the placenta in fetal programming: underlying mechanisms and potential interventional approaches. Clin Sci (Lond). 2007;113(1):1–13.

Basics of Genetics in Fetal Medicine

13

Genetics is the study of hereditary characteristics which are passed from one generation to another through genes. With growing understanding of the human genome, a lot has been deciphered of what was once considered a mystery. Yet, while this rapid expansion of knowledge and technology in genetics has helped us become better equipped with information to answer many clinical questions, it is the same ever-progressing science that makes us feel inadequate time and again as clinicians. There is a constant need to update oneself and more importantly, the developments in the science of genetics have taught us that expression of genes is different from mere presence of genes, and thus the actual answers are at much more complex levels than what appear at the surface.

In short, genetics intimidates the average ObGyn clinician, and yet without a basic understanding of genetics, one cannot hope to practice meaningful fetal medicine. This chapter in this book therefore aims at providing an "insight into genetics" to practitioners in ObGyn and fetal medicine. The description here is nowhere close be "complete" or "sufficient" as the field of genetics is unimaginably wide but the information given here is definitely "necessary" because without understanding these fundamental concepts, one cannot hope to address any genetic query from patients. Most clinicians find it difficult to comprehend the contemporary technical genetic jargon of genetic tests, and there is a need for overcoming this apprehension by connecting each concept to its basics. In this chapter, these genetic concepts have been presented in a simplified language as important points to facilitate such understanding.

For a start, we are aware that "genes" are carriers of information that describe or define our characteristics.

- Genes are strands of DNA (deoxyribonucleic acid) which carry information regarding which proteins will be formed in the body, and the flow of biological information is thus maintained in the sequence DNA → RNA → protein. If the information on the gene is wrong, the wrong protein will be formed and will lead to wrong functions.
- Chromosomes are structures that carry many genes. In fact, it may be appropriate to say that genes are "packed" into chromosomes so that their transfer from one cell to another can happen at the time of cell division.
- The number of chromosomes in a cell of an organism is specific and fixed for that species. As human beings, we have 46 chromosomes in our cells—23 pairs (22 autosomes and 1 pair of sex chromosomes—XX in female, XY in male). A depiction of all the chromosomes in the cell is known as karyotype. A karyotype is obtained from culture of amniocytes which allows these cells to multiply by mitosis. The culture is then arrested and the chromosomes are studied in "metaphase" after staining with "Giemsa" stain that causes a banding pattern

© Springer Nature Singapore Pte Ltd. 2022
C. Ratha, A. Khurana, *Fetal Medicine*, https://doi.org/10.1007/978-981-19-6099-4_13

known as G-banding. Individual chromosomes are identified and placed on the karyogram in descending order of size from chromosome pairs 1 to 23. The standard turnaround time for karyotyping on amniotic fluid samples is about 2–3 weeks.

Figure 13.1 shows a normal human karyotype obtained from the culture of amniocytes. Twenty-two autosomes are shown in pairs, while the 23rd pair depicting the sex chromosomes is hidden in concordance with the PCPNDT Act in India which prevents prenatal sex determination.

- Any abnormality in the "number" of chromosomes is called "aneuploidy" (Fig. 13.2). This may be a single chromosome being extra (trisomy, e.g., Down syndrome is "trisomy 21" as there are three chromosomes instead of the normal two in the 21st pair) or absent (monosomy, e.g., Turner's syndrome is seen when one X chromosome is missing). When an entire extra set of chromosomes is present, the condition is termed as "triploidy."
- Structural aberrations in chromosomes may be "deletions," "duplications," or "translocation" of certain regions. Deletions or duplications will affect the genes present in that region of the chromosome and hence will usually have significant impact on phenotype.
- Translocation means that a portion of one chromosome is detached and reattached to another chromosome (Fig. 13.3). Translocations may be "balanced" when there is no net loss or gain of chromosomal material or "unbalanced." Balanced translocations are usually compatible with a normal phenotype although carriers of such translocations may produce gametes carrying "unbalanced" chromosomal material, thus leading to adverse fetal outcomes like miscarriages or fetal abnormalities.
- There may sometimes be a "deletion" or "duplication" or "inversion" of a part of the chromosome, and this in turn can lead to a defect in the formation of proteins if these problems affect the area of the chromosome which carries the genes responsible for specific protein formation.
- In some cases, more than one cell lines may be detected and this is called "mosaicism," e.g., a certain percentage of cells may be euploid, while some cells may be aneuploid in the same fetus. Mosaicism poses a challenge in counseling as the phenotype may differ, and it is difficult to predict the severity of the affliction based on mere numbers. Such counseling should be done in consultation with a clinical geneticist who can help the parents arrive at an

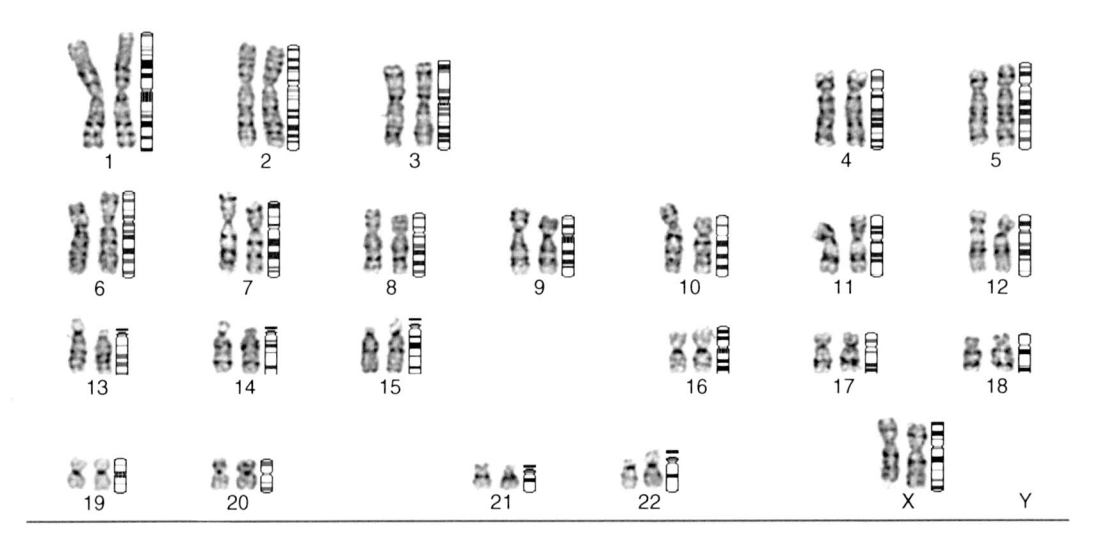

Fig. 13.1 Normal karyotype

13 Basics of Genetics in Fetal Medicine

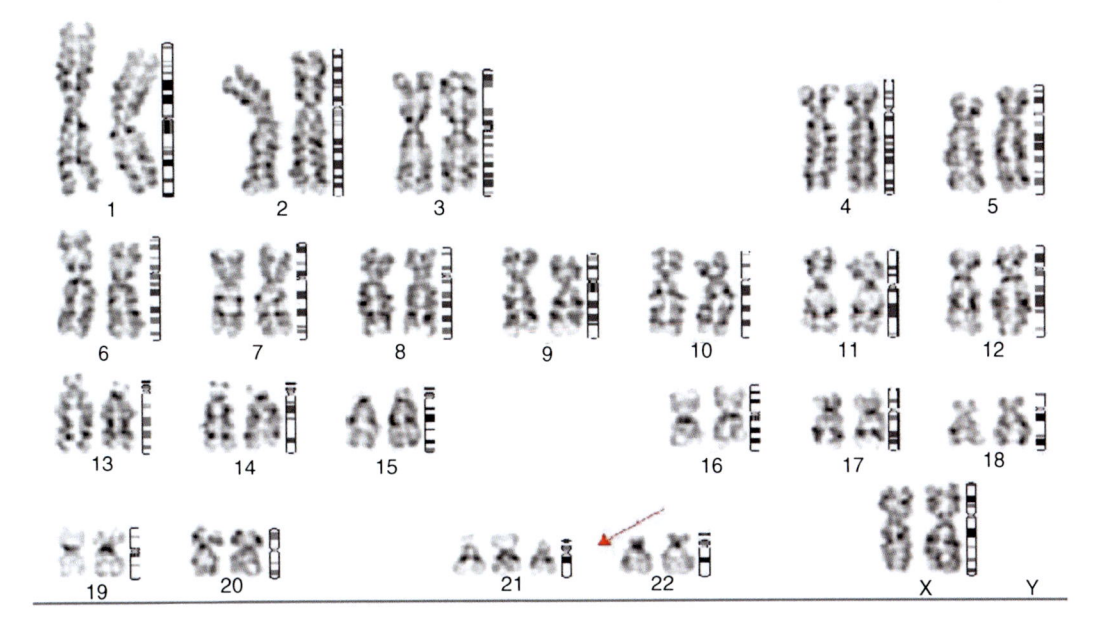

Fig. 13.2 Abnormal karyotype: trisomy 21

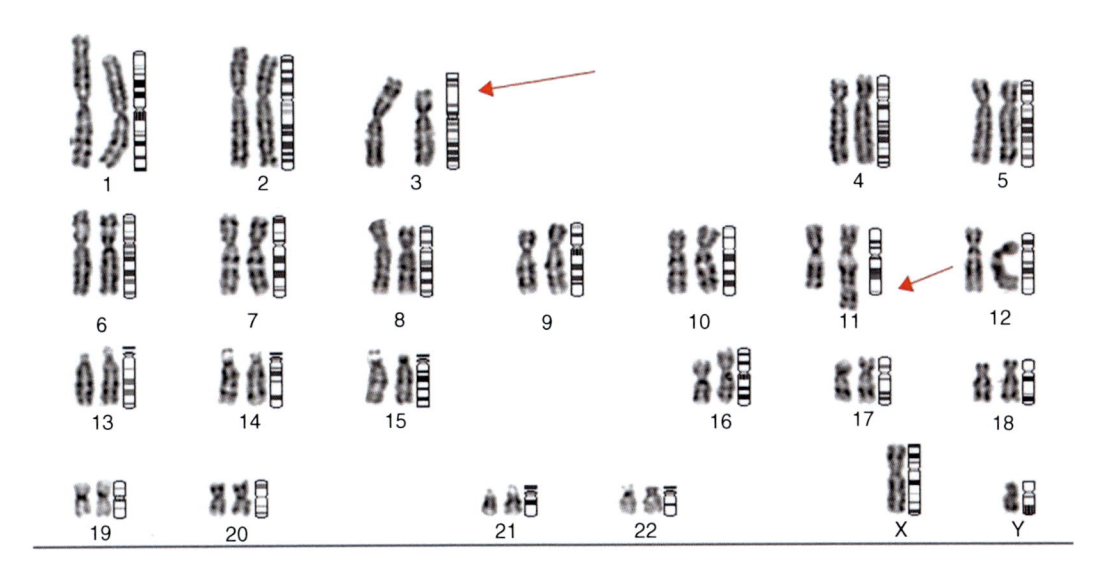

Fig. 13.3 Balanced translocation

informed decision regarding continuation or discontinuation of the pregnancy along with a clear plan for follow-up in future pregnancies.
- The abovementioned chromosomal abnormalities can be detected on a "karyotype" as shown in the figures above. The results of fetal diagnosis using conventional cytogenetic analysis by karyotype are dependent on the indication.

Sometimes, the abnormality in the chromosome may be smaller such that the "resolution" of the standard karyotype is not enough to detect problems of size smaller than 4–5 MB (mega bases)—such as a "microdeletion." This requires a higher-resolution study of the chromosomes—a technique which can scan the chromosomal regions up to 10—100 kB (kilo bases)!!

To understand this concept better, let us take a very simple day-to-day example. Checking chromosomes on karyotyping is similar to checking a rack of books on a library shelf—you check the number of books and can make out if a particular book is missing or extra or inverted or majorly damaged. However, just by looking at the rack, you may not be able to detect whether all the pages of each book are present and in correct order. For that you would require more intensive scrutiny like opening each book and counting its pages. This is what is done in a microarray where the chromosome is examined further closely and even a single missing page may be detected. This page, depending on which area of the book it belongs to, may or may not be "significant"—for example, a page which is a divider between two chapters and is missing may still allow the book to serve its function, but if the page containing a crucial chapter is missing, then the purpose of the book itself gets defeated. Similarly, changes in small parts of chromosomes may or may not be significant depending on the area they belong to, and this information is given in the report after the clinical geneticists analyze the microarray.

- This higher-resolution scanning of chromosomes to detect smaller changes in the "segments" of the chromosomes is called "microarray." In this test, "subkaryotypic" abnormalities are detected like microdeletions and microduplications which may be missed on a routine karyotype. Figure 13.4 shows the results of chromosomal microarray analysis which is normal, i.e., no clinically significant deletions or duplications or other chromosomal abnormalities in the given sample.

Due to the higher resolution of scanning the chromosomes, microarray yields more information as compared to conventional karyotype in evaluation of fetal anomalies and is becoming widely recommended as one of the first-line investigations in fetal structural anomalies, in evaluation of stillbirth, and in early miscarriages. The advantages in the latter two indications are that microarray can be performed on non-vital tissue also as it is a DNA-based analysis and does not need an active culture. In cases of stillbirths and miscarriages, culture failure of fetal cells would generally be the limiting factor for conventional karyotyping in the past leading to loss of vital information. As our understanding of fetal genetics is improving and the significance of this additional yield of information is being understood, cytogenetic microarray is being prescribed in amniotic fluid samples in cases where there are confirmed fetal structural anomalies out chromosomal problems beyond aneuploidies. The standard turnaround time for CMA on amniotic fluid samples is about 7–10 days.

In evaluation of childhood intellectual disability, cytogenetic microarray is now the recommended first-line test in genetic evaluation.

The results of CMA are either normal (Fig. 13.4) or abnormal/pathogenic (Fig. 13.5) or sometimes uncertain. The uncertainty arises due to detection of copy number "variants of unknown significance." Whatever copy number variants are detected on the CMA are compared with standard genetic databases to check if they are confirmed pathogenic variants or variants of unknown significance (VOUS). The VOUS definitely pose a challenge in counseling especially in prenatal cases, and therefore it is strongly recommended that such counseling be done in close coordination with a clinical geneticist who has access to a wide range of databases and follows the updated standard guidelines in reporting and counseling.

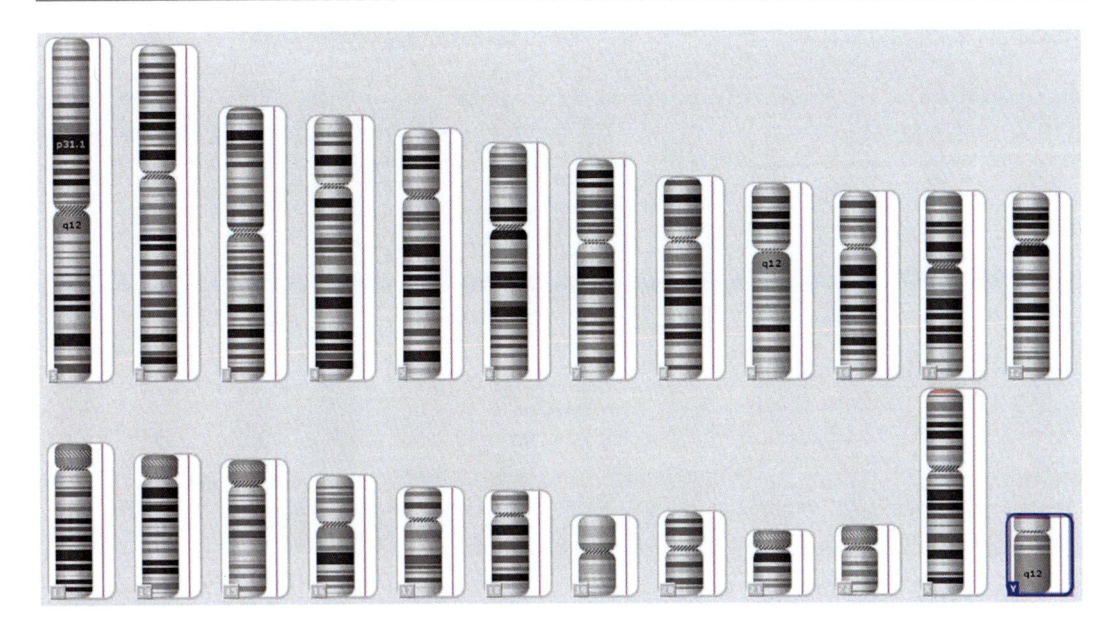

Fig. 13.4 Cytogenetic microarray: normal report

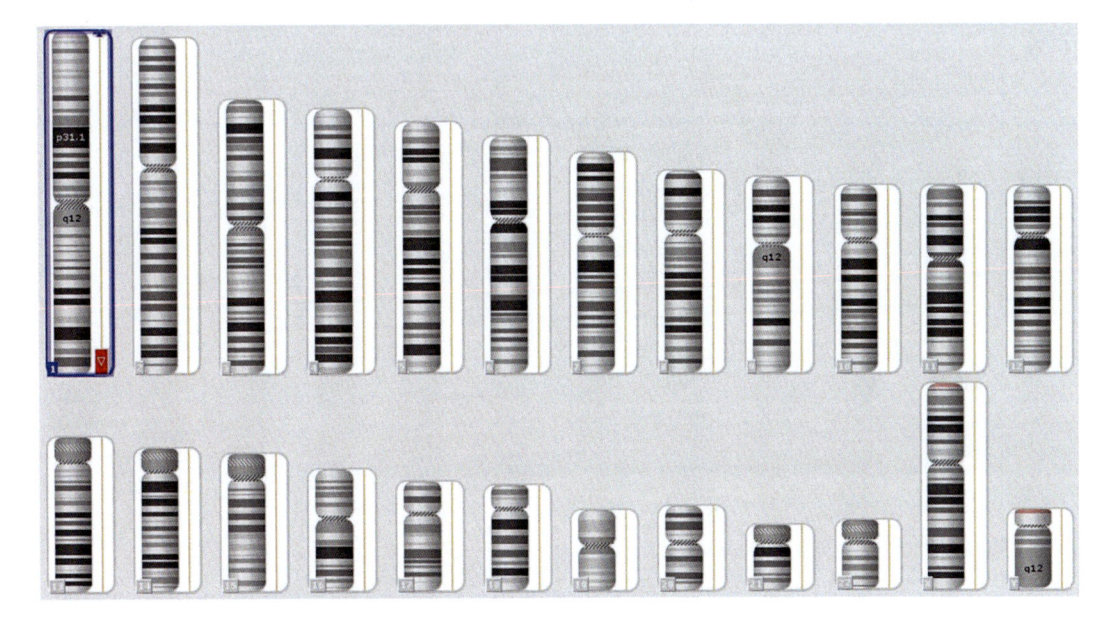

Fig. 13.5 Abnormal results on CMA

13.1 Fluorescence in Situ Hybridization (FISH)

This is a molecular technique for rapid detection of issues like aneuploidies and can yield results in 48–72 h which is significantly earlier than karyotyping or even microarray. FISH or fluorescence in situ hybridization involves use of probes that bind to specific areas of the fetal DNA and can thus be used to detect the number of chromosomes (useful in aneuploidies) or specific deletions or translocations. The probes are colored and they "hybridize" with cellular DNA (thus called FISH) resulting in a pattern as shown in

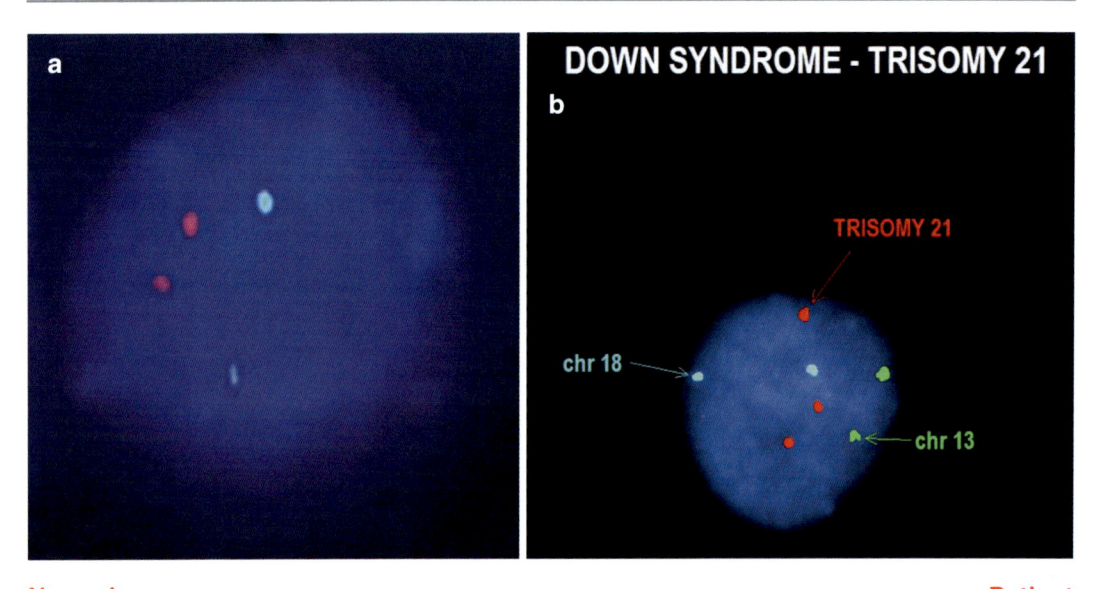

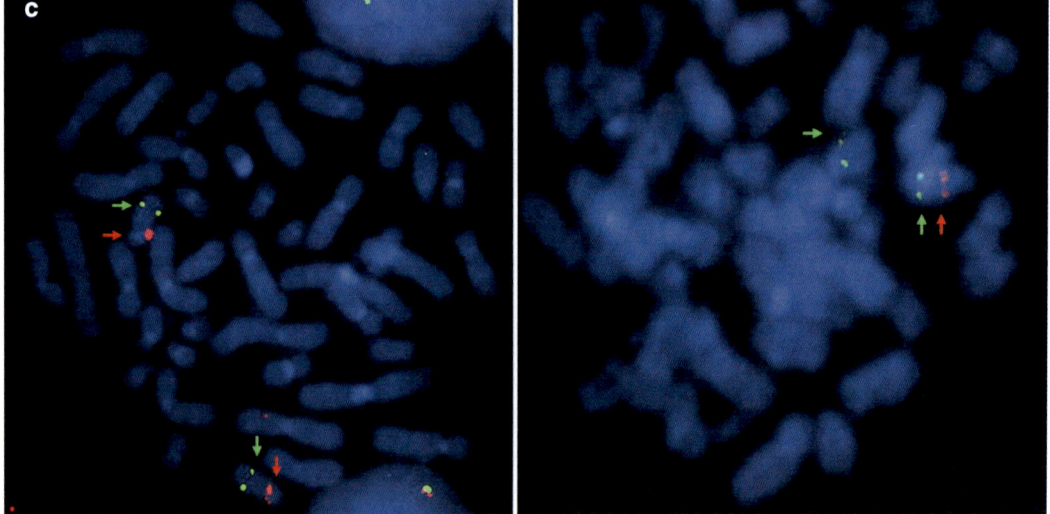

SNRPN (small nuclear ribonucleoprotein polypeptide N (15q11)-critical region
PML (Promyelocytic Leukemia) (15q24)-control region

Fig. 13.6 (a) Normal FISH. (b) Abnormal FISH—Down syndrome. (c) Comparative normal and abnormal FISH

Fig. 13.6. Normal FISH is shown in Fig. 13.6a, while abnormal FISH results are shown in Fig. 13.6b, c. When the nuclei of fetal cells are examined under fluorescent microscope, two spots, one for each of the two chromosomes, are visualized in normal subjects, while trisomies are revealed by the presence of an extra spot and monosomies by the absence of one spot.

13.2 Quantitative Fluorescent PCR (QfPCR)

Quantitative fluorescent PCR is another rapid diagnostic test for fetal aneuploidies, and it is based on the amplification of chromosome-specific DNA sequences (STR, short tandem repeats). Fluorescent primers are used to visualize the amplified segments and these can be quantified as peak DNA scanners. Normal euploid fetal cells are expected to show two peak areas (peak ratio 1:1) for each chromosome analyzed (Fig. 13.7), while trisomies are visualized either as an extra peak or as a 2:1 ratio peak between the two areas (Fig. 13.8).

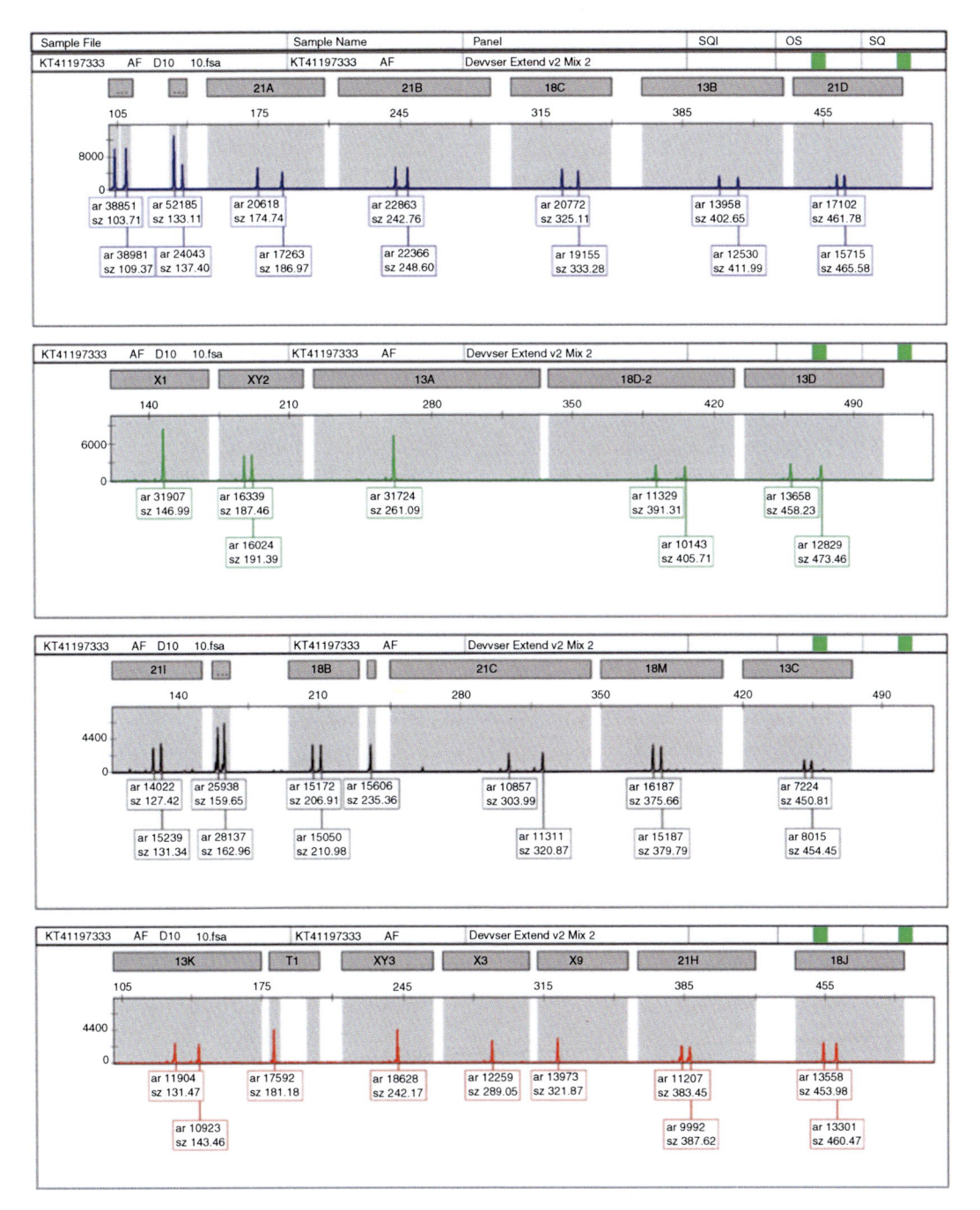

Fig. 13.7 Normal QfPCR

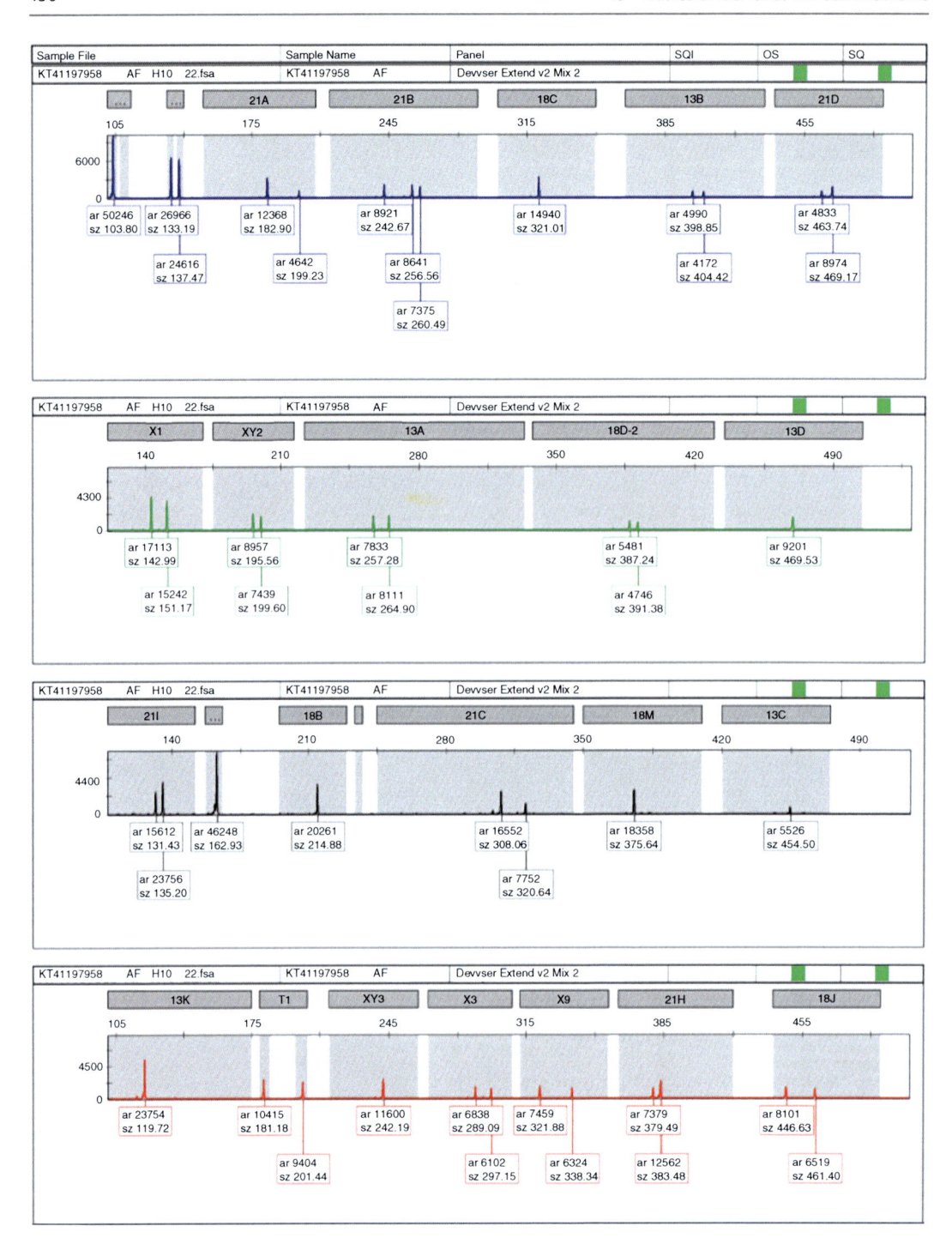

Fig. 13.8 Abnormal QfPCR—trisomy 21

QfPCR has some advantages over FISH in that it is able to report even on fewer fetal cells, and since the analysis can easily be automated, many samples can be processed at the same time, the whole process taking less than an hour.

13.3 Multiplex Ligation-Dependent Probe Amplification (MLPA)

Multiplex ligation-dependent probe amplification or MLPA is another rapid diagnostic test which is a variation of the multiplex polymerase chain reaction that permits amplification of multiple targets with only a single primer pair. The MLPA technique facilitates the amplification and detection of multiple targets with a single primer pair—it does not amplify the target DNA, but only the probes. Thus, many sequences can be amplified and quantified using just a single pair of primers. In comparison to other rapid diagnostic tests, MLPA requires a very small quantity of DNA, and it is fast, cheap, and simpler to perform. Figure 13.9 is a sample MLPA report and in current-day genetics, this technique has found many clinical uses.

MLPA has a variety of applications:

1. Aneuploidy detection
2. Mutations and SNP (single nucleotide polymorphisms) detection
3. Chromosomal characterization of cell lines and tissue sample
4. Detection of gene copy number
5. Detection of duplications and deletions in human cancer predisposition genes such as BRCA1, BRCA2, hMLH1, and hMSH2

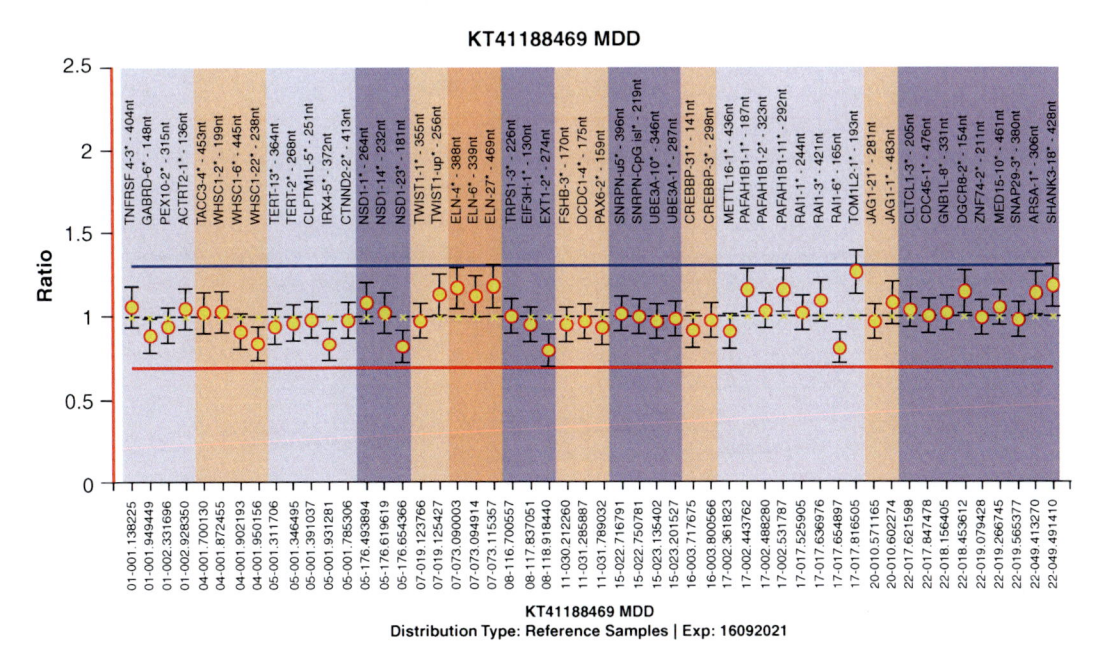

Fig. 13.9 MLPA results—normal

13.4 Clinical Exome Sequencing (CEX)

The human genome consists of many genes and every gene has "exons" which are the segments of DNA coding for proteins and "introns" which are the noncoding regions in the gene. All the exons of a person's genome comprise "whole exome" of the individual, while the clinically known exons could be grouped under "clinical exome." "Sequencing" is a process of reading the genetic material in an orderly manner to detect any mistakes in the expected pattern. The test is performed on DNA and large sequences are read to detect any possibility if errors like "point mutations" or "point deletions" may not have been detected otherwise. If we go back to the example of books in the library, if microarray was counting the pages, gene sequencing is like reading the lines of the pages. *Whole genome* sequencing would be like reading the entire book, *whole exome* sequencing would be like reading important chapters, and *clinical exome* sequencing could perhaps e compared to reading specific, marked, highlighted headings. These highlighted zones might be altered if several people gave their inputs and after a few more revisions, more areas might get highlighted. Similarly, the known regions of the genome today will be increased tomorrow once newer genes are identified so the scope of the "clinical exome."

Figure 13.10 is a sample report of clinical exome sequencing, and it reveals the presence of a "homozygous" genetic abnormality at a particular location of a gene which is classified as pathogenic because there is a known condition (in this case, Vici syndrome), associated with this particular variation, inherited in an autosomal recessive manner. This test has become a very important investigative tool for recurrent problems in families with background consanguinity and even otherwise where genetic conditions are suspected. In many cases, it helps unravel the so-called "unexplained" causes for problems like multiple children in a family with neurodevelopmental delay, recurrent neonatal deaths, and similar clinical situations. In some fetal anomalies with a normal karyotype or normal microarray, the possibility of "genetic" abnormalities remains, and in the absence of known handles, a clinical exome sequencing can help in looking at possible genetic aberrations. As with microarrays, the CEX is also expected to give results that are normal, abnormal, or uncertain. Application

---

CLINICAL EXOME SEQUENCING

CLINICAL INFORMATION

Fetus of ▮▮▮▮▮ presented with clinical indications of primary microcephaly, lisencephaly, colopoephaly and dilated third ventricle. Fetus of ▮▮▮▮▮ has been evaluated for pathogenic gene variations.

RESULT SUMMARY

Pathogenic variant causative of the reported phenotype was detected						
Gene and Transcript	Variant	Zygosity	Disease (OMIM)	Inheritance	Classification
EPG5 (-) (ENST00000282041.5)	c.420_421insTCTA (p.Val141SerfsTer20)	Homozygous	Vici syndrome (OMIM 242840)	Autosomal recessive	Pathogenic

No other pathogenic or likely pathogenic variants were detected in the screened genes as per the current literature and human genome variation database including Clinvar, 5000 Exome Global MAF and COSMIC.

Fig. 13.10 Clinical exome report

13.5 Targeted Mutation Analysis

of this test on fetal samples has to be considered very carefully. Empirical clinical exome on fetal samples is generally not recommended as it takes about 3–6 weeks (*depending on the lab services*) to get the results and in the absence of definite phenotype, variations of uncertain significance are difficult to understand or manage reasonably.

Clinical exome sequencing yields most fruitful results in cases with definite phenotype, and then the information is corroborated to allocate a genetic characteristic to that phenotype. Hence, it is more useful in evaluation of an index child with abnormalities or the parents of such a child for "carrier status" in the absence of the index sample. It is a good practice to discuss with a clinical geneticist and then only plan for such tests so that they can be appropriately interpreted and help in clinical management.

13.5 Targeted Mutation Analysis

Targeted mutation analysis is a method to directly test a very specific area within the gene where a known defect is expected to be found. Single gene disorders with known abnormalities, e.g., sickle cell anemia, spinal muscular atrophy, thalassemia, etc., can all be detected by targeted mutation analysis. This is a DNA-based test and is highly specific for the specific mutation we are looking for. It will identify any abnormality in that region alone and will not give any other information regarding the rest of the genome. Hence, the objective and limitation of such testing must be clearly understood. This is recommended in single gene disorders where parents are known carriers because the risk of recurrence of autosomal recessive conditions is 25% and autosomal dominant conditions is 50% in subsequent pregnancies. Ideally, parental carrier status must be established to justify the prenatal testing, but in some cases, if that has not been possible, prenatal diagnosis can be targeted based on the index sibling's report.

Figure 13.11 is a sample report of targeted mutation analysis for the sickle cell anemia gene.

Most obstetricians are intimidated by the myriad of genetic tests available and the novelty of genetic jargon which seems to be ever expanding. However, as you may have understood by now, the basics of genetics and its applications are simple, logical, and goal-oriented. Instead of getting carried away by the fancy of doing the latest or newest test for your patient, it is better to review the primary indication of testing and then plan a test appropriately. The following table (Table 13.1) effectively summarizes the contemporary genetic tests and their applications and limitations.

Previous child carrier for sickle cell anemia.

Test Performed – β Thalassemia Panel

Variants Detected

Variants identified	HGVS Name	Genotype	Clinical Significance
Hb S	HBB:c.20A>T	Homozygous (HbS/ HbS)	Sickle Cell Anemia
Hb S	HBB:c.20A>T	Heterozygous (/ HbS)	Sickle Cell trait
Hb S	HBB:c.20A>T	Heterozygous (/ HbS)	Sickle Cell trait

Fig. 13.11 Targeted mutation analysis report

Table 13.1 Summary of different tests available for genetic evaluation

	Aneuploidy	Large deletion/duplication/translocation	Micro deletion/duplication	Known point mutation	Many possible genetic mutations
Karyotype	Yes	Yes	No	No	No
Microarray	Yes	Yes	Yes	No	Not nonspecifically
FISH	Yes	May not detect if probe is not of that region	Only if probe is specific for that region	Only if probe is specific for that region	Not nonspecifically
QfPCR	Yes	May not detect if probe is not of that region	Only if probe is specific for that region	No	Not nonspecifically
MLPA	Yes	May not detect if probe is not of that region	Only if probe is specific for that region	Only if probe is specific for that region	Not nonspecifically
Clinical exome sequencing	No	May not detect if probe is not of that region	May not detect if probe is not of that region	Yes	Yes
Targeted mutation analysis	No	Only if probe is specific for that region	Only if probe is specific for that region	Yes	No

Key Learning Points in Basics of Genetics

1. Understanding basics of genetics is mandatory for a fetal medicine practitioner.
2. The possibilities of prenatal diagnosis by genetic techniques are rapidly increasing, and there is a dire necessity to keep oneself updated on the latest advances.
3. Although clinicians can understand the basics of molecular testing and genetic conditions, it is useful to consult a clinical geneticist while planning and interpreting genetic tests and their results.

Suggested Reading

Benn P, et al. Position statement from the Chromosome Abnormality Screening Committee on behalf of the Board of the International Society for Prenatal Diagnosis. Prenat Diagn. 2015;35(8):725–34.

Ranganath P et al. Genetic update for the next generation clinician 2017 (a compilation of articles from genetics clinics). Society for Indian Academy of Medical Genetics.

Van den Veyver IB. Recent advances in prenatal genetic screening and testing. F1000Res. 2016;5:2591. https://doi.org/10.12688/f1000research.9215.1.

Recurrent Fetal Problems: Looking for Solutions

14

In some unfortunate couples, pregnancy outcome is affected by problems in the fetus or the child after birth that recur in subsequent pregnancies and thus pose unique challenges. The classical problem of "recurrent pregnancy loss" is usually a condition of a pregnancy failure due to inability to sustain the fetus in utero largely due to maternal reasons and is largely an obstetric problem. When we talk of recurrent "fetal problems," we are considering an entirely different subset of problems where pregnancies may be affected by "fetal conditions" and in some cases may even go up to term asymptomatically, but the "fetal outcome" may be adverse—either manifesting in pregnancy, immediately in the neonatal period, or much later. Typical presentations may be:

1. Recurrent neonatal/childhood problems leading to neurodevelopmental delay and/or death
2. Recurrent fetal anomalies causing miscarriage or warranting termination of pregnancy
3. Recurrent fetal growth restriction or severe early onset maternal preeclampsia leading to early delivery and hence severe prematurity or in utero fetal demise

These cases become important in fetal medicine because they generally arrive at the fetal medicine clinic with huge files full of investigation reports and opinions from a variety of clinicians who have dealt either with the previous pregnancies or with the children at various stages of the illness. As each of the previous doctors has looked at only one aspect of the situation, their opinions are also limited in relevance to the entire case scenario when viewed in its totality. While every individual consultation in the past may be important at that situation and its advice appropriate for the limited issue being addressed at that point, they are like pieces of a jigsaw puzzle, and unless they are all put together in a coherent manner, the complete picture is often missed. Let us consider the following case as an example of the point being made here.

Case 1
Mrs X, 28 years old, consanguineous marriage (second degree), G3P2 L0 had two previous full-term deliveries at term. First child—male, 3 kg birth weight, and delivered vaginally—was "normal" for a month or so and then developed seizures, failure to thrive, and neurodevelopmental delay and died at the age of 3 years. Second child—baby girl delivered by elective LSCS at term (indication—to avoid possibility of "birth injury" which may be related to the outcome of the first child). This child was asymptomatic till 1 month of age but then developed the same symptoms as the first child and followed almost a similar timeline to her death at the age of 3 years.

Now she is 18 weeks pregnant and has been referred to fetal medicine clinic for the solution of her problems based on her history. The couple arrive at the fetal medicine clinic with a lot of hope that they will have a healthy baby this time!! This clinical scenario is not uncommon in fetal medicine clinics. We are now well equipped with wonderful scan machines and a lot of knowledge in fetal anatomy physiology, genetic, etc. as highlighted in the preceding chapters, yet this situation frustrates us due to our helplessness in providing a definitive solution in this scenario. You may be wondering why—and the reasons are many. Let us list out the problems in the given scenario:

1. There are two cases of deaths following severe morbidity in their children so the case is "recurrent."
2. We do not know the exact "cause" of the problem.
3. Both children were "structurally" normal with average weight at birth—therefore, a "normal" anomaly scan at 18 weeks or normal growth scans thereafter cannot reassure us in this pregnancy regarding the final outcome.
4. There is a risk of "recurrence" but we have no way to predict it as we do not know the exact cause!!

Once all these points are analyzed, the most obvious solution to our problems is knowing the exact cause of the past problems and then finding a method of ruling out that *cause* in this pregnancy. As both cases had an almost similar clinical presentation, the etiology is likely to be the same, and in a consanguineous couple where we expect both partners to have many similarities in the gene pool, this condition could be an autosomal recessive genetic disorder. Both parents may be asymptomatic carriers (heterozygous) of the disease-causing gene, and when the two disease-causing genes come together (homozygous)—at a theoretical recurrence risk of 25%—the child will manifest the disease. Therefore, in the given case in this pregnancy also, there is a theoretically 25% chance of recurrence of the disease. We know that fetal DNA testing can help us detect fetal genes—however unless we know our "target," the results of empirical genetic testing in the fetus can yield a lot of uninterpretable information. Moreover, we need to collect fetal cells through an amniocentesis which carries potentially an added and procedure-related risk of miscarriage. Hence, such invasive testing is only justified when we are sure that it will help us get a final result.

If we had the DNA of the previous children, that would be an ideal situation in order to establish the primary cause in the person first affected or the "proband"—in this case, the expected mutation in "homozygous "state. If that homozygosity is proven in the proband, then both parents could be checked to confirm that they too carry the same mutation in "heterozygous" state and we know that they are asymptomatic in this regard. Therefore, this proves that individuals who harbor a heterozygous mutation are asymptomatic carriers and those who are "homozygous" for the mutation are likely to be affected. This sounds logical but sadly in most such cases, the proband DNA is not available and hence such testing becomes impractical. Instead, we try to do an empirical search for mutations in the parents by "clinical" or "whole" exome sequencing. This test usually takes about 4–6 weeks to give results and only after these results, we can plan targeted prenatal testing.

The "frustration" about starting such a workup plan at 18 weeks is thus obvious because though we may be able to find the exact cause of the problem, we may even be able to establish the genetic status of the fetus, but in those 25% cases that are likely to be affected, termination of pregnancy is no longer an option in most clinical setups due to the advanced gestational age! The treatment options for such genetic conditions are extremely limited, and it seems ironical to finally know the reason for the suffering in the past and not being able to offer any solution at present.

This brings us to few important aspects on retrospective analysis of the case:

1. When a child has unidentified reasons for "failure to thrive" or "neurodevelopmental delay," possibility of genetic etiology should be kept in mind—especially in recurrent cases.

2. The pediatricians/pediatric neurologists need to be sensitized to the need for arriving at a genetic diagnosis if possible—ideally by involving a clinical geneticist.
3. In cases where parents have cost concerns and are unable to invest in major genetic tests, a simple cost-effective method of "DNA storage" in suspicious cases can be adopted which then can be used for genetic analysis anytime later.
4. Cultural practices can hinder the investigation of such cases. In many societies, where such mishaps are considered "inauspicious," families destroy all such data following the death of a child and sometimes change the doctors and do not reveal such history!! It is, therefore, very important to explain this possibility to the parents clearly and reiterate the need for preserving all clinical notes, pictures, and relevant information for future workup too. This practice can only change by better counseling and generating awareness about genetic conditions so that superstitions are replaced by rational behavior.

Case 2
Mrs Y, 29 years old, nonconsanguineous marriage, G6 P1L1 A3, is now 11 weeks pregnant. First pregnancy was terminated due to large cystic hygroma detected at 12 weeks; second pregnancy was a spontaneous miscarriage at 8 weeks; third pregnancy resulted in a full-term normal delivery of a structurally normal child; now 4 years with normal developmental milestones, fourth pregnancy was terminated due to multiple fetal defects (bilateral ventriculomegaly, absent stomach bubble, bilateral club feet, and unilateral cleft palate and lip) detected at the 16 weeks' scan; and fifth pregnancy was a spontaneous miscarriage detected at 10 weeks after cardiac activity was documented at 7 weeks. There is no significant history of maternal medical disorders, infections, or teratogenic drug intake. Ultrasound scan reports are available for all pregnancies but no further workup done in any of the previous cases.

Now, she has been referred to the fetal medicine clinic at 11 weeks for advice regarding fetal care in the present pregnancy. In this case, unlike the previous scenario, the pattern of presentation appears to be different in each pregnancy. The possibilities are that this may be just by chance with no relation whatsoever between the different pregnancies, but as clinicians, we do understand that recurrence of such problems needs further workup before we label it as "just by chance."

Ideally, if the previous affected pregnancies would have been investigated, we may have had information regarding the exact cause for each mishap, and then we would predict the chances of the present pregnancy being affected. However, in the absence of such information, we again have to pick up clues from the available resources and form a plan of care.

Upon analyzing the history in this case, we can make the following observations:

1. There is likely to be a "recurrent" pathology.
2. Unlikely to be infections—fetal infections generally do not "recur," and to consider the rare possibility of a different teratogenic infection each time, the history is not corroborative.
3. Each time the fetal presentation is different including early pregnancy losses too.

This brings us to consider the possibility of "chromosomal" rather than "genetic" etiology, and one condition which can explain such recurrence is if one of the parents is a carrier of a balanced translocation. Therefore, in such cases, parental karyotyping can be a reasonable investigation.

The parent who carries the balanced translocation in his or her karyotype is generally asymptomatic. However, this individual can form gametes with either normal, "balanced," or "unbalanced" rearrangements. While the "normal" or "balanced" gametes can lead to successful pregnancies, the "unbalanced" translocations contribute to a zygote which is incompatible with normal life and result in malformations and/or miscarriage. This concept has been discussed in detail in the chapter on the basics of genetics.

It is already a proven fact that chromosomal abnormalities contribute mostly to early pregnancy miscarriages. This is possible even with parents who have normal karyotype because the etiology of such aberrations is usually "nondisjunction" during the meiosis while the gametes are being formed. The chances of recurrence of miscarriage is considerably higher when any of the parents carry chromosomal translocations, and this can also result in variable fetal presentations like in the case above. Conducting a fetal karyotype in any case of multiple fetal malformations or unexplained miscarriage is thus a reasonable investigation in arriving at a final diagnosis regarding the cause.

In this case, we have no proven reason so far but each time fetus has presented with structural anomalies or a miscarriage. The pregnancy is now at 11 weeks of gestation so we can proceed for a detailed first trimester fetal scan and check the fetal structure. If any anomaly is detected, then a fetal karyotyping can be offered. If the scan is normal, a combined screening test for aneuploidies can be offered and the fetus can be reviewed at 17–18 weeks for a detailed midtrimester anomaly scan. It may be useful to discuss the possibility of parental karyotyping in the meantime because if indeed one of them is carrying a balanced translocation, then it becomes mandatory to check fetal chromosomes and offer a microarray even of scans and screening tests are normal. Scans detect structural normalcy and all chromosomal rearrangements do not manifest as detectable structural malformations. While inheriting translocations, subkaryotypic microdeletions may be caused which can only be detected by a microarray and sometimes these may have functional significance.

If the parental karyotype is normal and fetal scans and growth continue to reveal a structurally normal, average growing fetus, then the pregnancy can be continued with expectant antenatal care for both mother and fetus with serial surveillance.

Case 3
Mrs Z, 30 years old, nonconsanguineous marriage, G4 P1L0A2, is now 12 weeks pregnant. First pregnancy was a missed miscarriage at 12 weeks with a structurally normal fetus and second pregnancy was a fetal demise at 24 weeks with early onset FGR, large jellylike placenta, and high resistance flows in uterine arteries seen on scan at 20 weeks of gestation. The fetus had "echogenic bowel" reported on the anomaly scan and fetal karyotype was normal. In her third pregnancy, she again had early onset FGR and had developed severe preeclampsia at 24 weeks. She had to be delivered at 27 weeks due to rapid deterioration of maternal parameters—600 g male baby, succumbed to complications of extreme prematurity in the NICU on day 3. Fetus was structurally normal and had a normal karyotype.

She has now arrived at 12 weeks to the fetal medicine clinic in view of the previous history of "fetal losses" hoping for a solution in the present pregnancy. This is again a common scenario in the fetal medicine clinic, and only after a systematic "history taking" exercise, one realizes that the problem in this case scenario may not be totally of "fetal" origin.

Points to ponder in this case are the following:

1. Although the final outcome has been a fetal loss in each pregnancy in this case, the fetus has remained structurally and chromosomally normal but suffered intrauterine growth restriction probably due to severe placental insufficiency.
2. Such recurrent uteroplacental insufficiency points at the possibility of maternal causes leading to the vascular complications, e.g., maternal thrombophilias.

The evidence on the "causal" association of fetal loss due to maternal thrombophilias is yet to be firmly established, but there is a general acceptance that pregnancy complications can be a result of maternal antibodies or prothrombotic conditions. Altered levels of placental biomarkers have been proven in several studies on pregnancy outcomes with maternal autoimmune, prothrombotic conditions. It has also been shown that normal values of placental biomarkers in early pregnancy have a good negative predictive value for adverse pregnancy outcomes. However, since the physiological changes of pregnancy make the diagnosis of such conditions difficult, the ideal time to diagnose them is in the nonpregnant state. So in the given scenario, it would have been a good idea to have checked for such conditions in the "interconception" period. However, now that she is already at 12 weeks of gestation, it will be useful to offer her a comprehensive first trimester screening where in addition to fetal parameters, a maternal risk assessment for preeclampsia can be done by a combination of uterine artery Doppler, history, biophysical, and biochemical markers, and women at high risk for preterm preeclampsia can be offered low-dose aspirin from 12 weeks to 36 weeks to reduce the incidence and complications of the disease.

As illustrated in the above case, if the diagnosis of a prothrombotic condition could have been unequivocally diagnosed before pregnancy, then optimum thromboprophylaxis methods could have been instituted in a proper, evidence-based care scheme.

As clinicians, we are often confronted with situations that "should have been" or "could have been" worked up differently, but the hard fact is that patients present to us in any given scenario and we have to pick up pieces of clues and indicators from the available history and documents and frame the most reasonable care plan for the next pregnancy. In cases of recurrent fetal problems, cases present as either with confirmed diagnosis or with reasons to suspect some diagnosis. The following flowchart (Fig. 14.1) gives us a scheme of how to proceed such cases.

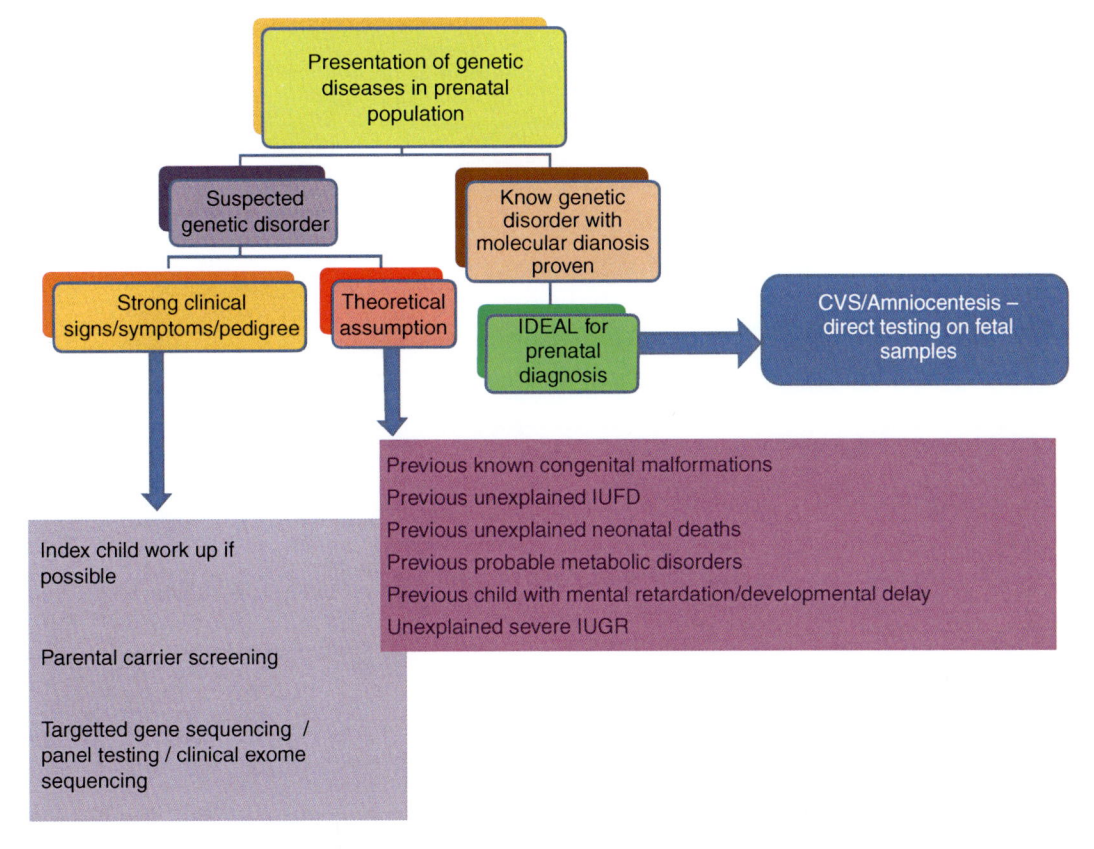

Fig. 14.1 Flowchart of care planning in cases of recurrent fetal problems

As is clear, the most important determinant of ensuring a good fetal outcome in a case with past fetal problems is the knowledge of what exactly is the cause of the previous problems—the "primary diagnosis." Only if this is known, the future plan of care can be truly "appropriate." In maternal causes, we realized that prepregnancy investigations are more helpful. Similarly, in fetal causes, the "index case" workup would yield vital information that can help us in the future. So the "golden window" for workup in cases of recurrent fetal problems is the "interconceptional period." So pediatricians, physicians, surgeons, or neurologists dealing with children with unexplained developmental delay or metabolic problems or congenital anomalies must suggest at least one visit to a fetal medicine specialist for a "prepregnancy" counseling. A complete prepregnancy workup can go a long way in improving the overall perinatal outcome in cases of recurrent fetal problems.

- Establishing the primary diagnosis requires a complete workup of the index case, and this must be considered even while caring for a pregnancy where the fetal prognosis is so poor that a termination is warranted.
- Termination of pregnancy should be associated with adequate fetal testing and storage of DNA if needed to facilitate future tests.
- Planning care in subsequent pregnancies with history of fetal problems is best done preconceptionally so a comprehensive preconception counseling and workup should be suggested in these cases.

We may not be able to cure everything in fetal medicine, but we can certainly care.

Key Points to Remember
- Fetal problems may be recurrent—either in a similar pattern or in differing patterns depending on the primary cause of the problem.
- The exact recurrence risk depends on the primary etiology.
- Genetic or chromosomal issues can be tested in a fetus but the best results are obtained only when the primary diagnosis is known.

Invasive Prenatal Diagnostic and Therapeutic Procedures

15

Prenatal diagnosis of fetal conditions by "invading" the gestational sac is done in cases where there is a need to evaluate fetal cells or fluids directly. These procedures are generally ultrasound-guided needle procedures performing which requires great skill and training. While conducting the procedure is considered technically challenging, the clinician must realize that conduct of the procedure itself is a small part in the entire scheme of fetal health management. The indication of the procedure, the decision of which tests are to be performed on the fetal samples, and the final interpretation of the results of these tests are actually the most important prognostic factors for any prenatal test. It is therefore important for the doctor to understand the fetal health issue in depth and be clear about how is a fetal sample testing going to help in the further management of the case before embarking upon an invasive prenatal test. These tests carry potential risks to the pregnancy—both to the mother and fetus—and hence need to be regulated by judicious protocols. In this chapter, we will discuss the common prenatal invasive procedures—both diagnostic and therapeutic.

Before we start discussing each and every prenatal invasive procedure, some common "checklist points" need to be scrutinized. This checklist is a quick reminder of all the important aspects of prenatal invasive testing and should be handy in every clinic for reference by the entire medical team—including nursing and support staff who help in the documentation and maintenance of

Table 15.1 Invasive prenatal procedure checklist

• Indication
• Pretest counseling
• Rhesus status check—anti-D for Rh-negative mothers
• Maternal HIV and Hep B screening
• Consent
• Legal forms (e.g., PCPNDT forms in India)
• Lab requisition forms
• Result analysis
• Posttest counseling

records. In some countries, prenatal tests come under specific legal sections and demand specialized documentation. These points are enumerated in Table 15.1.

15.1 Indication

The "indication" for any invasive prenatal tests is the pressing reason which justifies a potentially "risky" procedure in a pregnancy. This is by far the most important aspect while planning any prenatal invasive procedure. There has to be an unequivocally pressing reason to obtain a fetal sample for testing either the genetic or biochemical composition which is going to affect antenatal care or decisions regarding continuation of pregnancy.

Common indications for prenatal diagnostic procedures are to obtain fetal cells or DNA for karyotyping, genetic analysis, or biochemical analysis. Cases are selected based on preliminary screening tests such that those with high risk are offered invasive tests. Fetal abnormalities warrant chromosomal/genetic testing to rule out associated syndromes and establish prognosis. Some genetic conditions like sickle cell anemia, beta thalassemia, or some metabolic syndromes may be known in the family, and thus high risk of recurrence warrants prenatal testing.

Every case has to be individually worked up and if a justifiable indication exists, a prenatal invasive procedure can be planned.

15.2 Pretest Counseling

Prior to the procedure, the couple should be told about the purpose of the procedure (clear indication/severity of the disorder) and the potential complications, including technical problems that might necessitate a second procedure. The genetic risk versus the procedure-related risk and test accuracy should be weighed before deciding to undergo the test. They should be told about the time required before results will be available and the accuracy and limitations of the diagnostic test(s) planned, including possible inability to make a diagnosis. Alternatives that may yield the same or similar information but are less invasive options should also be discussed. It imperative to understand whether termination would be warranted following confirmation of the affliction and whether termination is acceptable to the couple. Since the clinician has a broad idea of the expected results, it is prudent to counsel hypothetically regarding all possible outcomes prior to undertaking the test so that the overall experience of the test is satisfactory.

15.3 Rhesus Status Check

Prenatal invasive procedures involve the possibility of increasing feto-maternal transfusion and therefore potentially can cause isoimmunization unless specific precautions are taken. It is most important not to do harm in any medical process.

The point about checking rhesus status has been placed separately to make sure that any clinician, whenever contemplating a prenatal invasive procedure, does not forget this point.

In rhesus negative women, a pretest indirect Coombs test must be done to assess her antibody status. If not isoimmunized, then appropriate dose of anti-D should be administered for postprocedure prophylaxis. It is important to date and document the dose given for future reference in that pregnancy.

15.4 Maternal HIV and Hepatitis B Screening

Mother to fetus transmission of HIV and hepatitis B is a palpable risk which increases in the setting of a prenatal invasive procedure. In case of HIV-positive women, adequate antiretroviral medications can be started to prevent fetal transmission. There are no specific methods of preventing mother to child transmission for hepatitis B, and hence in women positive for hepatitis B, appropriate counseling and case selection is important. The risks of fetal transmission have to be carefully weighed against the benefit of prenatal diagnosis.

15.5 Consent

The principles of consent for any medical procedure apply similarly for prenatal invasive procedures. A clear, written consent is mandatory prior to conducting any invasive prenatal procedure. The consent should be taken after a detailed pretest counseling with the patient being aware of the reason for the test, the expected results and plan of care thereafter, the risks entailed in the procedure, and the other clinical options including the specific conditions of avoiding the test. The clinician should provide the patient enough time to decide voluntarily whether to accept or decline the invasive test. A copy of this consent should be carefully filed in her clinical notes.

15.6 Amniocentesis

Amniocentesis is one of the most commonly performed invasive prenatal diagnostic procedures. This involves aspirating 10–20 ml of amniotic fluid through a transabdominal puncture of the amniotic cavity using a 20–22 G hollow needle. It can be performed safely any time after 15 weeks of gestation in the pregnancy. The ideal time for amniocentesis for prenatal diagnosis is 16–20 weeks as there are technical safety issues at earlier and later gestations. Amniotic fluid aspiration prior to 15 weeks of gestation has been associated with risk of talipes and fetal respiratory problems. After 16 weeks, the fetal membranes get well apposed with the uterine walls, thus eliminating the possibility of "tenting" of the membranes during entry of the needle, thus making the procedure safer. The other advantage is that the availability of fetal cells is adequate by this gestation making it an appropriate window to obtain fetal samples. Third trimester amniocentesis is associated with higher risk of the need for multiple punctures and blood-stained fluid although it does not increase the risk of emergency delivery.

A 22 G spinal needle is most commonly used to aspirate amniotic fluid through a transabdominal approach under real-time ultrasound guidance by continuous needle tip visualization (Fig. 15.1). Care is taken to avoid a transplacental route whenever possible and with appropriate skill and experience, the risk of fetal/cord injury is minimal. The aspirated fluid is straw colored and contains cells of fetal origin. Most of the cells floating in amniotic fluid are epithelioid although fibroblastoid and amniotic fluid-specific cells are also present. It is estimated that at 16 weeks, there are more than 200,000 cells/mL of amniotic fluid of which only 3–4 cells/mL are

Amniocentesis

- Aseptic precautions
- Avoid placenta
- Needle thickness 22G
- Continuous needle tip visualisation

Complications:
- Failed procedure/Dry tap
- Bloody tap
- Multiple punctures

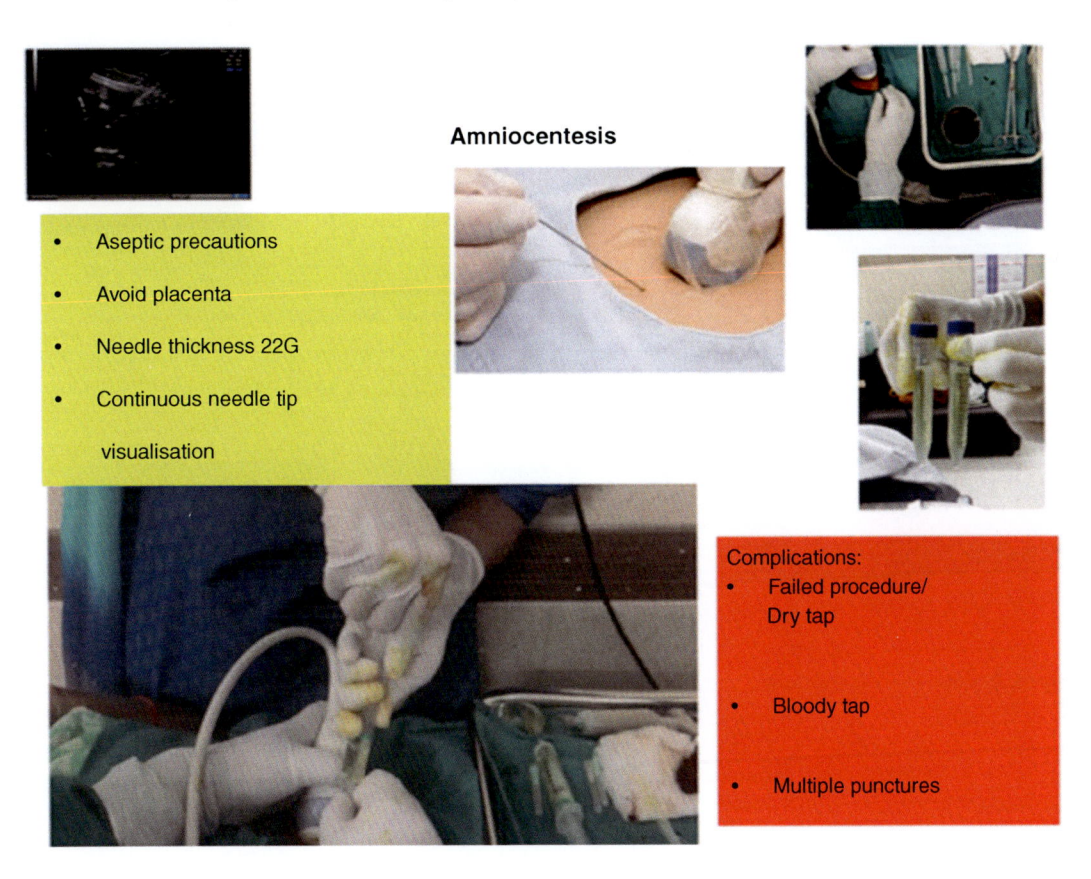

Fig. 15.1 Amniocentesis

capable of attaching to a culture substrate and yielding colonies. Before 15 weeks, there is a significant decline in cloning efficiency (fewer than 1.5 clone forming cells/mL fluid). This sample is sent to the lab in sterile falcon tubes, and as per the indication of the procedure, genetic, cytological, or biochemical testing can be performed to obtain the desired prenatal diagnosis.

Amniocentesis carries 0.1–1% added risk of miscarriage depending on the operator experience. Frequent complications are bloody tap, dry tap, or a failure to culture cells in the lab from the sample.

15.7 Chorionic Villus Sampling (CVS)

The placenta has cells of both maternal and fetal origin. In earlier gestations, the chorionic villi in the developing placenta can be used to obtain fetal cells and DNA. This procedure can be done any time after 10 weeks of gestation technically, but practically, it is done between 11 and 14 weeks after a detailed structural evaluation and aneuploidy risk assessment of the fetus. Since the sample obtained has solid tissue, a thicker needle is used for CVS as compared to amniocentesis. Usually, 18 G or 20 G disposable spinal needle of adequate length (7.5–15 mm) is used. The needle is passed through anterior abdominal wall into the substance of the chorion frondosum under continuous needle tip visualization under ultrasound guidance. Unlike amniocentesis where the needle is static in the amniotic fluid, in CVS the needle is moved up and down gently to break the villi, and a strong negative pressure suction by a 20 cc syringe is needed to aspirate the villi. Figure 15.2 shows the needle position and sample aspiration in CVS.

The earlier age of performance of CVS along with the technical details like use of a thicker needle for CVS is the reason for a marginally higher

Chorionic Villus sampling (CVS)

- Transabdominal access under USG guidance
- 18 G long spinal needle
- Chorionic villi aspirated and transported to lab in sterile media
- Sample used to extract fetal DNA and cells for prenatal diagnosis

USG guided needle aspiration of chorionic villi

Chorionic villi in collection medium

chorionic villi

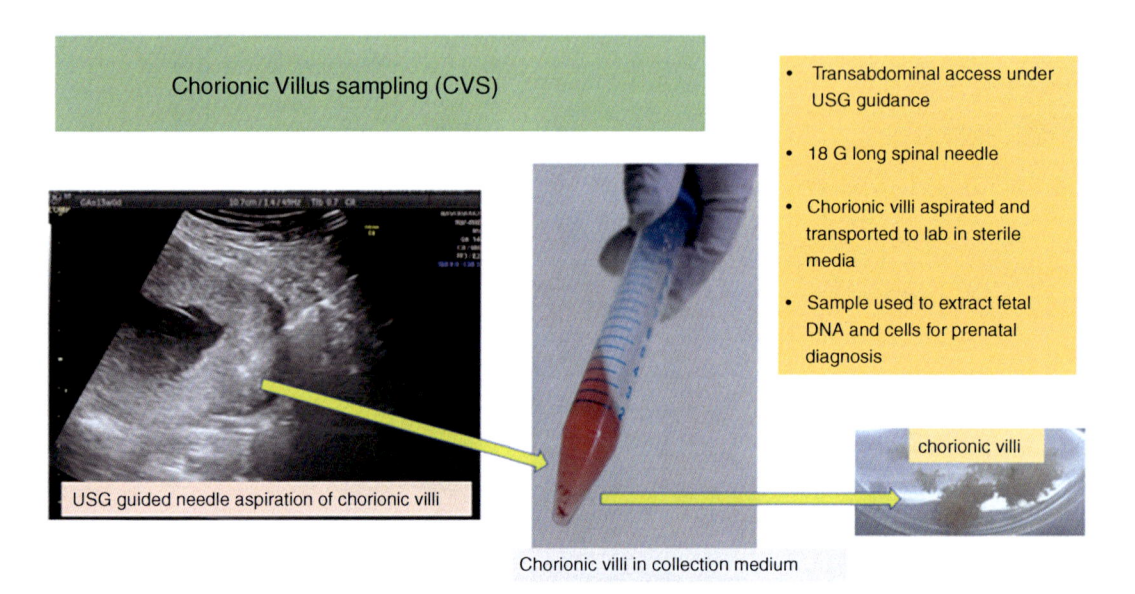

Fig. 15.2 Chorionic villus sampling

risk of miscarriage after CVS as compared to amniocentesis. Operator skill and experience is an important factor affecting the procedure-related risk of pregnancy loss. The distinct advantage of CVS is the earlier gestation age of performance allowing an earlier prenatal diagnosis. It is also known that the yield of fetal cells and DNA from CVS is much greater than 20 ml of amniotic fluid. However, the possibility of placental mosaicism, maternal cell contamination, and culture failure at CVS may necessitate repeat procedure in the form of amniocentesis in some cases.

15.8 Fetal Blood Sampling

Fetal blood sampling provides an unequivocal fetal sample for prenatal diagnosis. Fetal blood can be obtained by tapping the fetal umbilical vein in the cord either transplacentally near the cord insertion in an anterior placenta or in a free loop of the cord in posterior placenta. A 22 G long spinal needle is used. Extreme care is needed while performing this procedure as it carries a higher risk of fetal loss as compared to CVS and amniocentesis (Fig. 15.3).

Although the needle is thinner, the target is the umbilical cord, and there is a possibility of intrauterine bleeding from the cord or inadvertent puncture of the umbilical arteries leading to fetal bradycardia.

Fetal blood sampling is therefore done only for pressing indications where either amniocentesis is not possible like severe oligoamnios or prior to intrauterine transfusion to confirm fetal hematocrit and plan the exact volume of transfusion.

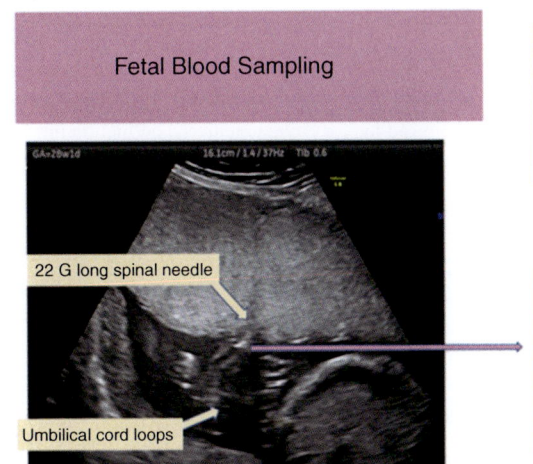

Fetal Blood Sampling

- Transabdominal access under USG guidance
- 22 G long spinal needle
- Fetal blood aspirated in 1-2ml heparinised syringes

- Transported in Heparin tubes for karyotyping
- For DNA based studies sample is transported in EDTA tubes as heparin insterferes with DNA extraction
- Common indications of FBS–fetal infective agents PCR, karyotyping, pre transfusion hematocrit estimation

Fig. 15.3 Fetal blood sampling

Table 15.2 Common invasive fetal therapeutic procedures

Procedure	Indication	Instruments/technique	Intended benefit
Aspiration of abnormal fluid collection in fetus	Pleural effusion Selected fetal cysts causing significant pressure effects	USG-guided needle aspiration using 22 G long needle	Relieving the pressure due to the abnormal fluid collection Assessment of the fluid to ascertain its nature and guide further treatment
Intrauterine blood transfusion	Fetal anemia	Transabdominal percutaneous USG-guided procedure with 20 G long spinal needle—intravascular or intraperitoneal	Increase the fetal hemoglobin and prevent risk of hydrops or IUFD
Selective fetal reduction	Fetal anomalies in twin pregnancies or high-order multifetal pregnancies	Fetal intracardiac KCl in cases of multichorionic pregnancies Interstitial LASER/radiofrequency ablation or bipolar cord cautery in monochorionic pregnancy	Reduce the abnormal fetus to help in the unhindered growth and development of the normal fetus Optimize the perinatal outcome of higher-order multifetal pregnancy by reducing it to twins
Placental anastomoses ablation	Severe twin-to-twin transfusion in MCA twins	Fetoscopy-guided LASER photocoagulation of placental anastomoses	Stop the physiological effects of the TTTS which would otherwise adversely affect both fetuses
Fetal endotracheal balloon occlusion	Congenital diaphragmatic hernia with risk of severe lung hypoplasia	Fetoscopy-guided balloon placement in fetal trachea with occlusion of the lumen	Maintain prenatal lung volume to minimize the risk of lung hypoplasia and improve the outcome of postnatal surgery
Open fetal surgery	Open neural tube defects in fetus	Hysterotomy for repair of fetal meningomyelocele followed by reposition of fetus in utero and closure of uterine incision	Prevent neurological damage due to tentorial herniation in ONTD

15.9 Invasive Prenatal Threapeutic Procedures

Some invasive procedures are done in the antenatal period with the aim of "treating" certain fetal conditions. Fetal therapy is a highly specialized area and a detailed discussion on this count is beyond the scope of this book. A synopsis of common procedures done for fetal therapy is presented in Table 15.2.

> **Key Learning Points in Invasive Procedures for Prenatal Diagnosis and Therapy**
> 1. Invasive prenatal diagnosis is a powerful method to obtain definitive information for fetal conditions.
> 2. All invasive procedures carry a procedure-related risk of pregnancy loss and hence must be undertaken after careful consideration and appropriate pretest counseling.
> 3. Appropriate documentation of the counseling, consent, and conduct of the procedure must be maintained as per local guidelines.
> 4. Invasive therapeutic procedures present several dilemmas in view of the guarded fetal prognosis, and all the factors must be discussed ideally in a multidisciplinary team setting prior to embarking on such a procedure.

Rhesus Isoimmunization and Fetal Infections

16.1 Rhesus Isoimmunization

Rhesus isoimmunization is a common clinical problem seen in maternal-fetal clinics. The rhesus blood group system is based on the presence or absence of "D-antigen" on the red blood cells (RBCs) of an individual. Women who are rhesus negative do not have the D antigen on their RBCs, while those who are rhesus positive do have this. Unlike the ABO blood groups, the antibody against the rhesus antigen (anti-D antibody) does not "naturally" exist in the system, and it is produced by rhesus negative individuals as a response to exposure to the D-antigen. This exposure to D-antigen to rhesus negative individuals can occur either by mismatched blood/blood product exposure or through feto-maternal hemorrhage in cases of a rhesus negative woman carrying a rhesus positive fetus.

When a woman is rhesus negative, she is "homozygous" negative as rhesus negativity is a recessive trait. If her partner is also rhesus negative, then all their kids will be rhesus negative and this will not cause a clinical problem. If, however, a rhesus negative woman is carrying the child of a rhesus positive father, the child may be rhesus positive or negative depending on the zygosity of the father and the assortment of genes. If the father is "homozygous" positive, all children borne by this couple will be rhesus positive, while if the father is "heterozygous," 50% children will be rhesus positive and 50% rhesus negative (Fig. 16.1).

Now when a rhesus negative woman carries a rhesus negative fetus, there is no mismatch, and no clinical problems are anticipated even if there is any feto-maternal bleed. However, if a rhesus negative woman is carrying a rhesus positive fetus, then the clinical outcome depends on whether or not she has anti-rhesus or anti-D antibodies. If she has these antibodies, then the antibodies can destroy fetal red blood cells causing fetal anemia and severe cardiovascular dysfunction in the fetus leading to hemolytic jaundice, hydrops fetalis, and eventually fetal demise. It is therefore important to remember the following facts about rhesus isoimmunization:

1. First pregnancy in a rhesus negative mother with a rhesus positive fetus is uneventful.
2. ANY pregnancy in a **nonisoimmunized rhesus negative mother** with a rhesus positive fetus is uneventful.
3. ANY pregnancy in **an isoimmunised rhesus negative mother** with a **rhesus negative fetus** is uneventful.
4. If **an isoimmunised rhesus negative mother** has a **rhesus POSITIVE fetus**, then fetus is at risk of anemia.

It is therefore imperative that for any rhesus negative woman, her anti-D antibody status MUST be checked at the time of first booking. EVERY rhesus negative woman MUST be offered an INDIRECT COOMBS TEST at booking. If she is rhesus negative, nonimmunized with

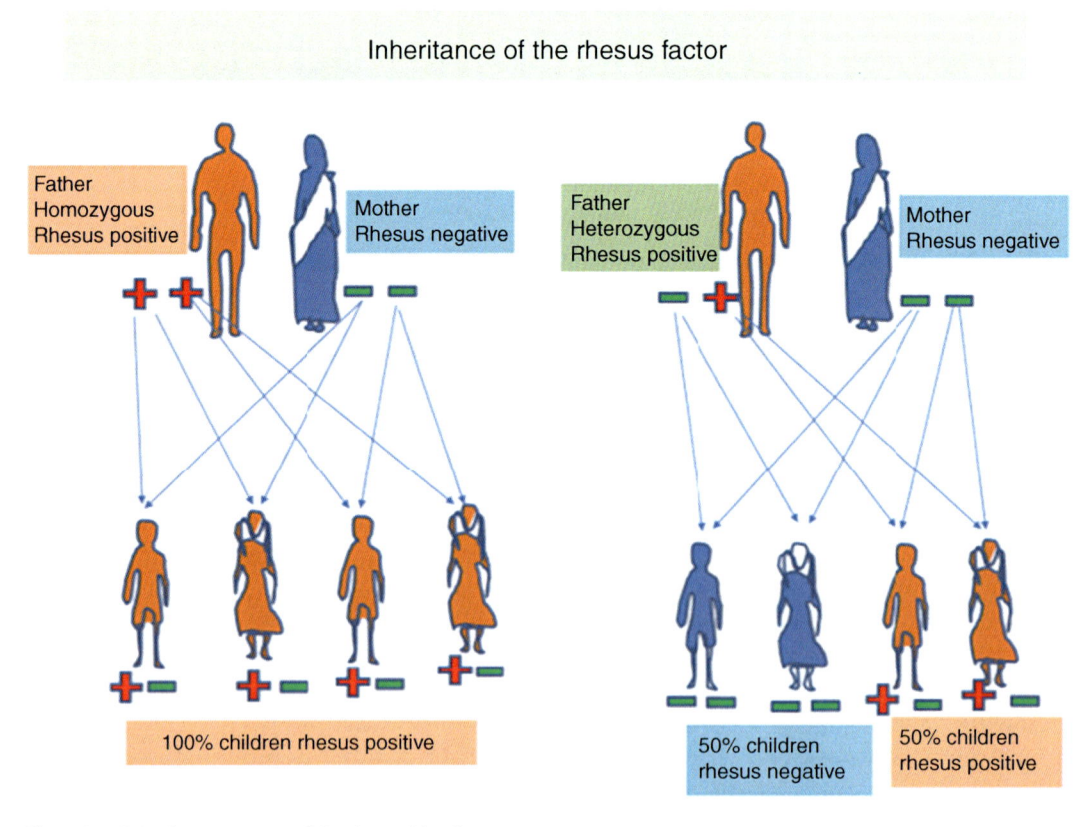

Fig. 16.1 Inheritance pattern of the rhesus blood group

Table 16.1 Indications to offer additional antenatal anti-D in rhesus negative women

1. Antepartum bleeding
2. Invasive procedures like amniocentesis, CVS, etc.
3. Maternal abdominal blunt trauma
4. External cephalic version
5. In cases of miscarriage/termination/ectopic pregnancy

a partner who is rhesus positive, ICT must be repeated at 28 weeks and routine anti-D prophylaxis may be given to prevent isoimmunization. This is repeated at 34 weeks and following delivery within 72 h if the baby is rhesus positive. Apart from routine antenatal anti-D, there are some indications for additional anti-D prophylaxis to unimmunized rhesus negative women when at higher risk of isoimmunization. Such conditions are listed in Table 16.1.

If a rhesus negative pregnant woman is found to be isoimmunised, then her fetus is at risk of hemolysis in case it is rhesus positive. Now establishing the rhesus type of the fetus through invasive testing is counterproductive as it can increase the fetomaternal bleed and worsen the isoimmunization. Noninvasive prenatal testing can help in establishing the fetal rhesus genotype and if this facility is available, it must be called for. If the fetus in utero is found to be rhesus negative, then we do not anticipate any problems in the current pregnancy and no specific monitoring is needed.

If however it is confirmed that the fetus of an isoimmunized mother is rhesus positive or if facilities to detect fetal rhesus type is unavailable, it is prudent to put the fetus under surveillance for detecting any adverse effects of the antibodies like fetal anemia. Quantifying the antibody titer in the mother has a limited role as any which way the final common pathway of fetal affliction is through fetal hemolysis and subsequent anemia so monitoring the same is easier and more productive. Fetal anemia can be detected by monitoring the peak systolic velocity (PSV) of the fetal middle cerebral artery (MCA) on Doppler examination. The MCA-PSV (Fig. 16.2) rises in cases of fetal anemia and the value can be plotted on nomograms for the corresponding gestational age. The method of conducting fetal MCA flow assessment has been described in detail in the chapter of fetal Dopplers in this book.

In cases of severe fetal anemia, it is usually above 1.5 MOM for that stage of gestation and warrants treatment in the form of fetal blood transfusion. Fetal blood transfusion is done using O negative, leuko-depleted, gamma-irradiated, packed RBCs with very high hematocrit. The high hematocrit allows for a lesser volume needed to be transfused for correction of fetal anemia. Further details on fetal transfusion are given in the chapter on fetal therapy. Following transfusion, the fetus is kept on serial monitoring and in rare cases, repeat transfusion may be needed after a few weeks.

Fetal blood transfusion is an example of successful fetal therapy and the outcomes in well-selected cases are very good. This intervention is lifesaving for the fetus and helps in prolonging intrauterine gestation till a stage where the risks of extreme prematurity are avoided. Delivery may be considered by 34 weeks if anemia recurs in a transfused fetus, but the final decision to deliver between 34 and 37 weeks will depend on the composite inputs from the neonatologist, fetal medicine specialist, obstetrician, and the parents.

Although treatment of fetal anemia is possible, there are inherent challenges, and it is best to prevent rhesus isoimmunization by optimum prophylaxis with passive ant-D immunization.

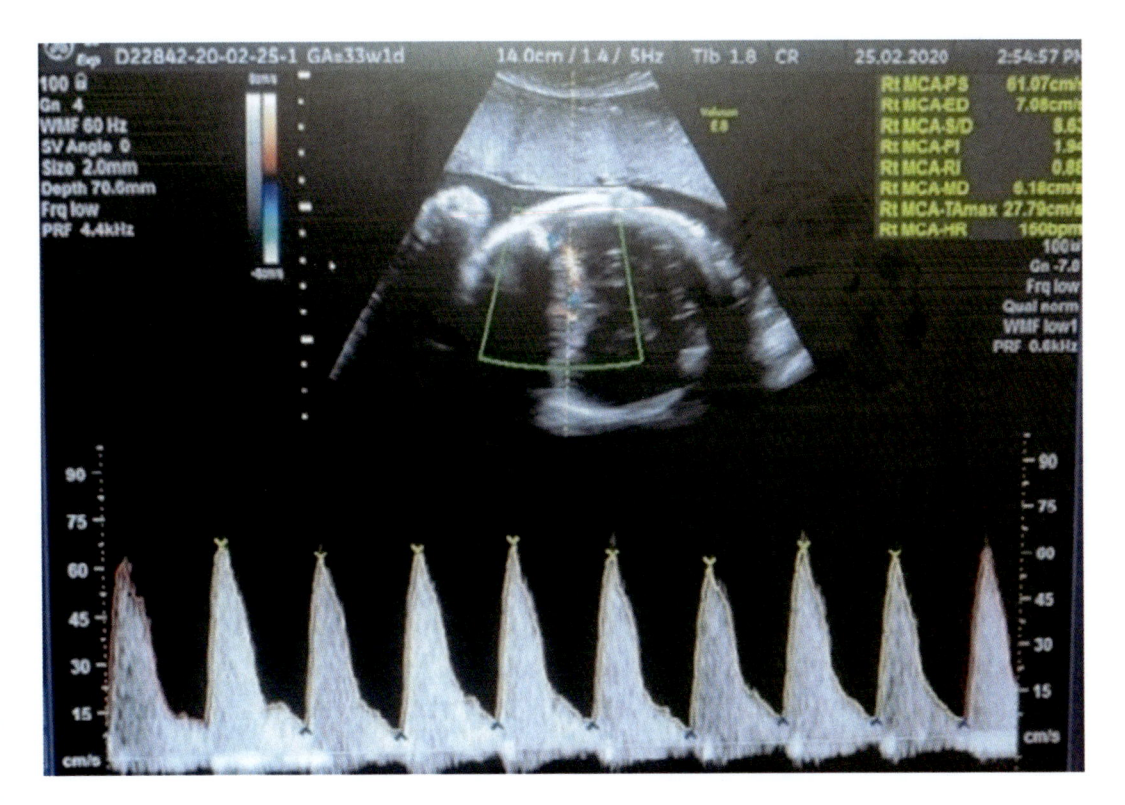

Fig. 16.2 MCA Doppler showing PSV

16.2 Fetal Infections

The fetus in utero can be infected by parasitic organisms that can gain entry into the fetal system through different routes as shown in Fig. 16.3. While transcervical or transamniotic infections do occur in special circumstances, their impact is usually manifested as chorioamnionitis and effects are systemic at the maternal level.

There are some specific "fetal infections" which are vertically transmitted through the placenta to the fetus in utero after a maternal infection in pregnancy. The primary infection in the mother or even the antibodies may not be detected unless looked for specifically as the mother herself remains asymptomatic in these conditions. The fetus, however, may be significantly affected by these conditions and show several changes that can lead to serious risks of morbidity as well as mortality. It is therefore important to be aware of the panorama of fetal manifestations as a sign of response to maternal infection.

An infection is caused by organisms like viruses, bacteria, fungi, and parasites which enter the body of the host and cause disease. The disease process involves specific tissue response leading to organ damage and dysfunction. Although there are many organisms that can cause fetal infections, the common concerns are always with infections of the "TORCH" group and few others such as parvovirus, varicella, Zika virus, etc.

As these infections are spread transplacentally, the chances of "infection" are less when the mother gets infected in the first trimester as the placental mass itself is less at that time as compared to the second or third trimester. However, if the infection does cross the placenta, the "effects" of the infection are more severe in the first trimester than later.

As stated earlier, the mother may remain asymptomatic while being the primary host of the infections that could affect the fetus, but the fetus may get severely affected depending on the kind of organism and the stage of pregnancy that the infection sets in. These fetal infections are diagnosed after some nonspecific stigmata of infective process are noticed on the antenatal

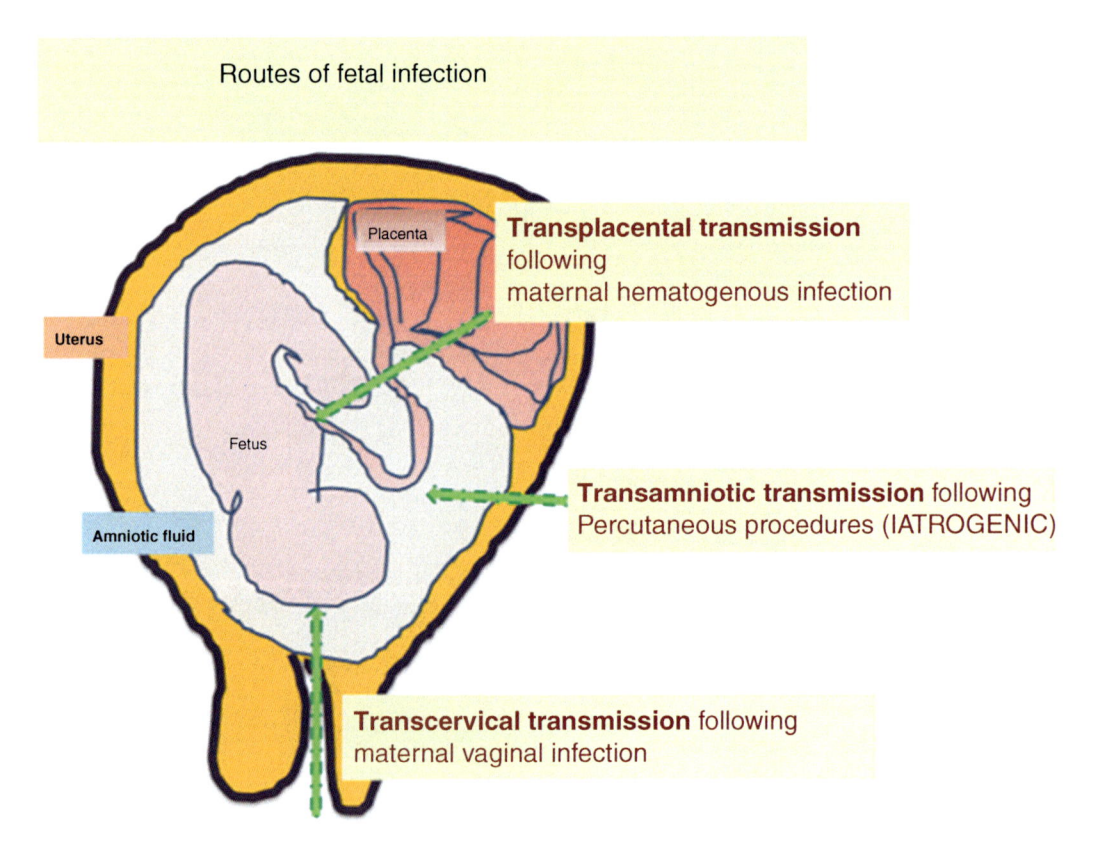

Fig. 16.3 Routes of fetal infection

ultrasound assessment. Table 16.2 lists some of the findings on fetal ultrasound which indicate a high possibility of fetal infection.

These signs are rather nonspecific and seen in most congenital infections. Whenever fetal infection is suspected, a preliminary maternal serology is done to assess maternal immune status for these infections and either rule out the possibility or determine which infection to be looked for in the fetus.

Maternal serology is done by assessing the IgM and IgG levels for the specific infection suspected. IgM is produced as an acute response to infection and usually indicates a recent infection. IgG is the second line of antibodies, indicating old infection and some degree of immunity—even for the fetus as it can cross the placenta. IgG avidity testing is an additional test that helps in timing the infection such that high avidity indicates an old infection, while low avidity indicates a recent infection—usually within 3–6 months. This helps in dating the timing of infection with the period of gestation and thus anticipating the effect on the fetus in the present pregnancy. The summary of maternal serology interpretation is given in Table 16.3.

Maternal serology is used as the first screening method to anticipate if there could be fetal infection in the current pregnancy after a suspicion is raised usually by ultrasound findings suggestive of infection or rarely when the mother has fever with rashes or lymphadenopathy in pregnancy.

The "gold standard" for diagnosing fetal infection is by isolating the pathogen or its specific nucleic acid from the amniotic fluid or fetal blood sample. Such a test understandably carries a good "positive predictive value" for fetal "infection" but does not always correlate with fetal "affection" as the fetal infection may be asymptomatic in few cases. One also needs to understand here that despite being "asymptomatic" of having no discernible ultrasound features of infection in fetal life, there may be long-term sequelae manifesting in childhood for fetuses infected in utero.

On the other hand, if the fetal sample tests negative for the infective agent, it does not rule out the possibility of infection as there may be technical limitations to detecting the infective agent in fetal samples. Sometimes the timeline of the infection is unclear due to nonspecific symp-

Table 16.2 Common signs of fetal infection on antenatal ultrasound

1. Fetal growth restriction
2. Oligo-/polyamnios
3. Large placenta with calcifications
4. Hyperechogenic fetal bowel
5. Fetal visceral calcifications
6. Fetal hepatosplenomegaly
7. Fetal brain changes (calcification/cysts/ventriculomegaly, etc.)
8. Fetal ascites/hydrops
9. Fetal anemia

Table 16.3 Interpretation of maternal serology testing regarding congenital infections

Antibodies	Indication	Expectation	Treatment
IgM negative IgG negative	No recent infection No past infection	Not immune	If vaccine available—can be given
IgM positive IgG negative	Recent infection for the first time	Expect severe sequelae if fetal infection	Treat primary infection if possible
IgM positive IgG positive	Recent infection with development of some immunity reinfection	Do IgG AVIDITY Low avidity—recent infection High avidity–old infection (>3–6 months)	AVIDITY test helps in timing the infection
IgM negative IgG positive	Past infection/immunity	NO TREATMENT NEEDED	NO VACCINE NEEDED

toms in the mother, and sometimes the serology may be "false positive" due to cross-reaction with other antibodies leading to negative results on fetal sampling. Repeating invasive tests for mere clarifications carries logistic limitations which clinicians will understand, and therefore the "diagnosis" of fetal infection is limited to the cohort of cases that show confirmed positive results of organism nucleic acid PCR or culture following fetal sampling.

The principles described above are applicable in general to most intrauterine infections with minor individual variations. Table 16.4 shows some individual details of the common congenital infections that are encountered in regular clinical practice.

Table 16.4 Overview of common congenital infections

Name of infective agent	Type of agent	Possible postnatal effects of fetal infection	Management and prognosis	Preventive vaccine
Cytomegalovirus	DNA virus of the herpes family	Sensorineural hearing deafness even in apparently asymptomatic cases and long-term neurological disability	NO effective treatment available in regular practice. Only under research settings, valacyclovir and hyperimmune globulin are being used	No
Toxoplasma	Parasite *Toxoplasma gondii*	Chorioretinitis and neurological disability	Spiramycin can reduce vertical transmission in pregnancy. Treatment of fetal infection in utero is by a combination of pyrimethamine and sulfadiazine	No
Rubella	RNA virus of *Togaviridae* family	Congenital cataract, hearing loss, neurological disability, and cardiac malformations	No effective treatment available. Infection in the first trimester may justify termination of pregnancy due to severe adverse effects	Yes
Herpes simplex virus	DNA virus	Direct teratogenicity is low although some cases of neurological abnormalities are known. Peripartum transmission can lead to ophthalmic and neurological sequelae	Acyclovir can be given to treat both primary and recurrent herpes infections in pregnancy	No
Varicella zoster	DNA virus of the herpes family	Rarely, fetus is affected with fetal varicella syndrome—limb defects, dermatological scarring, eye abnormalities, neurological disability	Acyclovir can be given to treat maternal symptoms. Passive immunity can be provided by immunoglobulin to minimize the effect of maternal infection	Yes
Parvovirus B19	Single-stranded DNA virus	Anemia with thrombocytopenia	Fetal blood transfusion (both RBC and platelets) can help prevent in utero hydrops and demise	No
Treponema pallidum	Spirochete *Treponema pallidum*	Congenital syphilis—many manifestations, e.g., skeletal abnormalities, corneal scarring, neurological disability, etc.	Benzathine penicillin	No
Zika virus	RNA virus of the *Flavivirus* type	Microcephaly and even in the absence of microcephaly, there may be neurological disability due to brain abnormalities that are part of the congenital Zika virus syndrome	No effective treatment known	No

As is evident from the preceding discussion, the suspicion of fetal infection when based on ultrasound findings and serology reports warrants a detailed counseling of the couple regarding all the possibilities including the uncertainty of the final outcome. It is often disappointing for the parents when the possibility of long-term sequelae is discussed even in the absence of ultrasound signs and yet it is imperative on the fetal medicine consultant to share the information. A multidisciplinary team approach helps in such situations including the obstetrician, neonatologist, and infectious diseases physician along with the fetal medicine consultant.

Key Learning Points
1. Rhesus isoimmunization is a preventable condition if appropriate precautions are taken in the rhesus negative pregnancies.
2. Universal blood group/Rh screening for pregnant women and ICT for rhesus negative women must be promoted.
3. Fetal MCA-PSV is an effective, noninvasive method of screening for fetal anemia.
4. Fetal blood transfusion in carefully selected cases is a lifesaving intervention for anemic fetuses.
5. Fetal infections are caused by transplacental transfer of the TORCH organisms following maternal infection which may be asymptomatic.
6. Suspicion of fetal infections is mostly based on typical ultrasound findings or in cases of maternal fever with rash.
7. Maternal serology helps suspect fetal infection although confirmation is by amniotic fluid PCR.
8. Individual infections carry different prognosis based on the organism and gestational age at the time of infection.
9. Some infections like rubella and varicella are preventable by immunization and preconceptional immunization is a good practice.

Suggested Reading

Mari G, Deter RL, Carpenter RL, et al. Noninvasive diagnosis by Doppler ultra-sonography of fetal anemia due to maternal red-cell alloimmunization. Collaborative Group for Doppler Assessment of the Blood Velocity of Anemic Fetuses. N Engl J Med. 2000;342:9–14.

ISUOG Practice guidelines. Role of ultrasound in congenital infection. Ultrasound Obstet Gynecol. 2020;56:128–51.

17 Potential for Assessing Maternal Morbidity in Fetal Medicine Clinics

The mother and the fetus are inseparable in pregnancy—in fact, the "separation" marks the end of pregnancy! So while "fetal medicine" is the study of health and disease conditions of the fetus, it is very important to realize that the maternal health and disease conditions can have a bearing on fetal health and vice versa.

Fetal medicine is definitely the science dealing with health issues of the fetus in utero, but the fact remains that these health issues are integrated with the mother as long as "fetal" life continues. There are some maternal health issues which may be predicted or detected due to the clinical assessment in fetal medicine clinics. In this chapter, we discuss some such maternal medical disorders like preeclampsia, hyperglycemia, and some autoimmune conditions.

17.1 Uterine Artery Doppler Studies Predict Risk of Preeclampsia

Preeclampsia is a pregnancy-specific syndrome which involves hypertension and proteinuria or maternal organ dysfunction. The exact etiology may have remained a matter of speculation through the past century, but the central role of impaired placentation in the disease is well established—whether this is the cause or effect of a primary pathology remains elusive to a final explanation.

In cases of impaired placentation, there is inadequate trophoblastic invasion of maternal spiral arterioles, and the uteroplacental bed remains a high resistance zone. Blood flow patterns through the uterine arteries are indicative of the distal resistance in the uteroplacental bed. In case of high resistance, the spectral flow pattern of the uterine artery shows impeded flow in diastole with high pulsatility indices. This is reflective of suboptimal placentation and is effectively predictive of the risk of preeclampsia in the mother in that pregnancy.

Uterine artery Doppler in the second trimester is usually done transabdominally. The ultrasound probe is moved laterally in the lower segment, and color Doppler is used to identify the uterine artery at the apparent crossover with the external iliac arteries (Fig. 17.1).

Then pulse wave Doppler is used to get a waveform which may be representative of good diastolic flow (Fig. 17.2) or high resistance flow (Fig. 17.3).

High resistance flows in the uterine artery have been associated with the risk of developing preeclampsia in the current pregnancy. Several studies have correlated the uterine artery Doppler parameters with the risk of developing preeclampsia and the predictability is definitely better in later gestations. The placentation is completed in two waves, and sometimes an abnormal flow in the first trimester may improve following the second wave of trophoblastic

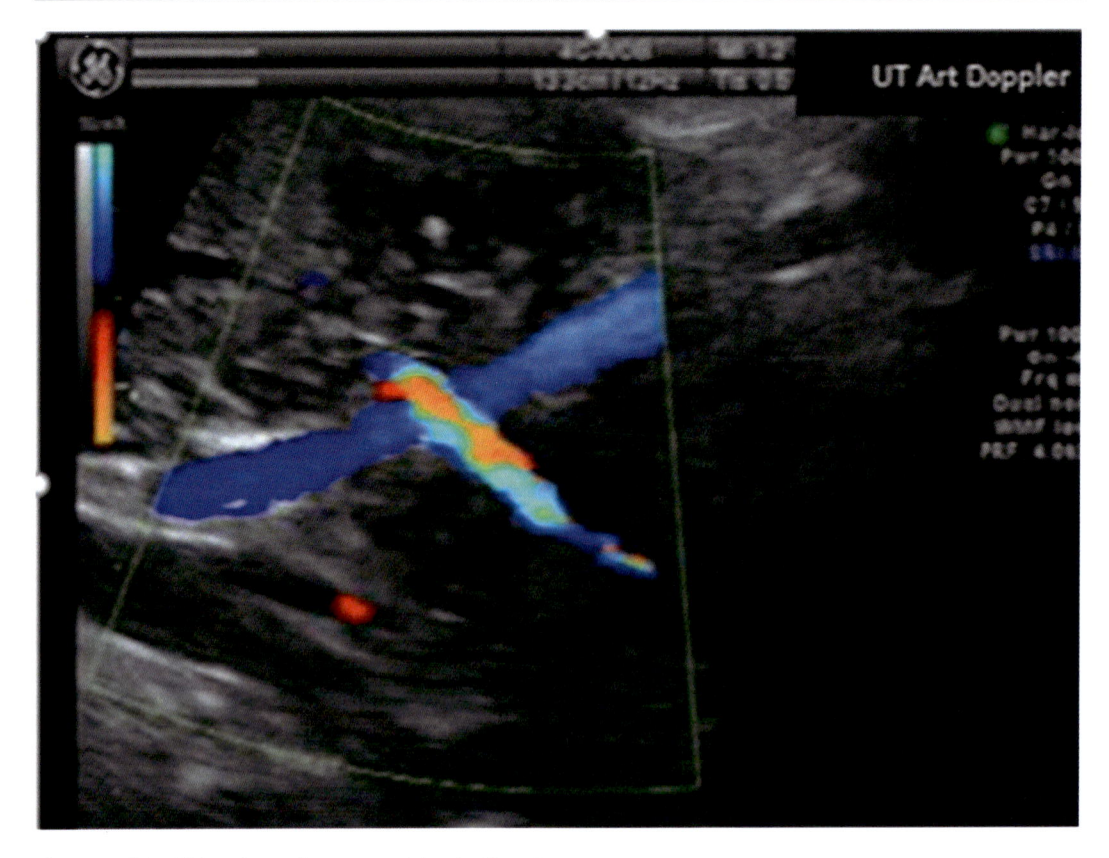

Fig. 17.1 Identifying the uterine artery with color Doppler

invasion—hence, the possibility of "false-positive" prediction is higher earlier on in pregnancy.

The ASPRE trial established that it is possible to effectively prevent preterm preeclampsia or delay the onset and severity of symptoms if prophylactic low-dose aspirin is started appropriately in the high-risk group before 16 weeks—or in other words, before the onset of the second wave of placentation. This has increased the importance of screening for preeclampsia in the first trimester. The Fetal Medicine Foundation, UK, has suggested a multimodality screening model which includes maternal mean arterial pressure, uterine artery Doppler, and biomarkers like PlGF (placental growth factor) in the first trimester to predict the risk of maternal preeclampsia. This algorithm allows the risk assessment in any pregnancy, and the "high-risk" group can be offered chemoprophylaxis (150 mg aspirin daily at bedtime started before 16 weeks and continued till 36 weeks of gestation) to reduce the incidence and severity of the condition.

17.1 Uterine Artery Doppler Studies Predict Risk of Preeclampsia 177

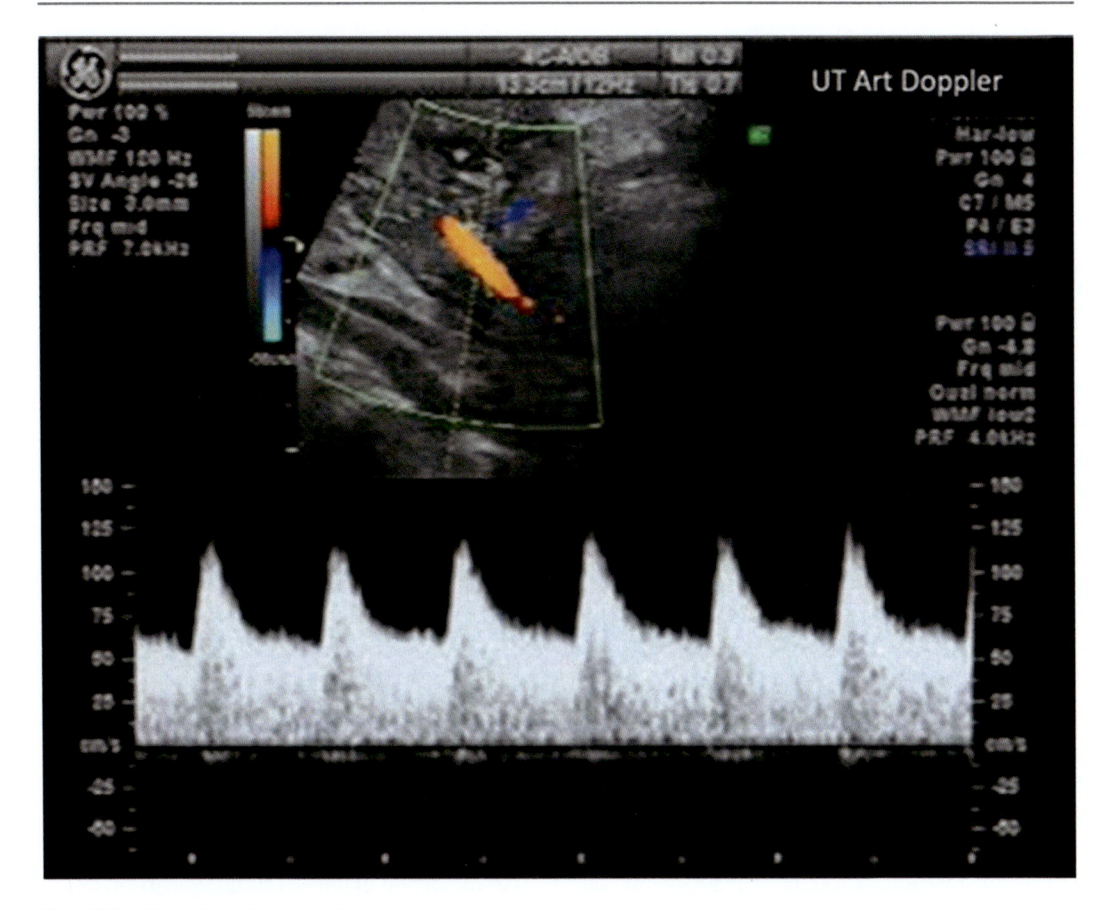

Fig. 17.2 Normal uterine artery flows

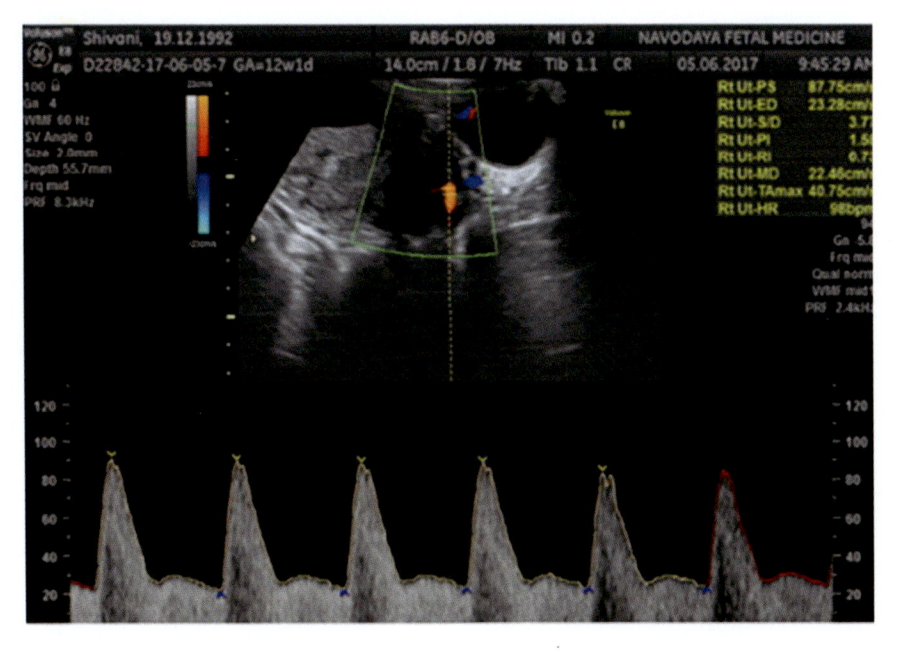

Fig. 17.3 High resistance flows in uterine artery

17.2 Hyperglycemia in Pregnancy

Pregnancy is known to be a diabetogenic state and women who have subclinical glucose intolerance may develop frank hyperglycemia in pregnancy. The current classification of hyperglycemia in pregnancy (HIP) includes two entities—diabetes mellitus in pregnancy (DIP), diagnosed before 20 weeks, and gestational diabetes mellitus (GDM), identified in the second or third trimester of gestation. Most obstetric units have their own screening protocols for GDM, and it is usually delayed until the late second or early third trimester of pregnancy, because the diabetogenic effects of pregnancy increase with gestation and, therefore, delayed testing maximizes the detection rate.

Sometimes, during a routine fetal assessment, detection of fetal macrosomia and/or polyhydramnios alerts the clinician toward the possibility of maternal hyperglycemia (Fig. 17.4). High levels of maternal glucose can pass through the placenta and lead to fetal hyperglycemia with fetal release of insulin, insulin-like growth factors, and growth hormone. This sequence eventually leads to increased fetal subcutaneous fat deposition and larger fetal size.

The clinical details of fetal macrosomia and polyamnios have been dealt with in separate chapters in this book, but here the mention of these entities is made to highlight that sometimes they could instigate a retrospective diagnosis of a maternal medical disorder during a routine fetal evaluation.

Such an incidental diagnosis is of paramount importance in GDM where appropriate glycemic control can help in optimizing both maternal and fetal outcomes of the pregnancy.

17.3 Maternal Autoimmune Diseases

Sometimes, during a fetal scan, congenital heart block or fetal anemia may be discovered leading to the discovery of presence of maternal antibodies as the etiology of these conditions. In most of these cases, the mother herself may be asymptomatic and her condition is diagnosed only based on suspicion during fetal evaluation. This chance finding also has significant impact on both maternal and fetal health.

An incidental diagnosis of fetal heart block in a structurally normal fetal heart raises the suspi-

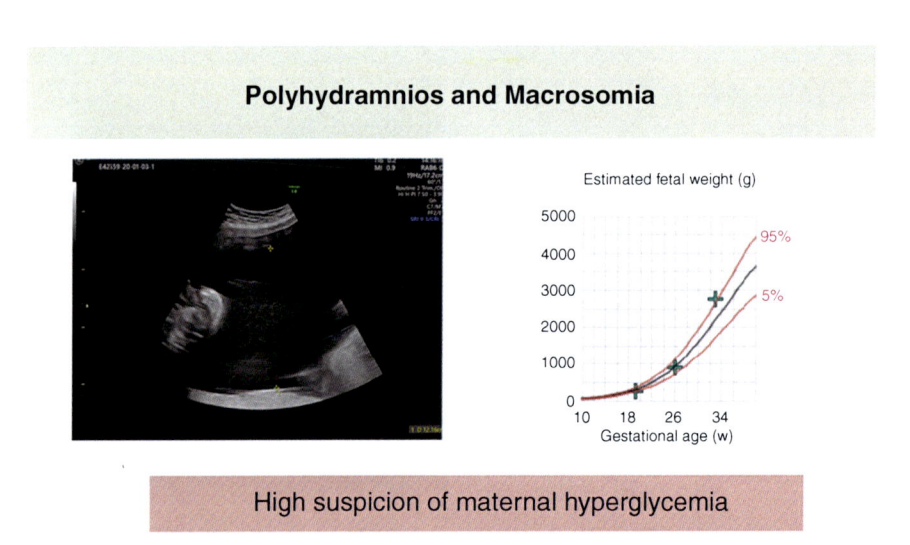

Fig. 17.4 Clinical features in fetus due to maternal hyperglycemia

17.3 Maternal Autoimmune Diseases

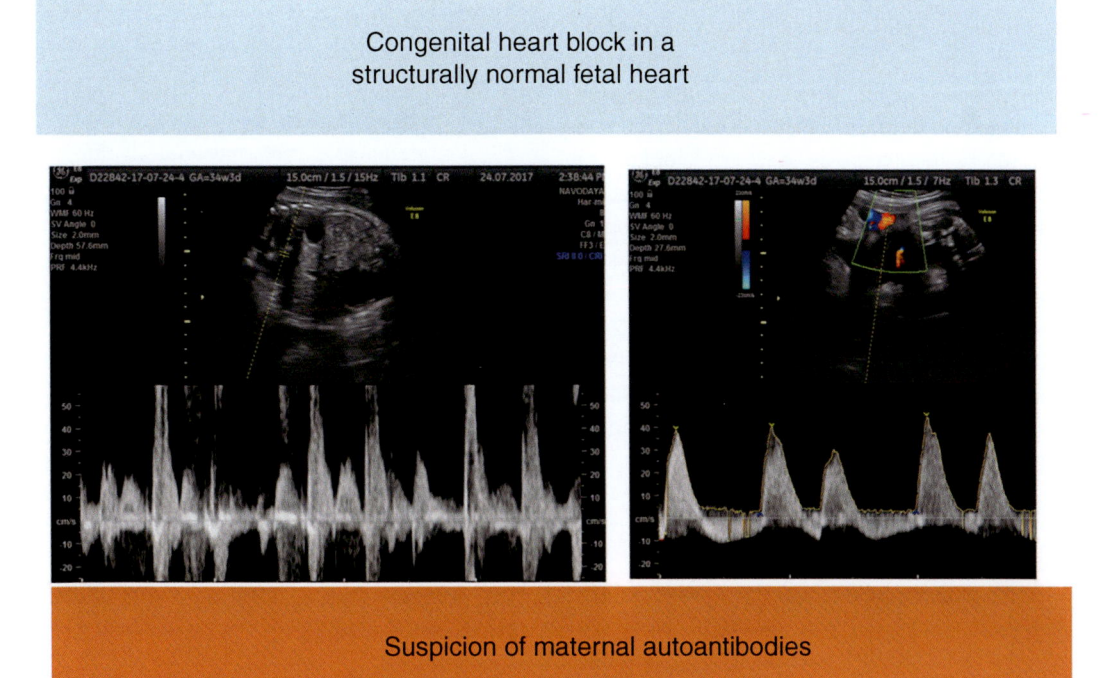

Fig. 17.5 Fetal heart block

cion of the presence of maternal anti-Ro/anti-La antibodies which can cross the placenta and lead to autoimmune-mediated congenital heart block (Fig. 17.5). This can be progressive leading to fetal hydrops and may ultimately be lethal to the fetus.

The anti-Ro/SSA and anti-La/SSB antibodies were initially related to patients with Sjögren's syndrome (SS) and systemic lupus erythematosus (SLE), but subsequent studies have shown that anti-Ro antibodies can be detected in many other autoimmune diseases. These diseases are usually multifaceted, complex entities with variable phenotypes, clinical presentations, and relapsing-remitting courses. Their primary diagnosis is therefore important as it has significant impact on the woman's health with long-term effects on multiple organ systems. Pregnancy provides an opportunity for this detection in asymptomatic women through findings in fetal evaluation.

The fetal prognosis of course depends on the stage of the pathology and gestational age at diagnosis. Early gestational age with advanced heart block is generally associated with high fetal mortality, while stage I CHB may sometimes be reversible with antenatal steroids and may lead to a live birth although postnatal issues may arise. These fetuses have a passively acquired autoimmunity that may be associated with serious neonatal complications like neonatal lupus or need for a pacemaker. Nevertheless, once maternal diagnosis is established and the mother is put under care of a rheumatologist, the outlook for future pregnancies improves due to optimal preconceptional care and planning.

Diagnosis of fetal anemia is possible by the raised fetal MCA peak systolic velocity (PSV) that has been discussed in detail in a previous chapter. However, sometimes an incidental finding of fetal anemia becomes the starting point of diagnosing maternal isoimmunization or parvovirus infection, while the mother may be asymptomatic otherwise. Maternal isoimmunization may be due to anti-D antibodies in rhesus negative women or due to atypical red cell antibodies which can be present even in rhesus positive women and often remain unsuspected.

Similarly, the diagnosis of severe fetal growth restriction with oligoamnios or even intrauterine fetal demise associated with significant uteroplacental insufficiency can lead to the diagnosis of maternal antiphospholipid antibodies or other forms of maternal thrombophilias.

There are few studies linking the possibility of myasthenia gravis in women who have fetuses affected with arthrogryposis multiplex congenita.

As the readers may have realized by now that many issues discussed in this chapter are repetitions of clinical issues dealt elsewhere in the book, the purpose of this repetition was to highlight that some maternal conditions may be unraveled only if the associated fetal issue is properly identified and worked upon. The course of the present pregnancy would depend on many factors, but definitely the course of future pregnancies can be optimized by adequate multidisciplinary care. Opportunistic diagnosis of maternal medical disorders provides an effective window to institute corrective medical and lifestyle measures so as to improve the woman's health in the long term.

Key Learning Points
1. Fetal medicine clinics also provide a method of detecting maternal problems as sometimes they may present indirectly in asymptomatic women.
2. Comprehensive maternal-fetal evaluation helps in identifying maternal morbidity which can be then addressed, thus minimizing long-term health risks for the mother.

Suggested Reading

Tranquilli AL, Dekker G, Magee L, et al. The classification, diagnosis and management of the hypertensive disorders of pregnancy: a revised statement from the ISSHP. Pregnancy Hypertens. 2014;4:97–104.

O'Gorman N, Wright D, Poon LC, et al. Multicenter screening for preeclampsia by maternal factors and biomarkers at 11-13 weeks' gestation: comparison to NICE guidelines and ACOG recommendations. Ultrasound Obstet Gynecol. 2017;49:756–60.

Rolnik DL, Wright D, Poon LC, et al. Aspirin versus placebo in pregnancies at high risk for preterm preeclampsia. N Engl J Med. 2017;377(7):613–22.

Hod M, Kapur A, Sacks DA, et al. The International Federation of Gynecology and Obstetrics (FIGO) Initiative on gestational diabetes mellitus: a pragmatic guide for diagnosis, management, and care. Int J Gynaecol Obstet. 2015;131(Suppl 3):S173–211.

Brito-Zerón P, Izmirly PM, Ramos-Casals M, et al. The clinical spectrum of autoimmune congenital heart block. Nat Rev Rheumatol. 2015;11(5):301–12.

Essentials of Counseling in Fetal Medicine

18

Counseling is one of the most important aspects of clinical practice in Fetal medicine. Counseling is the part where there is effective communication between the doctor and the patient after a particular fetal assessment is done. All clinicians will agree that unless this communication is done well, the final goal of "care" remains unachieved. Not only in fetal medicine, but also in every field of clinical medicine, effective doctor-patient communication is the crux of satisfactory treatment. Achieving great technical skills, using state-of-the-art machinery, and writing accurate reports are all very important accomplishments in fetal medicine practice, but unless you are able to explain the results to the most important stakeholders in fetal care—the parents—there remains a lacuna in the process which starts with lack of understanding the exact situation and may snowball into misconceptions and wrong decisions in pregnancy. Therefore, effective counseling—both "pretest" and "posttest" sessions—are vital in every fetal medicine clinic to ensure good fetal care.

18.1 Pretest Counseling

Every fetal evaluation test—be it an ultrasound scan or a serum screening test—MUST begin with a "pretest" counseling. If the parents are explained what is the test that they are about to undergo, the purpose of the test, and the possible outcomes, then they are much better equipped to handle the results and even in case of an adverse report, the anxiety levels are not unduly high.

Pretest counseling can be done at the same sitting as we mostly do for fetal scans or may be scheduled in advance for some specific procedures where the stakes are higher and the parents may need some time and further deliberation before they can reach a decision of whether or not to go ahead with a test or procedure. Supplementing oral advice with written information in the form of information leaflets is a good idea as sometimes parents are so stressed during the consultation that they may not understand or retain every piece of information that you have shared with them. If they take home leaflets, they can read them later and understand the situation better.

18.2 Pretest Counseling for Fetal Scans

It is good practice to do a pretest counseling for fetal scans. Prior to placing your probe on the mother, it would be very useful to spend a few minutes explaining the nature of the scan, what are the goals of the scan, the expected time frame, what can be seen, what cannot be seen, and the expected results. The fact that some part of the evaluation may require a transvaginal approach at times can also be mentioned at the outset to mentally prepare her for that possibility. It makes the patient feel as ease and she is far more relaxed during the session as compared to a situation where a doctor walks in directly without any priming and starts a technical scan with the patient very nervous and anxious about the happenings.

It is also important to explain that sometimes fetal position may not be favorable temporarily and we may have to let her go for a walk and review after sometime when the fetus may have turned into a better position. These points, however trivial they may appear, are important as some parents can get very nervous when you say a sentence like "I can't see the heart as baby is not moving inside"!! It may be an innocent statement of fact but carries unimaginable potential to unnerve your patient. Correct choice of words remains forever important, but timing a few such points in the pretest counseling will help you immensely in increasing overall patient satisfaction.

Many parents walk in for fetal scans expecting to be entertained by looking at the fetus in real time. While it is acceptable to allow them to experience this joy, what is most important is for everyone to realize that fetal scans are NOT a PR exercise—they have scientific indications and until those goals are achieved, a mere display of the fetal activity on screen is not going to lead us to the right consequence. Hence, doctors have to explain to the parents that first the clinical agenda has to be fulfilled, the technical checklist has to be completed, and only then we can "show" them the fetus for their satisfaction. Such pretest counseling will help gain their cooperation in allowing you to complete your clinical work without interruption and will also keep them prepared that we may find some issues which will then necessitate further discussion. If we do not prepare them prior to the scan, every little point can become a cause of major anxiety, frustration, and discontent with far-reaching consequences.

18.3 Posttest Counseling for Fetal Scans

Once the scan is complete and you have made the report, it is useful to meet the parents, explain the report, and address any of their concerns with regard to the scan. Even if everything is "normal" according to you, it is a good practice to mention the points evaluated on the scan and the limits of the scan. After addressing any particular query that they may have, the next time for fetal evaluation can be mentioned. If that is the last routine scan for this pregnancy, then the parents may be informed so and requested to revert with the outcome of pregnancy as it is equally important to follow-up the final results of your fetal evaluation and care.

In case there are any fetal "markers" or "anomalies" are found, then a detailed explanation of that specific issue and its impact on further fetal evaluation and the pregnancy in general has to be made. As discussed in previous chapters, all problems have specific care plans and multidisciplinary teams have to be constituted for executing those plans. The obstetrician remains the most important clinician in the care of a pregnancy, and in the event of any fetal problem, it is important to inform and involve the obstetrician about the alteration in fetal care. As such findings may be discovered in the middle of a busy clinical day and it may not be possible to arrange a joint multidisciplinary meeting right away, it is rational to do a preliminary counseling of the parents at the FM clinic, give them information leaflets, and arrange for a MDT meeting at a later date with all relevant subspecialists.

18.4 Pretest Counseling for Fetal Screening Tests

Screening tests, as defined earlier, are tests done on "apparently normal" people to pick out "low-risk" population that can be reassured and "high-risk" population that needs further testing and evaluation. It is therefore very crucial that *before*

18.4 Pretest Counseling for Fetal Screening Tests

undertaking any screening tests, the parents understand that the results may come "high risk" and this is *not* a diagnosis but only a probability of a problem and hence needs further investigation.

At this session, it may be useful to address the point that the screening test is being offered to her as part of a routine care process. Many women get very anxious the moment the doctor uses terms like "chromosomal abnormalities" and get defensive by stating that they do not have any such problems in the family or get nervous why suddenly there is this discussion about "problems." It is therefore useful to open the discussion on a positive note and explain that although everything looks normal at this stage of pregnancy, there are possibilities of problems in some cases and hence some tests are done to look for those women who have higher chances of these problems and such tests are called "screening tests." Most of the time, difficulties arise in the process of screening due to neglect of the "pretest counseling." These few extra minutes spent in explaining the rationale of a screening test to the couple goes a very long way in ensuring compliance and reasonable reactions to the results of the test (Fig. 18.1).

By "counseling" clinicians generally mean "explaining" the results of the fetal evaluation to the couple and sometimes their family members. Most doctors think of counseling as an act of "talking" to the patient, whereas if you look into

A	Allot a quiet and comfortable space in the clinic for counselling sessions
M	Meet the couple and introduce yourself
I	Introduce sensitively the reason for having this session
C	Check what are their concerns
A	Answer all their queries and explain the next possible steps
B	Be sure that they have understood
L	Leaflets with written information can be handed over for better understanding
E	Expect a decision regarding future care for the fetus — either right away or after they think over the issue

Fig. 18.1 AMICABLE checklist for counseling sessions

the actual meaning of counseling, it involves "listening" to the other person's concerns and then advising them further to help them reach a decision. It is important to realize in all fetal medicine consultations that we are not communicating with the "patient" per se. We are communicating with the mother or the parents about a baby yet to be born! As such, there is a rather abstract idea in most people about the existence of this fetus, and the attachment is so emotional that parents often find it difficult to individualize this fetus and discuss anything that could be a "problem" to the fetus! Most fetal medicine consultations start with a high baseline anxiety, and the onus lies on the fetal medicine doctor to moderate the emotional quotient and bring the discussion to a rational platform. It will be correct to state that appropriate counseling by the fetal medicine specialist can be "lifesaving" for a fetus!!

Key Learning Points
1. Counseling remains the cornerstone of effective clinical service—until your patient understands the course of management, the job of a doctor is unfinished.
2. Your patients may not remember exactly what you said to them but they will remember how you made them feel—if you are able to convey your intentions in planning her care, your patient will not lose faith in you.
3. Remember, most of the discontent in medical practice today is because of poor communication between doctors and patients—talking to your patient is not a waste of your time; it is the very purpose of your practice!

Printed by Books on Demand, Germany

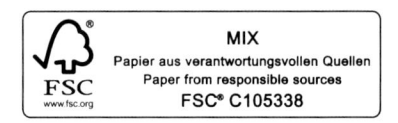